THE SYNAPTIC
ORGANIZATION
OF THE BRAIN

THE SYNAPTIC ORGANIZATION OF THE BRAIN

SECOND EDITION

Gordon M. Shepherd

PROFESSOR OF NEUROSCIENCE
YALE UNIVERSITY SCHOOL OF MEDICINE

New York   Oxford
OXFORD UNIVERSITY PRESS
1979

Copyright © 1974, 1979 by Oxford University Press, Inc.
Printed in the United States of America

Library of Congress Cataloging in Publication Data

Shepherd, Gordon M
  The synaptic organization of the brain.

  Bibliography: p.
  Includes index.
  1. Brain.   2.   Synapses.   3.   Neural circuitry.
  I.   Title. [DNLM: 1.   Brain—Physiology.
  2.   Neurons—Physiology. ·3.   Synapses.
  WL300.3 S548s]
  QP376.S48   1979   612'.82   79-899
  ISBN 0-19-502548-2   ISBN 0-19-502549-0 pbk.

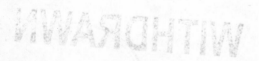

For Grethe

PREFACE

Knowledge of synaptic organization continues its vigorous growth, and I am grateful for the opportunity to update this account of it. The objective remains the same: to synthesize the results of research as they bear on the organization of synapses into circuits, and begin the task of elucidating the principles that underlie function.

The major development since the first edition appeared has been the coming of age of methods for studying the neurochemistry of synaptic transmission at the cellular level. Neurochemistry is now in the process of merging with neuroanatomy, electrophysiology, and biophysics in the multidisciplinary analysis of synaptic organization. This is reflected in this edition by the inclusion of new sections on neurochemistry in most of the chapters. In some cases it has been possible to provide summary diagrams correlating putative neurotransmitters with the main synaptic circuits of given regions.

Several new chapters have been added. The introductory material on synaptic physiology has been expanded, and there are now separate accounts of membrane potentials and neurochemical aspects. The sequence of systems under review now begins with a new chapter on peripheral ganglia, which have been intensively studied at the neuronal and synaptic level, and provide valuable models for multidisciplinary analysis. Another region attracting considerable interest has been the basal ganglia, lying as it does at the crossroads of neurochemistry and behavior. Finally, the chapter on the neocortex has been expanded into separate accounts of motor and sensory areas. I have tried to draw attention to some recent technical advances in the effort to sort out cortical circuits, as well as give some flavor of recent debates about concepts of cortical organization. All the chapters have been updated to include results obtained with new methods, especially immunocytochemistry, horseradish peroxidase labelling, 2-deoxyglucose mapping, neuronal modelling, and the monitoring of unit activity in behaving animals.

In this edition, as in its predecessor, I am only too aware of the risks that attend an effort to cover widely diverse areas of research. Brevity begets its errors of omission and commission; one hopes for a margin of clarity and understanding. The references have been chosen with care from a voluminous literature; I ask my colleagues' indulgence in the selections. The time for writing has been wrested from the life of the laboratory, and my intentions to cover such topics as the development and plasticity of synaptic circuits, as well as several other brain regions, were not realized.

My debts are many. Drs. W. M. Cowan, D. P. Purpura, J. E. Dowling, G. R. Strichartz, R. E. Burke, C. R. Michael, J. L. Price, W. T. Thach, Jr., H. R. Ralston III, and W. Rall read individual chapters of the first edition, and their counsels carry over into this one. Drs. T. V. Getchell, J. S. Kauer, F. R. Sharp, W. B. Stewart, N. R. Krieger, P. Greengard, M. C. Nowycky, U. Waldow, K. Mori, C. A. Greer, and R. K. Brayton have been my colleagues in recent research; their energies and ideas leaven much of what is recorded here. I am deeply indebted to Dr. Sol Erulkar, who read the entire manuscript and straightened out many matters of detail and emphasis. Dr. M. C. Nowycky also read the manuscript and proofs. All of these colleagues have had to contend with the brevity necessarily imposed on the coverage of each area, and the remaining errors are solely mine. I have made most of the original drawings, and take responsibility for errors in them too. Ms. Brenda Jones of Oxford University Press has been most patient in editing the manuscript, and the steady support of Mr. Jeffrey House has made it all possible.

Finally, I am happy to record my gratitude to the National Institute for Neurological and Communicative Diseases and Stroke, and to the National Science Foundation, for their support of my work and that of my colleagues in neuroscience. At a time when funding for basic research is so uncertain, the progress recorded herein, in many ways literally undreamt of a generation ago, provides perhaps some justification for the past and optimism for the future.

G. M. S.

Hamden, Connecticut
April 1979

CONTENTS

4. NEUROTRANSMITTER MECHANISMS   56

Molecular Nature of Synaptic Transmission, 56; Graded Release of Transmitter Quanta, 59; Steps in Synaptic Transmission, 60; Metabolic Pathways, 63; Dale's Principle, 65; Identification of Transmitters, 68; Neurotransmission and Neuromodulation, 69; Transport of Substances, 70; Energy Metabolism and 2-Deoxyglucose Mapping, 73; Synaptic Modification, 75.

5. DENDRITIC ELECTROTONUS   78

Steady-State Electrotonus, 79

Dendritic Length, 81; Dendritic Diameter, 82; Dendritic Branching, 85.

Transient Electrotonus, 87

Synaptic Potentials in Dendritic Trees, 88; Synaptic Potentials in Dendritic Spines, 91; Synaptic Interactions, 93.

Part 2
ORGANIZATION OF NEURONAL SYSTEMS

6. PERIPHERAL GANGLIA   99

Neuronal Elements, 100

Inputs, 101; Principal Neuron, 101; Intrinsic Neuron, 101; Neuronal Populations, 103.

Synaptic Connections, 104

Basic Circuit, 105

Synaptic Actions, 108

Neurotransmitters, 111

Dendritic Properties, 114

Parasympathetic Ganglia, 115

Carotid Body, 118

7. SPINAL CORD: VENTRAL HORN   121

Neuronal Elements, 122

Inputs, 122; Principal Neuron, 125; Intrinsic Neurons, 127; Neuronal Populations, 128.

Synaptic Connections, 130

Basic Circuit, 132

Synaptic Actions, 136

Recurrent Inhibition, 139; Types of Inhibition, 141.

THE SYNAPTIC
ORGANIZATION
OF THE BRAIN

1

INTRODUCTION

Most organs of the body are made up of cells that are relatively simple in form and either similar or, at least, obviously complementary in function. That the brain is organized in this way is by no means evident; the impression is rather the reverse. The brain seems to be made up of a bewildering complexity of parts, and the cells within the parts seem to be characterized by an inscrutable complexity of form, extent, and relationships with each other. This is true of the nerve cells, or *neurons*, which transmit nervous signals, as well as of the surrounding cells, or neuroglia, and the many types of sensory, muscle, and gland cells to which the neurons are functionally related.

The student of the brain is therefore faced with a severe challenge: What are the principles that govern the organization of neurons in the different parts? If the subject is to be a science, it must be built on this foundation. If neurons are indeed organized according to some common principles, are our present methods sufficient to identify them?; do these principles provide meaningful insights into the nature of brain functions?; and do they provide a useful basis for experiment and theory?

The function of any organ depends upon interactions between its constituent cells, and in the brain, interactions between neurons are the very essence of its function. These interactions take place through connections termed *synapses*. The study of brain function, therefore, must rest on a study of synaptic organization.

TRADITIONAL CONCEPTS OF SYNAPTIC ORGANIZATION

The traditional view of the synaptic organization of neurons in the brain is illustrated in Fig. 1.1. We see here a sensory cell of the dorsal root

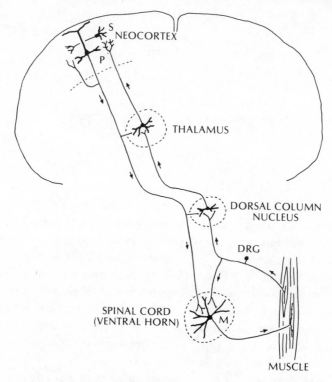

FIG. 1.1. Examples of local regions and some circuits formed through the long axons of principal neurons. M, motoneuron; DRG, dorsal root ganglion cell; P, pyramidal (principal) neuron; S, stellate (intrinsic) neuron.

ganglion (DRG), which receives stimuli in the periphery of the body and, through its long fiber, termed an *axon*, conveys signals to both the spinal cord and to higher centers. Within the spinal cord, the axon terminals make their specialized contacts—synapses—onto motoneurons, which are, by definition, the neurons that innervate the muscles. This is the classical reflex arc that was studied by Sherrington and formed the basis of his great book, *The Integrative Action of the Nervous System* (1906).

The sensory fibers also connect to cells in higher centers (dorsal column nucleus), which, in turn, connect to cells in the thalamus. The thalamus is the great gateway to the neocortex of the cerebrum. From the cortex, pyramidal neurons send fibers to many regions, including those along the sensory input route (as shown in Fig. 1.1). The longest fibers in the human brain reach all the way to the motoneurons in the spinal cord. In this manner are formed the complex loops and pathways that are the basis for delayed reflexes and conditioned responses, as well as the many kinds of motor, emotional, and intellectual behavior that originate within the organism itself.

Figure 1.1 illustrates that the brain consists of many local regions, or centers, and many pathways between them. At each center, the *input fibers* make synapses onto the cell body (*soma*), and/or the short branched processes emanating from the cell body (*dendrites*), of the cells contained therein. Some of these cells send out a long axon that, in turn, carries the signals to other centers. These are termed *principal, relay,* or *projection* neurons. Other cells are concerned only with local processing within the center. These are termed *intrinsic* neurons, *local* neurons, or *inter*neurons. An example of this latter type is shown in the cerebral cortex in Fig. 1.1. The distinction between a principal and an intrinsic neuron cannot be rigid, since principal neurons also take part in local interactions. It is, nonetheless, a useful way of characterizing nerve cells, which we will use throughout this book.

The principal and intrinsic neurons, together with the incoming input fibers, are the three types of neuronal constituents common to most regions of the brain. We will refer to them as a *triad* of synaptic elements. The relations between the three elements vary in different regions of the brain, and these variations underlie the specific functional operations of each region.

Figure 1.1 illustrates the fact that each type of neuron is distinctive; neurons in different centers are of different size, form, extent, and branching pattern. The varieties of neurons, and their probable relationships to each other, were first revealed by the histologists of the 1880's. Their principal tool was the Golgi method, which has the remarkable property of impregnating only a few neurons in any given region, but doing so in their entirety. Figure 1.1 is, in fact, a composite drawing of Golgi-impregnated neurons. Chief among these classical histologists was Ramón y Cajal, who may be regarded as the first architect of the nervous system. His great textbook *Histologie du Système Nerveux* (1911) was the most exhaustive and cogent account of the neural elements and circuits of the brain, as studied with the light microscope.

From Cajal and Sherrington and their contemporaries are derived the concepts of nervous organization that came to be regarded as classical. Chief among them are the following. The circuits of the brain are built up of individual neurons. Each neuron has three parts: cell body, axon, and dendrites. Neurons transmit to each other through synapses. Transmission at synapses is one way; hence, the concept of "dynamic polarization" (Cajal) of the neuron, the neuron receiving synaptic inputs at its soma and dendrites and sending impulses out through its axon. The axons diverge (by branching) and converge (by overlapping onto a single target neuron). A neuron "integrates" its various inputs; the motoneuron, for example, acts as the "final common path" (Sherrington) for synaptic inputs controlling the muscles.

Over the intervening years, these concepts have appeared to be confirmed and extended by the anatomical and physiological studies of the long-distance pathways in the brain. Although never elevated to the status of a "central dogma" (wisely, as we shall see), they nonetheless have been widely accepted as the functional framework of the neuron doctrine. As such, they have been the basis of thinking not only in neuroanatomy and neurophysiology but also in psychology and the behavioral sciences, the clinical neurological sciences, and neural modeling, to say nothing of countless popular expositions of brain function.

SYNAPTIC ORGANIZATION OF LOCAL REGIONS

This body of principles was a remarkable achievement, particularly in view of the fact that it was based largely on deductions from the shapes of neurons and that proof for synaptic connections was lacking. The principles were derived almost exclusively from studies of principal relay neurons, with their obvious fiber connections to distant regions. Even in his original article on the neuron, Waldeyer (1891) explicitly pointed out that little could be said about the functional significance of dendrites or of neurons whose axonal arborizations were entirely local. Thus, it is probably fair to say that, from the start, the organization of local brain regions has never been adequately included within the framework of functional concepts built up around the neuron doctrine.

With the passage of time, progress in understanding the organization of local brain regions was very slow. For many regions, little could be said about the sites of synapses made by long axons, whether onto the principal neurons or the intrinsic neurons contained therein. Within a region, one could only speculate about the connections made by the intrinsic neurons. In most regions, there was little direct evidence about the physiological actions of particular synapses. The notion of inhibition was absent from the thinking of Cajal and of many who followed him. Finally, consistent definitions of an axon and a dendrite could not be agreed upon in the face of the enormous variety of processes exhibited by different neurons.

To all this was added the problem that local regions appeared to be distinctly different. Different types of neurons were present in each region, and specialized methods were necessary for studying them (i.e., visual stimuli for studying the visual regions, auditory stimuli for studying the auditory regions). This made it all the more difficult to perceive similarities in the connections and properties of neurons, which would provide a basis for principles of organization common to all regions.

These matters awaited evidence that could only be gained by improved methods, specifically, the use of microelectrodes, which can record from single, clearly identified nerve cells, and the electron microscope, which can reveal internal fine structure and give proof of synaptic connections. Both methods were introduced to the study of the brain in the 1950's, but the data they provided were not closely correlated until the 1960's. To these two essential tools have been added the power of the computer to analyze data and construct neuronal models, and a burgeoning armamentarium of biochemical methods that has brought the analysis of neurotransmission to the level of the single neuron and single synapse. It is thus only in very recent years that results bearing directly on the long-unanswered questions about the synaptic organization of neurons in local regions of the brain have become available.

These results have been consistent with some of the classical notions, but inconsistent with others. Most unexpected have been the findings of synapses from axon to axon and from dendrite to dendrite, of a wide variety of functional properties of dendrites, and of synaptic interactions that take place without the mediation of nervous impulses. For most students and workers in the field, the brain was already complicated enough; to assimilate these new complexities was to be asked to pile Ossa on Pelion.

In sifting the new evidence two points have begun to emerge to provide a basis for a rational synthesis. One is that the concept of the single neuron as a functional unit—receiving information by way of its dendrites and sending information out by way of its axon—is much too limited and, in many cases, inaccurate. The new findings, particularly with regard to dendrites, indicate that a single neuron may contain many functional units in terms of its individual synaptic input-output relations and its dendritic compartmentalization. Also, any given neuron is only one small fragment of larger functional units made up of multineuronal assemblies.

The other point that has begun to emerge is that the local regions are not so different from each other as formerly appeared to be the case. At the synaptic level, particularly, similarities in structural patterns and functional properties have been found amid the welter of detail. The importance of identifying these similarities is that it is only against the background of what is common to different regions that the significance of their differences in structure and function can be assessed. This is no more than a truism that applies to all fields of scientific inquiry.

These considerations have indicated that we are moving toward a re-definition of the basic units of function in the nervous system. It is conceivable that the synapse and the ensembles of circuits built up from it provide the reproducible operational units for nervous organization. The issue has been raised (Shepherd, 1972b) and debated (Rakić, 1975; Pearson, 1976; Peters, Palay, and Webster, 1976; Bullock, 1976; Shepherd, 1977, 1979; Calvin and Graubard, 1979; Mountcastle, 1978). There are also indications that much of the computational language of the nervous system is in the form of local potentials controlling individual synapses (Rall and Shepherd, 1968; Pearson, 1976; Schmitt, Dev, and Smith, 1977), and that complex aggregates of local synaptic circuits may constitute the neural substrates of higher brain functions (Schmitt et al., 1977). There is thus a keen and growing awareness of a revolution not only in our knowledge of synaptic organization but also in our understanding of the principles of organization and their relation to behavior.

PLAN OF THE BOOK

In this book, we will attempt a systematic comparison of those parts of the mammalian brain that have been most thoroughly studied. Our approach is therefore one of *comparative neuronal systems*. It is also *multidisciplinary* in that it draws on the coordinated evidence from anatomy, physiology, neurochemistry, and biophysics. It focuses on the *structure-function relations* of synapses, since it is in the different kinds of junctional organization between neurons that our knowledge has undergone its most rapid increase, and this is where understanding must start, if one is to build up principles of organization at higher levels.

We shall begin by briefly reviewing the structure of neurons and synapses and their functional properties. We will consider some essential properties of synapses, particularly the conductance changes related to synaptic actions, and the neurotransmitters which control these changes.

The relation between structure and function depends to a large extent on the dynamics of electrical current flow in the neuronal processes. Because of the complexities of dendritic branching, this has been one of the greatest problems in the analysis of synaptic interactions. The solution to this problem, largely due to the work of Wilfrid Rall, has been one of the most important developments of recent years. The methods are mathematical and biophysical in character and have not been readily available to a wide range of students. We will discuss some of the essential features involved in their application at the level of synaptic organization.

Figure 1.2 indicates the parts of the brain that will be studied in this book. Most of them are known even to the beginning student. As a prelude, we begin with peripheral ganglia, the simplest and most accessible of synaptic systems. The spinal motoneuron is next, as the classical subject for the study of central organization. The olfactory bulb is then introduced; its study has provided some of the clearest evidence about local synaptic organization, as well as support for concepts that go beyond the classical motoneuron model. The retina and cerebellum each have distinctive and stereotyped structures; together with the olfactory bulb, they are the best understood of the local regions of the brain. The thalamus has also received much attention; it forms a natural bridge to a consideration of the telencephalon. Within the telencephalon, the basal ganglia occupy a key position. At the highest level, it is possible to consider all three types of cortex in the evolutionary scale: olfactory, hippocampal, and neocortical (both sensory and motor areas).

In each chapter, the same sequence will be followed: First, a description of the main types of neuronal elements; second, a description of the major types of synaptic connections between the neurons; third, a summary of organization in terms of a basic circuit diagram, with a discussion of the cardinal aspects of the organization of that region; fourth, the dynamics of the local circuits in terms of the main types of synaptic actions; fifth, the evidence for neurotransmitters; and sixth, a consideration of the dendritic properties crucial to the synaptic interactions. Keeping to this sequence will, it is hoped, make it easier for the reader to compare the different regions.

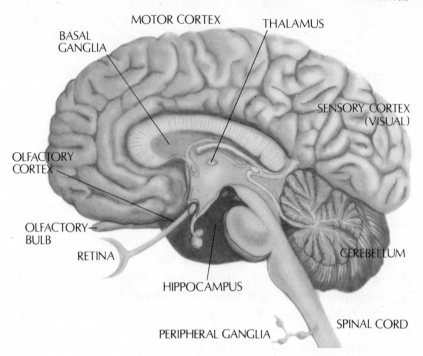

FIG. 1.2. Local regions for which synaptic organization will be described in this book.

DIMENSIONS The dimensions of nerve cells and their processes are important factors in the study of synaptic organization. The classical histologists who studied Golgi-stained neurons were primarily interested in describing the marvelously varied shapes of neurons and the distributions of the processes, and they paid relatively little attention to dimensions. Cajal, for example, provided no scales for the diagrams in his monumental survey of neuronal architecture (Cajal, 1911). In modern studies of fine structure with the electron microscope, there has been a similar tendency to emphasize the shapes of processes and terminals and the patterns of synaptic connections. The application of methods for analyzing electrical current flows, however, requires precise figures for the dimensions of axonal and dendritic processes. Such figures are necessary, not only for understanding synaptic integration in neurons of a given region but also for comparing the organization of different regions.

A scale for lineal (distance) measurements is provided in Fig. 1.3. Just

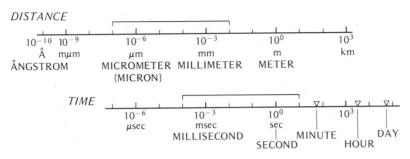

FIG. 1.3. Scales (logarithmic) for distance and time. Brackets, ranges relevant to the synaptic organization of local regions.

as we live our daily lives in a world of inches and feet (or centimeters and meters), so the student of synaptic organization lives in a world of micrometers and hundreds of micrometers. As shown in Fig. 1.3, a micrometer (μm) is one-millionth part of a meter, one ten-thousandth part of a centimeter, or one-thousandth part of a millimeter. Its colloquial name is "micron" and it will be the common currency of our descriptions in this book.

In comparing dimensions in different parts of the brain, the student is never more frustrated than by the multiplicity of scales and magnifications that so often confront him. We will try to ease at least this much of the burden by the use of only two scales in the later chapters. For the diagrams of neuronal elements, all magnifications will be $\times 55$; i.e., 5.5 mm in the diagram equals 100 μm actual length. For diagrams of synaptic connections, all magnifications will be 100 times this, or $\times 5500$; i.e., 5.5 mm in the diagram equals 1 μm actual length. By this systematic approach, some dramatic and important differences in size between processes of different regions will be brought out.

Figure 1.3 also provides a temporal (time) scale for measurements. What the micron is to the dimensions of synaptic organization, the millisecond (one-thousandth of a second: msec) is to the time course of synaptic actions. As it turns out, the time courses of synaptic actions are too varied to permit their representation on only one time scale, so the student must pay particular attention to the scales in comparing recordings of synaptic actions in different regions. The number of different time scales has, in any case, been held to a minimum to facilitate comparisons as much as possible.

The dimensions of space and time involve only the simplest concepts of quantitation, yet the student will find that their usefulness as tools in the analysis of synaptic organization requires a facility that comes only with practice.

Part 1

PRINCIPLES OF STRUCTURE AND FUNCTION

2

AXONS, DENDRITES, AND SYNAPSES

The study of synaptic organization requires, first, the identification of the structures that take part in synaptic connections, and we will, therefore, begin with an overview of the current knowledge of the parts of the neuron and the different kinds of synapses. The identification of neuronal parts turns out to be quite difficult because of the extraordinary variety of forms neurons and their processes assume. The types of neurons represent almost every imaginable extreme, and even within a type it is fair to say that no two neurons are exactly alike. In an attempt to make sense of this bewildering variety, the classical histologists divided neuronal processes into *axons* and *dendrites*, on the basis of external shape, extent, and branching pattern. This distinction is clear cut only in certain simple cases, however, and, ultimately, our definitions must be based on fine structural criteria. The brief description that follows may be supplemented by the accounts of Peters et al. (1976), Bodian (1972), and Akert et al. (1972).

PARTS OF THE NEURON

The nerve cell, like all other cells of the body, is bounded by a *plasma membrane*. In cross sections of electron micrographs at low magnification (as in the diagrams of fine structure in this book) the membrane appears under the electron microscope as a single dark line, about 80 Å thick (i.e., just less than one one-hundredth of a micron). At higher magnifications it can be seen that there are, in fact, two dark lines with a light space between them. This gives the membrane a three-layered structure, with inner and outer leaflets.

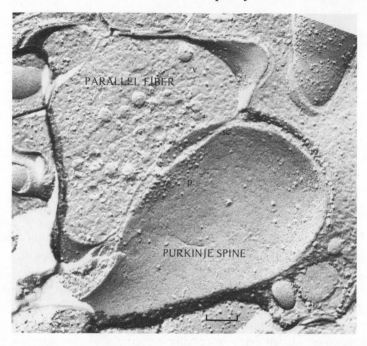

FIG. 2.1. A freeze-fractured specimen of synaptic terminals in the cerebellum. The line of cleavage is such that one sees the inner surface of an outer leaflet of a Purkinje cell dendritic spine; it also cuts across a synaptic terminal of a parallel fiber. Note the vesicles (v) in the presynaptic terminal, the widened synaptic cleft (sc), and the accumulation of small particles (p) in the postsynaptic terminal membrane. Bracket 0.1 μm. (From Landis and Reese, 1974.)

The plasma membrane is vividly revealed by the freeze-fracturing technique, in which a tiny block of tissue is frozen and then fractured by a swift blow with a sharp blade (Akert et al., 1972). A micrograph of a specimen prepared in this way is shown in Figure 2.1. The lines of cleavage are not between the membranes of the two neighboring neurons, but between the inner and outer leaflets of the same membrane. As can be seen in Figure 2.1, the fracture line jumps from one membrane to the next, or cuts entirely through a process, in its course through the tissue. In this view, the fracture line has cut through a synapse between a pre- and postsynaptic process. There is a collection of intramembranous particles on the inner surface of the outer leaflet of the postsynaptic membrane. Later, we will see how this correlates with the morphology of this type of synapse and its physiological action.

The three-layered structure comprises the *unit membrane*, common to all animal cells, which is thought to consist of oriented lipid and protein complexes. In all cells of the body this membrane controls the interchange of substances between the cell and its environment. In nerve cells it is, additionally, the site of origin of the electrical activity that is the basis of nervous signals. There is as yet no evidence for differences in membrane structure in different parts of the neuron. Hence, identification of neuronal parts must depend upon other criteria.

The fine structure of different parts of the neuron is summarized in Fig. 2.2, which shows a representative neuron surrounded by schematic drawings of electron micrographs of the various parts.

CELL BODY   The cell body (soma) by definition is the part of the neuron that contains the *nucleus* (see Fig. 2.2). As in all cells, the nucleus contains the genetic material of the neuron. The size of the cell body varies widely in different neurons, from 6 μm to 100 μm or more in diameter. The size of the nucleus similarly varies. It tends to fill nearly all the cell body of smaller cells, leaving only a narrow rim of cytoplasm. Larger neurons, on the other hand, tend to have relatively more cytoplasm.

The cytoplasm surrounding the nucleus, the *perikaryon*, contains a widespread system of membranes, the *endoplasmic reticulum* (ER), and numerous small particles, the *ribosomes*. The latter are the principal sites of protein synthesis in the cell. The distribution of the ribosomes is the basis for a fundamental distinction between ER that is covered with closely adhering ribosomes (granular, or rough, ER) and ER that has no adhering ribosomes (agranular, or smooth, ER).

In some parts of the perikaryon, the rough ER is organized into aggregations of pancake-like folds, or cisternae. These are called *Nissl bodies*, which are regarded as nodal points in the ER for the synthesis of structural and secretory proteins, including substances that play a role in synaptic transmission.

The smooth ER, on the other hand, is specialized in places to form stacks of cisternae and assorted vacuoles, the *Golgi apparatus*, implicated in the turnover of vesicle membranes and the packaging of secretory substances involved in synaptic transmission.

Mitochondria are scattered throughout the perikaryon. In vertebrate neurons, they range from 0.1–0.5 μm in diameter and up to several

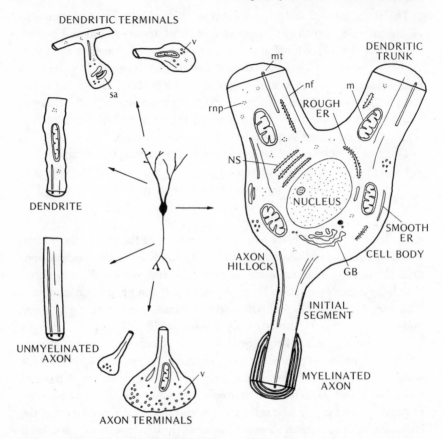

FIG. 2.2. Diagrams of the parts of the neuron. A principal neuron (as stained by the Golgi method or by intracellular injection of dyes), shown at center, is surrounded by schematic drawings of fine structure (as viewed in the electron microscope) of the different parts. ER, endoplasmic reticulum; GB, Golgi body; NS, Nissl substance; mt, microtubule; nf, neurofilament; rnp, ribonucleic particles; sa, spine apparatus; v, vesicles; m, mitochondria.

microns in length. They are often found in the vicinity of Nissl bodies, where, as in other cells of the body, they supply energy for metabolism.

Two elongated structures within the perikaryon are *microtubules* and *neurofilaments*. Microtubules are 200–300 Å in diameter. At high resolution, neurofilaments have a light core, hence, they also appear as tubules. Both these elements, singly or in aggregates, weave their way through the perikaryon. Microtubules are composed of protein and are thought to be involved in several functions, including cell division, the shaping of cell processes during development, and intraneuronal transport of substances; they may also have contractile properties. Neurofilaments are also thought to be protein. Their function is enigmatic, beyond the obvious one of imparting some structural rigidity. One possibility is that they are involved in intraneuronal transport.

A third type of fibrillary structure is the *microfilament*. This is approximately 50 Å in diameter, and composed of actin. It is present in axonal and dendritic growth cones, as well as in glia and other types of cells, and is believed to be responsible for the movements of neuronal processes that underlie morphogenesis.

Vesicles should also be included among the constituents of the perikaryon. They may be found singly here and there or in small clumps near the border. In the latter case, they form part of the presynaptic apparatus of a synapse from the cell body to a neighboring neuron. They will be described in detail later in this chapter.

Other types of organelles within neurons include subsurface cisterna; various types of large vesicles, including lysozymes; multivesicular bodies; and various inclusion bodies.

All the main internal structures of the perikaryon described above are common to animal cells, in general, with the exception of neurofilaments. An interesting finding is that the distribution of internal structures appears to be distinctive for some types of neurons. This suggestion that neurons with distinct geometrical shapes may have distinct patterns of internal organization within their perikarya is well worth further study. The significance of the differences between neurons is not yet clear; there is no correlation, for instance, between Nissl body occurrence and neuronal size.

AXON HILLOCK   We can now begin to consider the types of processes that arise from the cell body. In neurons that have an axon, the axon is often seen to arise from a cone-shaped region of the perikaryon or a large dendrite, the *axon hillock*. As shown in Fig. 2.2, the hillock is characterized by decreased density of ribosomes and other organelles and funneling of microtubules and neurofilaments; the former are typically grouped in fascicles. An axon hillock is particularly characteristic of large neurons with large axons, but it is by no means clear that an axon hillock, as characterized above, is present in all neurons, and especially in the smallest neurons with the finest axons.

INITIAL SEGMENT In neurons that give rise to a myelinated axon, the *initial segment* is that portion between the axon hillock and the point at which myelination begins. As indicated in Fig. 2.2, it is characterized by a thin layer of dense material underneath the plasma membrane, the so-called dense undercoating. Microtubules continue, singly or in fascicles, from the axon hillock into the initial segment. A few ribosomes may be present, but the other organelles of the perikaryon are absent. The initial segment is characteristic of neurons giving rise to myelinated axons, although it is absent in the Purkinje cell of the cerebellum. It is also doubtful whether the initial segment can be considered to be present, as an entity, in the smallest neurons giving rise to unmyelinated axons.

AXON The long single nerve process that extends from the axon hillock and initial segment is, by definition, an axon. The axon, thus, can always be identified if it has this origin. The fine structure of the axon is characterized by neurofilaments, microtubules, mitochondria, and smooth ER; generally, ribosomes are few or absent. The relative number of these structures depends on size. Large axons (up to 20 μm in diameter in the vertebrate brain) tend to contain many neurofilaments but relatively few microtubules. In small axons, however, the ratio is reversed. In the thinnest axons (0.1 μm) only a few microtubules may be present.

The criteria for identifying an axon include the sheaths that surround them. In their course through either the periphery or the brain, axons are enveloped by the processes of satellite cells, called Schwann cells. The Schwann cells enwrap the larger axons in many layers of plasma membrane; these tightly layered membranes are called *myelin*. In general, the larger the axon, the thicker the myelin, up to a hundred layers or so around the largest axons. Along its length an axon is enwrapped by a series of Schwann cells. The place where two Schwann cells meet is free of myelin for a micron or so, and this region is called a *node of Ranvier*. At the node, there is an undercoating of the plasma membrane similar to that of the initial segment. The internodal distance is characteristically 1 mm or so. As we shall see, myelin is a specialization that provides for rapid impulse transmission from node to node.

Although myelination is the most important distinguishing characteristic of large axons, the finest axons (below about 1 μm diameter) are unmyelinated. Fine axons predominate in the brain, in many pathways between regions and within regions, and other criteria for axon identification are therefore needed when such axons are viewed at a distance from their cell bodies. As we shall see, it is difficult, in electron micrographs of the neuropil of local regions, to distinguish fine axons from fine dendritic processes.

AXONAL BRANCHES   Axons characteristically have branches that distribute the signals traveling in them to more than one destination. The branches take several forms. An axon may simply divide into two branches of equal diameter; an example is the axon of the granule cell of the cerebellum. An axon may give off a relatively large branch, referred to as a *collateral*. Such a branch may arise during the long-distance course of the axon, as, for example, the collateral from the axon of a DRG cell to the spinal cord (see Fig. 1.1). Or a collateral may arise locally within the region of origin. Such a branch may have a generally lateral orientation, or it may run backwards within the region, in which case it is called a *recurrent collateral;* an example is shown in the cortical pyramidal cell in Fig. 1.1. Recurrent collaterals are important components in the synaptic circuits of local regions.

It is often stated that axons maintain their diameters during their course, in contrast to dendrites, which typically taper—and that axonal branches arise at right angles from their parent fibers, whereas dendritic branches arise at acute angles. Although these features are found in many neurons, they tend to be associated with neurons in which axon and dendrite are most differentiated, the one from the other; they are unfortunately less useful in identifying neuronal processes that are not so clearly differentiated.

The fine structure of axonal branches is generally similar to that of the parent fiber, being characterized mainly by variable numbers of microtubules. In axons that give rise to synapses as they pass by their target neurons (*en passage*), groups of vesicles are present in relation to synaptic sites; an example is the parallel fiber of the cerebellum.

DENDRITES   We have already mentioned some of the ambiguities of identification of neuronal parts. The problem becomes most difficult with regard to dendrites.

The simplest case we can consider is that of a principal neuron (note again the several examples in Fig. 1.1). All principal neurons have, by definition, a long axon. In these neurons, any process that is not the axon arising from the axon hillock and initial segment may be defined as a dendrite. The stout trunks of dendrites have much the same internal structure as that of the cell body from which they arise. Deiter's original term "protoplasmic prolongations" (1865) can, therefore, be said to have been right on the mark. Microtubules are prominent in the dendritic trunks, often present in orderly arrays, whereas neurofilaments are few; this is the reverse of the ratio for large axons. As in the soma, vesicles may be found, either scattered or in presynaptic aggregations.

This simple definition of dendrite, as a process that is not an axon, would appear to be general enough, but, unfortunately, it runs afoul the fantastic variety of neuronal processes. It does not even apply to all principal neurons. In invertebrates, for example, the cell body characteristically gives rise to a single process, which becomes the axon, and which also gives off a number of branches to the local region before projecting to distant regions. Our present knowledge is not sufficient to enable us to conclude whether the single process and the local branches are axonal or dendritic, and the usual practice is therefore to refer to them noncommittally as "processes" or "neurites".

In the vertebrate brain, the DRG cell (see Fig. 1.1) is a variety of principal neuron that has become specialized in the mammal for long-distance transmission between the periphery and the spinal cord. In this specialization, its central "axon" and peripheral "dendrite" have fused into one long fiber. The fact that the peripheral process is embryologically a "dendrite" but structurally an "axon" has presented a terminological dilemma unresolved to the present day.

The problem is even more difficult for intrinsic neurons; they are involved exclusively with local interactions and, therefore, do not require an axon for long-distance transmission. As a result, some intrinsic neurons have a morphologically identifiable axon, whereas others do not. In the latter case the definition of a dendrite as any process that is not the axon of a particular cell will not do, since the particular cell does not have an axon to begin with. The granule cell of the olfactory bulb and the amacrine cell of the retina are examples of this type of "anaxonal" neuron. In such cells, the common-sense approach is to call these processes dendrites on the basis of their similarity to dendrites of other neurons or else to use the noncommittal term "process."

These are only a few illustrations of the problem attending the definition of dendrite, as distinct from axon. They by no means exhaust the list. A further complication, for example, is the fact that myelination is not exclusively associated with axons; myelin is also found around cell bodies and dendrites in certain instances, as we shall see in the olfactory bulb. A myelinated structure, therefore, cannot be said to be, by definition, an axon; conversely, an unmyelinated structure may be either an axon or a dendrite.

It is often stated that the presence of ribosomes is a distinguishing characteristic of dendrites, but it is becoming clear that this generalization has limited usefulness. It has yet to be established that ribosomes are lacking in all the short unmyelinated axons of the brain. On the other hand, many processes that, by other criteria, would be accepted as dendritic contain few or no ribosomes.

As one proceeds from the dendritic trunk, through the larger to the smaller dendritic branches, one encounters occasional membranous cisternae and variable numbers of microtubules. A small branch may have lighter- or darker-staining background material and may contain a few ribosomes or none at all. Vesicles may be scattered about or found in presynaptic groups. In the smaller branches mitochondria become especially prominent, usually slender, and sometimes much elongated; their lengths may reach as far as 20 μm. By the time one reaches the smaller dendritic branches, the internal structure is not significantly different from that of axons and axonal branches of comparable size. In some cases, a more irregular contour and a more variable orientation aid in identification. But both the axonal and non-axonal (i.e., dendritic) processes of nerve cells are too variable to admit of generalization with regard to shape and extent.

TERMINALS After dividing into smaller branches, axons end in terminals of various descriptions, from simple enlargements (buttons, boutons, knobs, end-feet) to elaborate claws, mossy terminals, and other complicated configurations. Dendritic branches also terminate in a variety of ways, as simple enlargements (varicosities, knobs, spines, gemmules), as cilia or other fine elongated processes, as claws, and even as sheets. Apart from these specific shapes assumed by different terminals, no general statement can be made about their internal fine structure. Of the organelles we have considered, ER and ribosomes are usually scarce, mitochondria are usually plentiful, and microtubules and neurofilaments are variably present. Vesicles are usually (but not always) the most conspicuous component of terminals; they are either scattered or accumulated in dense clouds within the terminal cytoplasm. In addition, vesicles are organized in smaller groups in relation to synaptic contacts, as will be described in the next section.

Traditionally, electron microscopists have used the presence or absence of synaptic vesicles as the criterion for distinguishing an axon from a dendritic terminal when identifying profiles seen in electron micrographs; according to the functional interpretations of the neuron doctrine, axon terminals contain synaptic vesicles and dendritic terminals do not. The discovery of presynaptic dendrites, however, has rendered this criterion untenable. *A terminal cannot be identified as axonal solely on the basis of the fact that it contains synaptic vesicles.* In some cases, a relatively high density of vesicles is characteristic of axonal terminals; in others, the presence of a distinguishing organelle such as a spine apparatus (an aggregation of cisternae) indicates a dendritic spine. But, in general, the terminals of axons and dendrites form a single, very broad class. It may be noted that this is not at all inconsistent with the classical term "telodendria" for the terminals of axons.

A point perhaps worth noting is that the term "terminal", strictly interpreted, refers to the geometry of a process, i.e., the end of a branch or an excrescence from a branch. Presynaptic loci characteristically occur in geometrical terminals, but enough has been said here to indicate that they may also occur along the branches of an axon, along the branches and trunks of dendrites, and at the cell body. Terminal as an appellation for any presynaptic locus is firmly fixed in the literature, however, and we will use it in this more general sense, as well as in the stricter geometrical sense.

It may be concluded that the division of neuronal processes into axon and dendrite can be made only for the largest processes of principle neurons and certain intrinsic neurons. The smaller processes of all types of neuron overlap too much in their morphology to allow simple generalization. To deal with the practical problem of analyzing synaptic organization, the electron microscopist, confronted with a single view of a central region, must seek supplementary evidence in order to differentiate between the processes and identify the synapses and cell types from which they arise. Techniques which provide such evidence include: se-

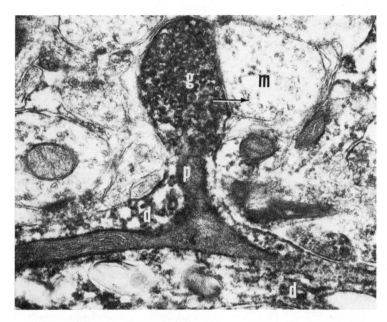

FIG. 2.3. Localization of the GABA-synthesizing enzyme GAD (glutamic acid decarboxylose) in a granule cell dendrite (d), pedicle (p), and spine (g) in the rat olfactory bulb. The spine stains darkly for the reaction product, in contrast to an unstained dendrite of a mitral cell (m). A dendrodendritic synapse connects the granule cell spine to the mital cell dendrite. (From Ribak et al., 1977.)

rial reconstructions of many sections to give a three-dimensional view, close correlations with Golgi-stained material, study of neurons that have been stained intracellularly, and observations of neurons undergoing selective degeneration.

The fact that synapses use different transmitters has provided powerful tools for identifying terminals; the methods include uptake of radioactively labelled substances and immunocytochemical techniques. The latter involve the making of antibodies to given transmitter enzymes or substances and attaching probes, such as fluorescent compounds or horseradish peroxidase, to them so that the reaction sites can be visualized. A characteristic result is illustrated in Fig. 2.3, taken from the olfactory bulb; a granule cell dendritic spine, positive for the enzyme which synthesizes the transmitter GABA, has a synapse onto another, nonreactive, process, a dendrite of a mitral cell. This method not only is an effective

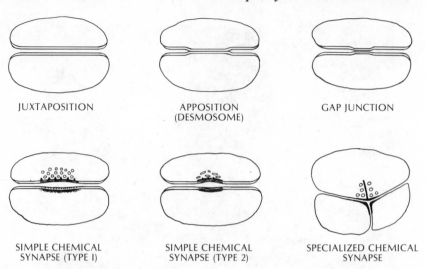

JUXTAPOSITION   APPOSITION   GAP JUNCTION
                       (DESMOSOME)

SIMPLE CHEMICAL   SIMPLE CHEMICAL   SPECIALIZED CHEMICAL
SYNAPSE (TYPE I)   SYNAPSE (TYPE 2)   SYNAPSE

FIG. 2.4. Types of junctions between nerve cells.

means for identification of terminals, but it provides the opportunity for making close correlations between neuronal structure and synaptic morphology, putative transmitters, and physiological actions.

TYPES OF SYNAPSES

In reviewing the fine structure of neuronal parts, we have avoided considering, as far as possible, the organelles that are related specifically to synapses. The reason for this has already been indicated, that if one follows classical concepts and uses the orientations of synapses as the basis for distinguishing between axon and dendrite, one may be led into error. Let us therefore consider synaptic morphology independently of neuronal morphology and then bring the two together.

MEMBRANE JUXTAPOSITIONS   There are several types of structural relations one neuron can have with another. The simplest is a juxtaposition of their membranes, the two being separated by the ubiquitous extracellular space (cleft) of about 200 Å. This is illustrated schematically in Fig. 2.4. Some of the fine unmyelinated axons (e.g., olfactory axons, parallel fibers of the cerebellum) have this membrane-to-membrane relationship with each other. It also occurs throughout the neuropil of the local regions of the brain, between dendritic processes or between closely packed cell bodies, as well as between neurons and their satellite cells. Juxtaposition of membranes provides for several possible functions, including ionic or metabolic effects, mediated by extrusion, and uptake of substances into and out of the intervening extracellular cleft. It may also provide for electrical interactions between neurons under some conditions; the site at which such an interaction occurs is an *ephapse*.

MEMBRANE APPOSITIONS The next stage of relatedness between neurons is a specific apposition of their membranes. This occurs at sites where (1) the two membranes come close together or are fused and/or (2) the membranes appear more dense. Such sites are found between cells throughout the body. Depending on details of structure, they are called occluding junctions, desmosomes, tight junctions, gap junctions, septate junctions, zonulae adherens, etc. (see Peters et al., 1976). They vary widely in size and form, ranging from small spots to long strips or patches. Such junctions provide for several possible functions: simple adhesion; transfer of substances during metabolism or embryological development; restriction of movement of substances in the extracellular compartment. An instance of the latter function is provided by the *tight junctions* between the cells that line the blood vessels and ventricles of the brain. The two outer leaflets of the unit membrane of these junctions, as illustrated in Fig. 2.4, are completely fused, to form a five-layered complex. These tight junctions restrict the movement of substances in the extracellular space and are responsible for the so-called blood-brain barrier.

An important type of membrane apposition in the nervous system is the so-called *gap junction*. Here, the outer leaflets are separated by a gap of 20–40 Å, to form a seven-layered complex (Figs. 2.4 and 2.5). In several cases, the presence of these junctions has been correlated with the physiological finding of a low-resistance electrical pathway between two neurons (see Reese and Brightman, 1969; Bennett, 1973). On this basis they have been categorized as *electrical synapses*. The junction varies in diameter from 0.1–10 μm. At high resolution, dense material is seen beneath each apposed membrane, and it can be shown that the membranes are part of two systems of channels, the one continuous with the extracellular space, the other connecting the two cells. Electrical synapses are a common form of interneuronal connection in lower vertebrates (Bennett, 1973); they have also been found at several sites in the mammalian brain (see next chapter). Gap junctions are found between

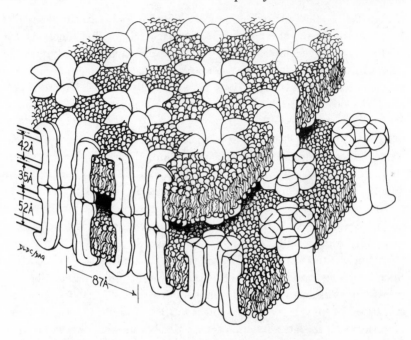

FIG. 2.5. Schematic diagram of a gap junction (electrical synapse). Channels provide for intercellular exchange of low molecular weight substances and electric current. Some gap junctions pass current in only one direction (rectifying junctions). Channel walls are composed of six protein subunits which span the lipid bilayer of each plasma membrane. Because of the gap between the membranes, extracellular substances can percolate between the channels. (From Makowski et al., 1977.)

many types of cells in the body besides neurons. In addition to electrical coupling, their possible functions include those mentioned above for closely apposed membranes.

CHEMICAL SYNAPSES The most complicated type of junction in the nervous system, and the type considered to be the most characteristic, is the chemical synapse (see Fig. 2.6). It differs morphologically from other types of membrane appositions in being strongly oriented, or polarized, from one neuron to the other. This polarization is determined mainly by two features: (1) an unequal *densification* of the two apposed membranes and (2) the presence of a group of small *vesicles* near the synaptic site. In certain cases (e.g., the neuromuscular junction), it can be shown un-

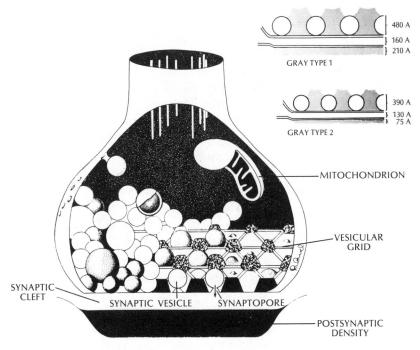

FIG. 2.6. Schematic diagram of presynaptic nerve terminal, with main constituents as labeled. Inset in upper right shows some characteristics of Type I and II synapses (pleomorphic vesicles usually seen at Type II synapses are not included). (From Akert et al., 1972.)

equivocally that transmission is from the vesicle-containing process to the other process, and one has, therefore, the terminology of a *presynaptic* process and a *postsynaptic* process, respectively.

Synapses were first identified in the electron microscope by Palay and Palade (1955). Gray (1959), working on the cerebral cortex, obtained evidence for two morphological types. There is a growing consensus that, despite many local variations and gradations between the two, this division has some validity. The two types are illustrated in Figs. 2.4 and 2.6. The distinguishing features may be summarized as follows. Type I: synaptic cleft approximately 300 Å; junctional area relatively large (up to 1–2 μm in extent); prominent accumulation of dense material next to the postsynaptic membrane (i.e., an asymmetric densification of the two apposed membranes). Type II: synaptic cleft approximately 200 Å; junc-

tional area relatively small (less than 1 μm in extent); membrane densifi-
cations modest and symmetrical.

Following the recognition of these types, evidence was obtained (see
Uchizono, 1965) that, in many parts of the brain, type I synapses are
associated with large spherical vesicles (diameter approximately 300–600
Å) which are usually present in considerable numbers. Type II synapses, on the other hand, are associated with smaller (100–300 Å diameter) vesicles, which are less numerous and which, significantly, take on
various ellipsoidal and flattened shapes. The distinction between round
and flat types of vesicles is by no means a sharp one; in many synapses a
vesicle simply tends to the one shape or the other.

These two morphological features (symmetry of membrane density
and shape of vesicles) have provided a convenient means for characterizing synapses, and we will use the terms type I and type II in this sense
to describe synapses in different regions of the brain.

The recognition of these two types of synapse has provided anatomists
with a most useful tool to unravel the synaptic organization of local brain
regions. Much of this usefulness has been based on the premise that all
the synapses made by a given neuron onto other neurons are either of
one type or the other. This is commonly called the *morphological corollary
of Dale's Law*, Dale's Law being usually understood as stating that a given
neuron has the same physiological action at all its synapses. As we will
see in the next chapter, this is neither what Dale, in fact, put forward
nor what electrophysiology reveals. Nor has it been proved that the
morphological corollary has universal validity; in the cochlear nucleus,
for example, there is evidence that an auditory axon makes both types of
synapses onto the same postsynaptic neuron (Kane, 1973). In the regions
of the brain under review here, the premise that all the synapses made
by a given neuron are of the same type has been generally assumed and
thus far substantiated.

Many neuroanatomists have been skeptical of the validity of the two
types of synapse on the basis of the fact that the flattening of vesicles has
been shown to depend on the osmolarity of solutions used in preparing
the tissue for electron microscopy (Valdivia, 1971). But, in a sense,
everything the electron microscopist sees is a distortion of the true dynamic living state. The interpretation of electron micrographs, and of
any preparations of anatomical specimens, must be made with this con-
stantly in mind. That the recognition of the two types of synapse has

been the basis for remarkable progress in the understanding of the synaptic organization of the brain may be regarded as sufficient reason for using it as the basis for our review of present knowledge.

These two types of synapse provide relatively small areas of contact between neurons. They may be characterized as *simple* synapses. They are typical of the contacts made by small terminals, both axonal and dendritic, and they are also the type of contact made by most cell bodies and dendrites when those structures occupy presynaptic positions. It is probably fair to say that they make up the majority of synapses in the brain. This, in itself, bespeaks an important principle of brain organization, that the output of a neuron is fractionated, as it were, through many synapses onto many other neurons and, conversely, that synapses from many sources play onto a given neuron. This is an essential aspect of the complexity of information processing in the brain.

In addition, there are, in many regions, much more extensive contacts with more elaborate structure that may be characterized as *specialized synapses*. The neuromuscular junction is an example in the peripheral nervous system. In the central nervous system, we find an example in the retina, where the large terminal of a receptor cell makes contact with several postsynaptic neurons; within the terminal, the synaptic vesicles are grouped around a special small dense bar. This arrangement is shown very schematically in Fig. 2.4 and is described in detail in Chapter 9.

One may also characterize the terminal structures in the geometrical sense, as previously defined. A terminal may be small and have a single synapse onto a single postsynaptic structure, as shown in most of the diagrams of Figs. 2.4 and 2.7. These may be characterized as *simple terminals*. On the other hand, a large terminal, with complicated geometry, may be characterized as a *specialized terminal*: examples are the neuromuscular junction and the basket cell endings around the Purkinje cell. In many regions of the brain, large terminals have synapses onto more than one postsynaptic structure; the receptor terminal in the retina mentioned above is an example. Another example is the large terminal rosette of the mossy fiber in the cerebellum, which has as many as 300 synaptic contacts onto postsynaptic structures (see Fig. 2.7).

Within the brain are all possible combinations of synapses and terminals. Simple synapses may be established by any of the parts of the neuron: terminals, trunks, or the cell body. Simple synapses may also be

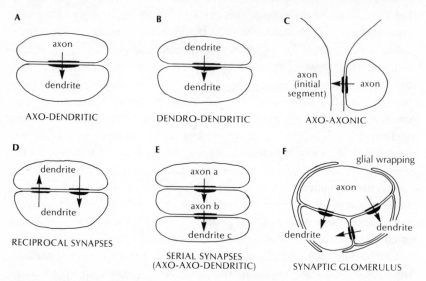

FIG. 2.7. Types of synaptic arrangements.

made by specialized terminals, as in the case of the mossy fiber of the cerebellum. On the other hand, specialized synapses may be made by small terminals, as in the spinule synapses of the hippocampus, and, finally, specialized synapses may arise from specialized terminals, as in the case of the retinal receptor.

PATTERNS OF SYNAPTIC CONNECTIONS   Synapses are also categorized by the kinds of processes that take part in the synapse. Thus, for example, a contact from an axon onto a cell body is termed an *axosomatic* synapse, whereas that onto a dendrite is termed an *axodendritic* synapse [Fig. 2.7 (A)]. Similarly, a contact between two axons is termed an *axoaxonic* synapse (C, E), and a contact between two dendrites is termed a *dendrodendritic* synapse (B).

   A single synapse seldom occurs in isolation in the brain; it is usually one of a number of synapses that together make up a larger pattern of interconnecting synapses. The simplest of these patterns is that formed by two or more synapses situated near each other and oriented in the same direction, i.e., they are all axodendritic. A more complicated pattern is one in which there is a synapse from process (a) to process (b), and another from (b) to (c). Such a situation is diagrammed in Fig. 2.7

(E). These are referred to as *serial* synapses; examples are axoaxodendritic sequences and axodendrodendritic sequences.

Another pattern has a synapse from process (a) to process (b), and a return synapse from (b) to (a). This is diagrammed in Fig. 2.7 (D). It is referred to as a *reciprocal* synapse. If the two synapses are side by side, they are called a *reciprocal pair*. The dendrodendritic synapses between mitral and granule cells in the olfactory bulb are of this type. If the two synapses are far apart, a *reciprocal arrangement* results. Finally, there are patterns of synaptic connections between tightly grouped clusters of terminals, called synaptic glomeruli (F).

The first synapses identified by electron microscopists were simple contacts made by simple terminals, of the axosomatic and axodendritic type. Since these simple arrangements were in accord with the functional concepts of the neuron doctrine, as summarized in Chapter 1, they came to be regarded as "classical" synapses. The axoaxonic and dendrodendritic types were identified later, as were the serial and reciprocal arrangements and the various types of specialized synaptic contacts and terminals. Since these synapses, terminals, and patterns did not fit classical concepts, the practice grew up of referring to the simple synapses as "conventional" and to all the other synapses as "unconventional" or even "nonusual."

In the brain, as in society, such terms carry inevitable overtones of moral opprobrium, and it is wisest to avoid them. Suffice it to say that there is probably no more certain sign of the obsolescence of an idea than the practice of labeling as "unconventional" those facts that do not fit it. The nervous system does not put these labels on its synapses. We may conceive that, in any given region, it is faced with specific tasks of information processing, and it assembles the necessary circuits from the available neuronal components. That many of the ways by which these components are connected do not fit classical concepts is reason to revise the concepts. A first step in that direction is to characterize synapses in terms of their relative complexity and specific patterns of connection, as we have attempted to do in the discussion above.

VESICLES Synaptic vesicles are a subject in themselves. They come, in the felicitous phraseology of Palay (1967), like chocolates, in a variety of shapes and sizes, and are stuffed with different kinds of filling. Small vesicles (200–400 Å in diameter) are the most common; they are the ones we have discussed in regard to type I and type II synapses. At some synapses, there is evidence that acetylcholine is bound to, or contained within, the vesicles; such synapses are, therefore, called cholinergic. At other synapses, the vesicles appear to be associated with certain amino acids. These are the putative transmitter substances that are released by the presynaptic terminal when it is activated and that mediate the synaptic action onto the postsynaptic membrane, as will be described in the next chapter.

Another type of vesicle is medium sized (500–900 Å in diameter) and contains a dense granule; these vesicles are associated with monoamines. Large vesicles (1200–1500 Å in diameter) are characteristically found in neurosecretory cells, for example, in the nerve endings of hypothalamic neurons which send their axons to the pituitary. A large, dense droplet within these vesicles contains a polypeptide hormone, which is released in response to the appropriate behavioral stimulus. A neuron, or indeed a single terminal, may contain more than one type of vesicle, possibly for transport and storage, or for immediate release at the synapse.

This very brief account only scratches the surface of the subject of synaptic vesicles, and the reader is referred to Peters et al. (1976) for further details. The main point to be made here is that the vesicles are structural evidence of the fact that chemical synapses constitute a variety of neurosecretory apparatus. Like other secretory mechanisms, they are activated by specific stimuli, have specific targets, and exert particular actions on those targets. The dynamics of these mechanisms are the subject of the next chapters.

3

SYNAPTIC POTENTIALS AND ACTION POTENTIALS

If neurons are remarkable for their variety of forms they are no less notable for their range of functions. Prominent among these are embryological growth and development, metabolism, response to injury or denervation, internal transport of substances, humoral secretion and reception in some cases, and last but not least, the transmission, integration, and storage of information. Our study of synaptic circuits is mainly concerned with those types of information processing that take place by means of relatively rapid electrical and chemical changes. These are the basis for the ongoing activity of nearly all forms of animal life, and are essential threads in the fabric woven by the other functions.

Rapid processing of information is mediated by the neuronal membrane potential and the changes wrought in it by synaptic potentials and action potentials. The biophysical and neurophysiological mechanisms of these potentials are treated in numerous standard texts (cf. Katz, 1966; Kuffler and Nicholls, 1976). We shall summarize these mechanisms very briefly, our intent being to emphasize only those aspects that are needed to understand the relation between functional properties and different parts of the neuron within the context of synaptic organization. We shall see that this gives a somewhat new perspective on what we know and do not know about the essential nature of the nerve cell.

MEMBRANE POTENTIAL

It is customary to represent functional properties of the neuronal membrane in terms of a model for a single locus. We consider therefore a locus,

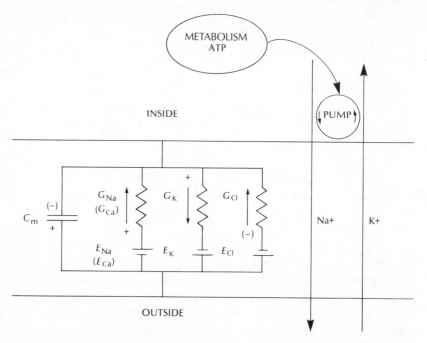

FIG. 3.1. Equivalent electrical circuit for a patch of neuronal membrane. C_m, capacitance; G, conductance channels for Na^+, K^+, and Cl^-; E, driving forces for ionic movements. G and E for Ca^{2+} indicated in parentheses. To the right, metabolic pump for maintaining ionic gradients across the membrane.

or "patch" of membrane, and represent its electrical properties with a simple circuit, as in Fig. 3.1. In this circuit, there is a capacitance (C_m), due to the lipids in the membrane. There is also an electrical resistance (R), which is divided into conductance channels (Conductance (G) = 1/Resistance) for the flow of ions. In series with the ionic conductances are batteries representing sources of electrochemical potential, which serve as the driving forces to move the ions through their channels.

A battery may obviously have one of two polarities across the membrane, to move positively charged ions inward or outward. The inward-directed battery (E_{Na}) represents the force that drives sodium ions (Na^+) through their conductance channel (G_{Na}). The outward-directed battery (E_K) represents the force that drives potassium ions (K^+) through their conductance channel (G_K). A third battery with its conductance channel is present for chloride ions (Cl^-). This battery moves the negatively charged chloride ions inward, and therefore has the same polarity as the K battery, since they both tend to make the inside more negative (less positive) than the outside. The third battery will be considered further when we take up synaptic potentials. Figure 3.1 can be expanded to include other ion species; for example, Ca^{2+} moves inward across the membrane through conductance channels that may be either distinct from, or similar to, those for Na (see parentheses in Fig. 3.1).

The driving forces for the ions derive from the differences in concentrations and charge across the membrane. As in all cells of the body, there is a relatively high concentration of Na outside the cell and a relatively high concentration of K inside. The batteries, therefore, represent the tendencies of the ions to move passively down their electrochemical gradients. The point at which the passive ion flow is balanced by the charge across the membrane capacitance defines the value of each battery. Since this is a point of equilibrium (i.e., no net flux of ions across the membrane) we refer to E as the *equilibrium potential* for a given ion. A common value for E_{Na} is $+50$ mV, for E_K is -75 mV.

At rest there is an excess of positive charge on the outside of the membrane capacitance and an excess of negative charge on the inside. This is due to a higher permeability to K than to the other ions, and the presence of impermeable macromolecules with negative charges in the cytoplasm. As a result, positive charge moves to the outside, bringing the membrane toward the potassium equilibrium potential. This creates the resting *membrane potential* (V_m), which is a characteristic of all cells of the body.

We are now in a position to ask what value the membrane potential may have. This will be set by the equilibrium potentials and the relative permeabilities for the separate ions; V_m is the weighted average of their contributions. In squid axon and vertebrate muscle fibers the permeabilities of K and Na have been found to be in the ratio of 20:1. The membrane potential accordingly has a value of approximately -70 mV, depolarized slightly from E_K ($1/20$th of the difference between E_K and E_{Na}). This is the traditional textbook value of the membrane potential. However, recent studies of different neurons have reported a range of values. For example, membrane potentials of about -45 mV have been found in invertebrate neurons, and values of -20 to -40 mV have been found in cells of the vertebrate retina. Lower values such as these are believed to be due primarily to larger resting permeabilities to Na ions. In contrast, glial cells are

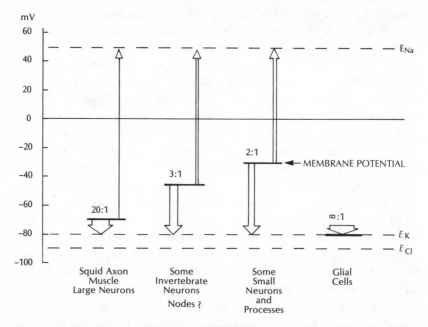

FIG. 3.2 Relative Na and K permeabilities and associated resting membrane potentials in different types of cells and processes (see text).

dominated almost completely by their permeability to K ions. These different cases, and the relative contributions of the ionic permeabilities to each, are illustrated diagrammatically in Figure 3.2.

These findings introduce a new concept, that the resting membrane potential is an important variable in the physiological repertoire of the neuron. We shall have opportunity to appreciate the significance of this variable when we consider synaptic mechanisms later in this chapter, and when we discuss the organization of sympathetic ganglia and the retina. The membrane potential may vary not only in different neurons but also in different parts of the same neuron. There are indications that it may be high in large cell bodies and axons, but relatively low in small axons, small neuronal processes and terminals, and nodes of Ranvier (cf. Fig. 3.2). This adds to the heterogeneous character of the individual neuron, and we must be prepared to take this factor into account in assessing the function of any neuron or neuronal part.

It remains to note that since the membrane potential depends on the different concentrations of ions on either side of the membrane, it tends to run down as the ions leak across through their conductance channels. The differences are maintained by the fact that the permeabilities are relatively low (i.e., the membrane has a relatively high resistance), and by the fact that associated with the membrane is a metabolic "pump" that extrudes Na and takes in K (see Fig. 3.1). The pump requires ATP for its energy, and is the functional link between the electrical properties of the membrane and the metabolic system of the cell. Depending on the coupling ratios between Na and K ions, the pump can make its own contribution to the resting membrane potential; this will be discussed further in relation to the mechanism of the action potential (see below). One can expect that variations in coupling ratios and associated energy metabolism also occur in different neurons and local parts of a neuron. Based on studies of ouabain binding, it has been estimated that there are 750 pumping sites per μm^2 in the unmyelinated fibers of the vagus nerve, and 4,000 sites per μm^2 in squid axon. The sites are thus extremely tightly packed; these figures are an order of magnitude greater than the densities of Na conductance channels (see below).

SYNAPTIC POTENTIALS

From the point of view of synaptic organization it is logical to consider next the ways by which the membrane potential can be changed at the junctions between cells.

ELECTRIC FIELDS   The simplest mechanism for effecting a change in the membrane potential is through the flow of current from a neighboring cell. Consider the situation diagrammed in Fig. 3.3 (A). An active site exists in the upper cell which causes current to flow inward at that site (as for example by the inward flow of Na ions). Associated with this is an outward flow of current to complete the circuit through neighboring membrane. The precise mechanism for this will be discussed later, and in Chapter 5, Dendritic Electrotonus. For the present we recognize that as the current emerges from the membrane it can flow directly back to the active site through the low-resistance extracellular space (solid arrow), or it can pass through the high-resistance membrane of the neighboring cell (dotted line). Naturally it will prefer the path of low resistance, but a tiny amount will pass through the membrane. If the points of entry and exit are sufficiently separate, there will be a net flow of current at each point, and one can record a corresponding tiny change in the membrane potential.

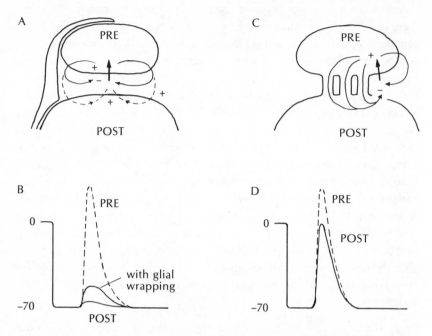

FIG. 3.3. Types of electrical interactions. (A) Field potential effects through membrane juxtapositions. (B) Representative recordings from pre- and postsynaptic processes in A. (C) Current flows through gap junction (electrical synapse). (D) Representative recordings from C. Note much larger loss in transmission in B than D.

Representative recordings for this case are illustrated in Fig. 3.3 (B). While this seems like a very inefficient mechanism, it can be enhanced in several ways. A large number of tightly packed active processes will heighten the effect, as could occur in the case of unmyelinated axons running together; olfactory nerves and cerebellar parallel fibers are possible sites for this. Large populations of synchronously active cells in the cerebral cortex generate currents sufficient to give rise to the waves of the electroencephalogram (EEG); this might also involve field effects between the cells, particularly between their dendrites. A glial wrapping can restrict the extracellular current flow and increase the amount crossing neighboring membrane (see Fig. 3.3 A,B); this has, in fact, been demonstrated for one of the input terminals onto the Mauthner cell (Furukawa and Furshpan, 1963; Korn and Faber, 1979).

An advantage of this type of interaction is that it requires no extra energy. The disadvantages are that the effects are minimal, diffuse, and nonspecific without structural constraints; and the membrane potential changes are rigidly locked to the original activity.

ELECTRICAL SYNAPSES Effective electrical coupling between cells is achieved through low-resistance connections—the gap junctions described in the previous chapter. The intercellular channels at these junctions have a very low resistance to current passing between the two neurons, and at the same time they prevent loss by leakage to the extracellular space. Thus, a potential change in a presynaptic terminal may be transmitted to a postsynaptic terminal with little attenuation, as shown in Fig. 3.3 (C,D). Experimentally this is the direct test for the presence of an electrical synapse, and was first reported by Furshpan and Potter (1959) at a synapse between two nerve fibers in the crayfish. In the central nervous system this test is not usually possible (but see Bennett, 1977), and one must rely on indirect evidence. This includes the presence of small unitary short-latency depolarizations during antidromic volleys (representing the electrically transmitted spikes from neighboring neurons), the lack of collision between these depolarizations and a directly evoked spike in the cell, and the lack of reversal potential (see next section).

Three sites have been found in the mammalian brainstem where these criteria seem to be met, and where gap junctions have been identified. These are illustrated in Fig. 3.4. In the mesencephalic nucleus of the fifth cranial nerve there are electrical synapses between cell bodies and between cell bodies and initial axonal segments (A). In the vestibular (Deiter's) nucleus the synapses occur between cell bodies and axon terminals. A spike initiated in one cell is transmitted to a neighboring cell as a short-latency depolarization by current flow through the axon terminals and branches, as shown in (B). In the inferior olive, dendritic spines are interconnected by electrical synapses. The spines also receive chemical synapses, and it has been suggested that when they are active they shunt current away from the electrical synapses, thereby uncoupling the cells. The postulated mechanism is illustrated in Fig. 3.4 (C,D). The reader is referred to the review by Llinás (1975) for further discussion of these interactions.

The salient features of electrical synapses derive from the nature of the

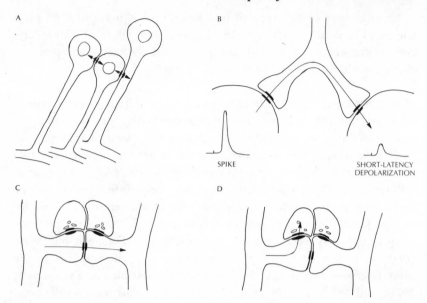

FIG. 3.4. Three examples of electrical synapses in the mammalian brain. (A) Mesencephalic nucleus of Vth cranial nerve (Baker and Llinás, 1971). (B) Deiter's nucleus (Korn, Sotelo, and Crepel, 1973). (C, D) Inferior olive (Llinás, Baker, and Sotelo, 1974). See text.

direct connections. They operate quickly, with little or no delay. They can provide for current flow in both directions, although they can also offer more resistance in one direction than the other (rectification). They provide a means of synchronization of populations of neurons. Their actions can be fixed and stereotyped in the face of repeated use, and less susceptible to metabolic and other effects than chemical synapses (see Nicholls and Purves, 1972; Bennett, 1973).

CHEMICAL SYNAPSES   The predominant type of synapse in the mammalian brain is the chemical synapse, operating through the release of a transmitter substance from the presynaptic to the postsynaptic terminal. The response of the postsynaptic terminal is called the *synaptic potential*.

Synaptic potentials may be either depolarizing or hyperpolarizing, as illustrated in Fig. 3.5. We consider first the depolarizing synaptic potential. As shown in A, the postsynaptic response consists of a net *inward* movement of positive charge. This can be brought about by a relatively

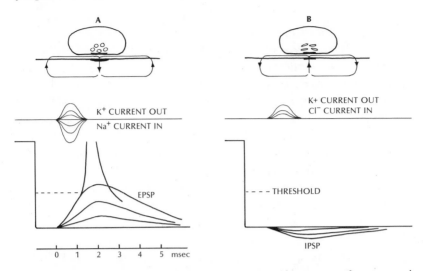

FIG. 3.5. Basic types of action at chemical synapses. *Above*, pre- and postsynaptic terminals, with net positive current flows shown by arrows for depolarizing (A) and polarizing or hyperpolarizing (B) actions. *Middle*, time course of ionic current flows; note that they are simultaneous rather than sequential, as in the case of the action potential. *Below*, recordings of postsynaptic potentials typical for an EPSP (A) and IPSP (B).

nonspecific increase in conductance to both Na^+ and K^+, and possibly other ions such as Ca^{2+}; it is as if a shunt had momentarily been placed across the membrane. The membrane moves toward an equilibrium potential near zero, the actual value depending on the ions involved and the ratios of their permeabilities.

We shall have more to say about the mechanisms underlying the synaptic potential in the next section and in the next chapter. For the present we note that the ion flows are simultaneous, and vary with the amount of transmitter substance liberated by the presynaptic terminal. The synaptic potential is therefore a graded response, in contrast to the all-or-nothing character of the action potential (as discussed later). Synaptic membrane is thus not "active" in the same sense that impulse-generating membrane is, and the two must not be confused.

Synapses that depolarize the membrane are necessary for bringing about generation of impulses, and these responses were therefore termed *excitatory postsynaptic potentials* (EPSPs) by Eccles and his associates in their pioneering microelectrode studies of the motoneuron (Eccles, 1964).

As we shall see, the terminology needs to be qualified somewhat in the light of recent knowledge about the organization of synapses.

The second basic type of synaptic potential is diagrammed in Fig. 3.5 (B). The action of the transmitter substance is to open conductance channels for a net *outward* movement of positive charge. The equilibrium potential for this ion flow is at a relatively polarized level of -80 to -90 mV; it can be brought about by an increased conductance for outward movement of positive charge (K^+) and/or inward movement of negative charge (Cl^-). These ion flows therefore tend to hold the membrane near its resting potential, or somewhat hyperpolarized. As in the previous case, this synaptic potential is a graded response. Since synapses of this type tend to keep the membrane from depolarizing, and hence work against the initiation of impulses, they are termed *inhibitory postsynaptic potentials* (IPSPs).

We recur to the question of terminology. "Excitatory" and "inhibitory" have classically been defined in relation to impulse initiation, but we shall see that some neurons do not have impulse-generating properties. In these neurons the synaptic response is not converted into impulses; rather, the potential itself is responsible, either directly or through electrotonic spread, for activation or suppression of local synaptic output. How do the terms apply to this situation? Here we note a remarkable consistency; as far as is known, transmitter release only occurs by means of membrane depolarization (cf. Hodgkin, 1972). To the extent that this generalization is true, we can therefore extend the definitions as follows: an EPSP is excitatory because it leads to impulse generation and/or synaptic transmitter release; an IPSP is inhibitory because it opposes impulse generation and/or transmitter release.

SYNAPTIC INTEGRATION It is largely through the interaction between excitatory and inhibitory synapses that the competition for control of the membrane potential in different parts of the neuron is carried out. This competition lies at the heart of the study of the dynamics of synaptic organization. The principle goes back to Sherrington (1906); following him, the process by which different synaptic inputs are combined within the neuron is termed *synaptic integration*.

The interaction of a single EPSP and IPSP serves as a paradigm for synaptic integration in central neurons, and it will be useful at this point to grasp certain essentials. Let us assume an excitatory synapse

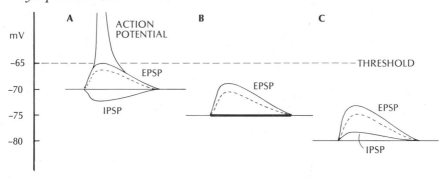

FIG. 3.6. Integration of EPSP and IPSP at different resting membrane potentials. Illustrates that IPSP conductance change reduces EPSP at all resting levels, but IPSP polarity changes in relation to E_K and E_{Cl}.

and a nearby inhibitory synapse, the activation of which individually produce an EPSP and IPSP, respectively, as shown in Fig. 3.6 (A). Assume now that the two are activated simultaneously. The effect of the IPSP is to reduce the amplitude of the EPSP, away from the threshold for impulse initiation, as is shown in Fig. 3.6 (A). The dotted line traces the resulting transient; it represents the "integrated" result of the two synaptic potentials.

Now it is commonly thought that this process of integration is a matter of simple algebraic addition of the two opposed synaptic potentials; to wit, "depolarization plus hyperpolarization equals membrane potential." However, this simple formula does not have general validity. As shown in Fig. 3.6 (B), when the resting potential is at the inhibitory equilibrium potential, no IPSP is recorded, but there is still a reduction of a simultaneous EPSP, due to the shunting effect of the increased inhibitory conductance. And when the resting membrane is more polarized [Fig. 3.6 (C)], the IPSP is in fact depolarizing (toward the inhibitory equilibrium potential), yet its effect is still to reduce the EPSP by virtue of the increased conductance. The essential inhibitory action is therefore not a hyperpolarization of the membrane, but rather an increase in ionic conductance that drives the membrane potential toward the equilibrium potential for those ions.

It is thus the opposition of synaptically activated conductances and ionic currents that controls the relative amounts of depolarization and hyperpolarization of the membrane potential. In addition, one must con-

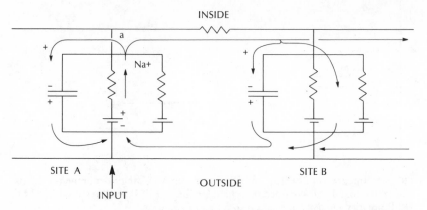

FIG. 3.7. Current flows underlying the depolarization of membrane patches. Initial input (as from an EPSP, applied current or local potential) causes *inward* current flow of positively charged Na ions. At (a), current can flow in two directions: *outward*, to depolarize membrane capacitance, or *longitudinally* and then *outward* to depolarize capitance of neighboring membrane patch. Thus membrane depolarization is brought about by both inward ionic current and outward capacitative current. Note that external current flow completes the circuit.

sider the geometrical relations between excitatory and inhibitory synaptic sites in a dendritic tree, and the electrotonic flow of current through the dendrites, as described in Chapter 5. Synaptic integration thus involves a complex interplay between ionic conductances and neuronal geometry.

IONIC CURRENTS   It will be useful at this point to consider more closely the relation between an ionic conductance change and the resultant change in membrane potential. For an example we take the case of a brief increase in conductance to Na ions. As shown in Fig. 3.7, Na$^+$ moves inward through its conductance channel at the active site (A). In the electrical circuit, the current reaches a point on the inside where it can travel in two directions. Some current passes onto the inner surface of the membrane capacitance, where it deposits positive charge that depolarizes the membrane. Some passes along the inside of the nerve cell to the next patch of membrane (B), where it can follow three paths: onto the membrane capacitance, through the membrane resistance, or further along the fiber. Ultimately all the current must pass out across the membrane and pass back along the outside of the cell to the negative pole of the Na battery.

Careful study of the diagram and current flows will help answer two questions that are often puzzling to the student. The first is, how can inward and outward current both depolarize the membrane? As can be seen, this is because inward current at an active site and outward current at a neighboring site both have the same effect, of putting positive charge on the inside of the membrane capacitance. The same reasoning applies to the relation between oppositely directed current flows and hyperpolarization.

The second question is, what are the time relations between the current flows and the potential changes? When the flow is rapid the potential response is slower, because charge is transiently stored on the membrane capacitance. The amount of slowing depends on the time constant (τ_m) of the membrane, given by the product of the membrane capacitance (C_m) and membrane resistance (R_m): $\tau = RC$. The relation between the rapid synaptic current flows and the slower synaptic potentials is shown in Fig. 3.5. For very slow or constant changes in conductance, a steady state exists in which the capacitance becomes an open circuit and can be ignored, and the spread of current to the neighboring site is determined solely by the resistance along the paths.

These relations between current and potential underlie most of the physiological properties of nerve cells. For instance, the diagram of Fig. 3.7 applies equally to the case of activation of an action potential and its propagation by local currents, as we shall see later. The slowing of potential responses and the decay of potential spread are both governed by electrotonic properties, as described in Chapter 5. The diagram also emphasizes a point that is especially germane for synaptic organization. At any site on a nerve cell there can be two pathways for interactions: internally with other parts of the same cell, by means of electrotonic spread or impulse generation, or externally through synapses onto neighboring cells.

CONDUCTANCE-DECREASE SYNAPSES Transient increases in conductance are the mode of operation at the neuromuscular junction and at many synapses onto central neurons. However, recent studies of sympathetic ganglion cells, retinal receptors, and certain invertebrate neurons have shown that some synapses may operate by an opposite mechanism,

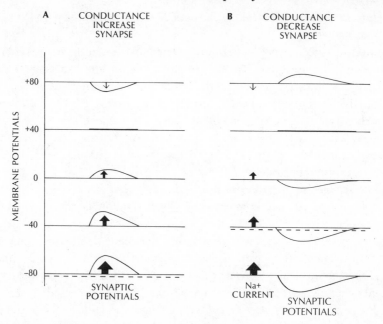

FIG. 3.8. Comparison of conductance-increase (A) and conductance-decrease (B) synapses. Synaptic potentials shown at different levels of controlled membrane potential. Arrows indicate direction and intensity of Na current flow. Dotted lines indicate resting potentials.

a decrease of a conductance. We are now in a position to describe briefly this type of synaptic action.

Let us recall that ion flows across the membrane depend on two factors: the conductance and the electrochemical gradient. Experimentally, if we move the membrane potential toward the equilibrium potential for an ion, the gradient decreases. At the equilibrium potential there is no net flow of the ion, and if the membrane potential moves further, the current through that channel actually reverses in direction. The experiment is illustrated in Fig. 3.8 (A). The traces represent recordings of synaptic potentials due to Na^+ conductance increases, at different holding potentials. The arrows indicate the directions and relative strengths of Na^+ current flow. Since the synaptic potentials have opposite polarities on either side of it, the equilibrium potential is also referred to as the *reversal potential*.

Now consider the case illustrated in Fig. 3.8 (B), which differs in two respects. First, the conductance for Na$^+$ in the resting membrane is increased. The membrane potential is therefore at a lower level (e.g., -40 mV, as indicated by the dashed line), due to the depolarizing effect of the inward leak of Na$^+$. Second, the effect of the synapse is to *decrease* the Na$^+$ conductance. This leaves the membrane to move toward the equilibrium potential of the ions to which it is more permeable, i.e., K$^+$ and Cl$^-$. The synaptic potential is therefore *hyperpolarizing*. The potentials decrease and reverse around the Na$^+$ equilibrium potential, but with opposite polarities to those shown in A.

In some cells this hyperpolarizing response functions as an IPSP, as in sympathetic ganglion cells (Chapter 6); in other situations, its function is not yet clear, for example, in the retina (Chapter 9). In addition to the conductance decrease, we may note other special properties. A hyperpolarization is achieved by selective control of an ion that depolarizes the membrane. The decreased conductance raises the resistance of the membrane, thereby increasing the membrane time constant and slowing the potential response. Associated with this, these synaptic potentials tend to have slow time courses. With respect to integrative mechanisms, an IPSP produced by this means does not have the current-shunting effect we noted in connection with Fig. 3.6.

It will be appreciated that if a hyperpolarization can be produced by turning off the conductance to Na$^+$, a depolarization could be produced by turning off the conductance to K$^+$. Nature has not missed this opportunity, and slow EPSPs produced by this mechanism have been found. They will be further discussed in Chapter 6.

Recently, it has been suggested that some synapses may act by a mechanism other than a conductance change in the postsynaptic membrane (Krnjevic, 1970). It is envisaged, instead, that an amino acid (glutamate, for example) released by the presynaptic terminal attaches to a carrier (protein molecule?) in the postsynaptic membrane. The attachment greatly increases the affinity of the carrier for Na, and the entire complex is then driven across the membrane by the Na gradient. The net transfer of cation depolarizes the membrane, resulting in an EPSP. For such a synapse, the upper curve in Fig. 3.5 would still describe the time course of Na movement, but by carrier rather than conductance change, whereas the EPSP response would be described as before by the lower curve. Whether or not this can be proved to be the mechanism at a given central synapse, it is of general interest because there is evidence that similar mechanisms operate elsewhere in the body, as in the uptake of amino acids from the digestive tract (cf. Schultz and Curran, 1970).

ACTION POTENTIAL

In our opening discussion of the parts of the brain (Fig. 1.1), it was pointed out that one of the necessary functions of neurons is that of transfer of signals over long distances, from peripheral receptors to the brain, from the brain to muscles and glands, and between different parts of the brain. This long-distance transfer takes place over long axons by means of *action potentials* or *impulses*. We will describe the mechanism of the action potential as it has been revealed in studies of the largest long-distance axons and then discuss short axons and dendrites.

The characteristics of the action potential are well known (see Katz, 1966; Hodgkin, 1968), and the essentials are illustrated in Fig. 3.9. A small stimulus, in the form of a depolarization of the membrane, causes a conformational change in a membrane protein which controls the permeability of Na channels. The change itself can be detected as a current, the *Na gating current* (Armstrong, Bezanilla and Rojas, 1974; Keynes, 1975). Na ions then flow inward, causing the membrane to rapidly depolarize from the resting value of -70 mV to $+40$ mV or so, following which it rapidly returns to the resting value. Below *threshold*, a stimulus elicits only a *local response* or no response; above threshold, the membrane goes through its stereotyped depolarization response independent of stimulus intensity. Hence, the membrane response is "all or nothing." It is *active*, in that the response reflects a property of the membrane rather than simply the stimulus itself. It is a highly nonlinear property.

The essence of this mechanism is that it is regenerative; in this respect it resembles an explosive gas mixture, certain electronic devices, and numerous other physical and chemical systems. The generally accepted model of this mechanism in nerve is that of Hodgkin and Huxley (1952) for the giant axon of the squid. In simplest terms, the model consists of a positive feedback relationship between Na conductance and membrane depolarization, such that the initial threshold depolarization leads to increased Na conductance and Na ion influx, which causes further depolarization, and so on. This cycle, once initiated, proceeds until the membrane reaches the potential at which there is no more driving force for the Na ions; this is the equilibrium potential for Na ions (E_{Na}), about 50 mV inside positive. As this point is reached, Na conductance is turned

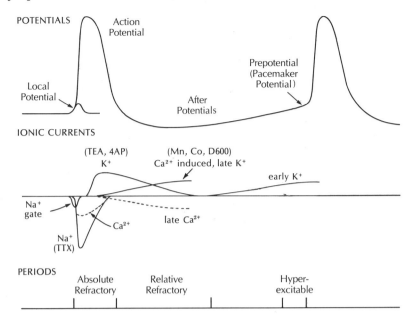

FIG. 3.9. Membrane potentials, ionic current flows, and the excitability cycle controlling the generation and frequency of impulses. Ionic currents in (B) based in part on Baker, Hodgkin, and Ridgeway, 1971; Connor and Stevens, 1971; Meech, 1972; Barrett and Barrett, 1976, and others. Slow Ca curve represents conductance change and/or ion accumulation. Inward currents below, outward currents above. Blocking agents indicated in parentheses: 4AP, 4-aminopyridine; Mn, manganese; Co, cobalt (see text). Time courses are only schematic; time scale compressed during interspike interval.

off (sodium inactivation), and a slower increase in K conductance begins. The E_K is slightly hyperpolarized relative to the resting membrane potential; hence, the K ion current (together with sodium inactivation) helps return the membrane potential to resting level. The directions of these current flows are indicated in Fig. 3.1, and their time courses in Fig. 3.9.

The regenerative all-or-nothing property can now be seen as the necessary mechanism for long-distance signal transmission. A patch of membrane undergoing this potential change generates current that acts to depolarize its neighboring patch (cf. Fig. 3.7). This patch then goes through exactly the same cycle, and so on, down the length of the axon. The action potential at the end of the axon is identical to that at the beginning; there has been no transmission loss. There have been small exchanges of Na and K along the way, which are restored by the ionic pump. When we speak of *active spread, nervous conduction,* or *impulse propagation,* we mean explicitly transmission by this action potential mechanism.

How then is information transferred over long axons by these identical signals? The answer, of course, is that, in the single fiber, it can only be carried as a *frequency code,* reflecting the time intervals between successive impulses. The cycle of generation of a sequence of impulses is illustrated in Fig. 3.9. An action potential is followed by a slower change, an *afterpotential,* which, in turn, merges with a *prepotential* from which the next action potential arises. Distinct changes in membrane excitability are associated with each period. During the action potential, the membrane is *absolutely refractory* to further stimulation. During the afterpotential, the membrane is busy pumping back ions, and the threshold is raised, i.e., it is *relatively refractory* to another stimulus. During the ensuing prepotential, however, the membrane is hyperexcitable. In cells that spontaneously generate impulses, the prepotential is also referred to as a *pacemaker potential.*

The conductance changes underlying this cycle of events have been studied in recent years using substances that selectively block different ion channels. For example, tetrodotoxin (TTX) blocks the voltage-sensitive sodium permeability, whereas tetraethylammonium (TEA) selectively blocks potassium permeability. The sodium inactivation mechanism can be blocked by the application of pronase, a proteolytic enzyme. Several types of calcium currents have been identified, using special proteins (e.g., aequorin) that emit light in the presence of ionized Ca. These types include early Ca entry (through Na channels), and delayed entry through a specific Ca channel. The relative contributions of Ca movements to the action potential can vary in different neurons, and in different parts of the same neuron (axon, cell body, dendrite; see below). The role of Ca in neurotransmitter release is discussed in the next chapter.

Figure 3.9 shows in a highly schematic fashion some of these ion movements and their relations to the time course of changes in membrane potential and excitability. The timing of an impulse is thus a complex outcome of a number of factors: membrane potential, underlying conductances, excitability cycle, the natural pacemaker properties of the membrane, and the background level of depolarization. The relative frequencies of spontaneous and induced impulses are crucial to the transfer of information by frequency codes.

In transmitting impulses over long distances, speed may be of the essence (as in the muscle reflexes discussed in Chapter 7), and it is enhanced by two factors. One factor is that the larger axons are myelinated; thus, conduction proceeds not continuously in these axons, but jumps, as it were, from node to node. This is *saltatory conduction*. When patches of excitable membrane are thus separated, the separation obviously must not exceed the distance over which current flow along the axon will be sufficient to activate the impulse mechanism. Thus arises the concept of *safety factor*, the excess of current beyond that required for theshold stimulation. The safety factor is normally high, but it becomes an important variable affecting information transfer under conditions of high-frequency transmission (i.e., through partially refractory membrane), fatigue, anesthesia, injury and disease, and propagation at axonal branch points.

The other factor is that the conduction rate increases with the increasing diameter of the axon; current flows more easily from patch to patch, in accordance with the properties of electrotonus to be discussed in the next chapter. For myelinated axons, the conduction rate, in meters per second, is approximately six times the diameter in microns. In unmyelinated axons, the velocity appears to vary with the square root of the diameter. From the largest myelinated axons of 20 μm diameter down to the finest unmyelinated axons of 0.2 μm, the conduction velocities range from about 120 m/sec down to less than 1 m/sec. There is, thus, about a hundred-fold range of impulse conduction velocities in axons. For the amusement of the intuition, it may be noted that these rates translate to a range of some 200 down to 2 miles per hour (see also Fig. 4.8).

ACTION POTENTIALS IN THIN AXONS Thus far we have considered the impulse mechanism in terms of the classical action potential of the giant axon (diameter 0.5–1 mm) of the squid. But, as Alice might have said, there are no squid axons in the brain. Studies of peripheral nerves show that the general model is applicable to the active membrane at the nodes of myelinated axons. However, variations must be expected; for example, the impulse at the node of Ranvier appears to be generated almost exclusively by Na currents and Na inactivation, there being an apparent lack of K channels at this site (Chiu et al., 1979). The model is believed to apply generally to axons in the central nervous system. But that is an assumption that must be tested. This is particularly true for the thin unmyelinated axons that make up the majority of axons in the brain and that are the most relevant to synaptic organization.

These axons are the least accessible to experiment, but recent work has begun to reveal their properties. There is evidence, for example, that the density of Na conductance channels in the membrane is surprisingly low. A figure of only 2–3 channels/μm^2 has been estimated for fish olfactory nerves and 27 channels in vagal unmyelinated fibers (Colquhoun, Henderson, and Ritchie, 1972); by comparison, the density in squid axons is of the order of 500/μm^2 (Levinson and Meves, 1975). Since the fish olfactory axons have diameters of 0.2 μm, it appears that there is only one channel for every micron or so of length. This has conjured up the vision, to J. M. Ritchie and his co-workers, of a kind of "microsaltatory" conduction taking place from channel to channel along these very thin fibers.

Compared to large axons, a thin fiber has a radically increased ratio of surface membrane to internal volume, and this places a far greater and more immediate burden on the energy-requiring ionic pumps we mentioned above. It has been shown that "following just a few impulses in unmyelinated axons, there are well-defined changes in: the high-energy phosphate compounds required for the recovery process; the electrical activity that reflects the operation of the sodium pump; oxygen consumption; and heat production" (Greengard and Ritchie, 1971). Unmyelinated axons, consequently, are very dependent on an adequate glucose supply, for use as fuel or possibly as a precursor of energy-providing acetylated compounds.

The nature of the ionic pumping mechanism has been intensively studied. It is a characteristic of unmyelinated fibers that the action potential is followed by a large hyperpolarizing afterpotential, which has been correlated with the rise in internal Na ion. It was first thought that, during this afterpotential, the ionic pump simply ejects one Na ion for every K ion taken in and is, therefore, electrically neutral. There is growing evidence, however, that, to a more or less degree, the Na ion is actively extruded. This results in a net movement of electrical charge across the membrane and, hence, an active contribution to the membrane potential. Such a pump is termed *electrogenic* and is thought to be present in several kinds of nerve cell and nerve process, vertebrate and invertebrate, as well as in a variety of body cells (e.g., muscle cells, red blood cells) (see Greengard and Ritchie, 1971). This pumping mechanism is important not only for impulse conduction and recovery, but also, in some cases, for synaptic transmission, as was discussed above.

What of the potassium that appears just outside the membrane during the action potential? It has been found that during the ensuing hyperpolarizing afterpotential, the sensitivity of the membrane to K ion is greatly increased over normal. Therefore, we have this additional factor to consider as a means of interaction between nerve cells and between a nerve cell and its surrounding glial cells. The effect of K^+ on synaptic transmission will be discussed in the next chapter.

ACTION POTENTIALS IN SHORT AXONS Thin axons may be long axons, arising from principal neurons and carrying impulses to distant regions; these are the kind of axons that have been the subjects of the studies mentioned above. But thin axons also arise from intrinsic short-axon cells and distribute within their local region. In such cases, the axon may be very short; we will encounter examples (e.g., the thalamus) of axons only a few hundred microns in length, shorter than the dendritic branches of many neurons. Now, if we consider the likely assumption of an impulse duration of 1 msec and a conduction rate of 1 mm/ msec, it is immediately evident that the wavelength of the impulse may be greater than the length of the axon. This implies that, at its peak, the impulse would be spread almost equally through most of the length of the axon. This is quite different from the case of the thin axon that projects outside a region, in which case the wavelength of the impulse is only a fraction of the length of the axon. Because the two cases appear so different, it is possible that the impulse in a very short axon may have a significance beyond simple propagation. This will serve to highlight the point that we, in fact, have very little direct information about the physiological properties of the axons of short-axon cells.

ACTION POTENTIALS IN DENDRITES The properties of dendrites in central neuropil have received a good deal more attention than the properties of short axons. But as long as methods were not available for direct study of activity in central neurons, these properties were only the subject of speculation. An ancient line of thought held that dendrites provide for vegetative functions only. When the action potential in axons came under study, it became fashionable to consider that impulses were the sole means of signal transfer in all parts of central neurons, including their dendrites (see Forbes, 1922). The pendulum swung the other way when the early intracellular studies of Eccles and his collaborators (Eccles, 1953) showed that motoneuron dendrites do not normally generate impulses; these studies and those of Bishop (1957) and others seemed to give credence to the idea that dendrites mainly supported graded activity.

It is only recently, with the introduction of microelectrode recordings combined with intracellular staining techniques and biophysical models, that direct evidence for dendritic properties could be obtained. With these techniques, the question of active versus passive properties of dendrites has become one of the central concerns of neurophysiologists. In reviewing the evidence in later chapters, we will see that spread of signals through some dendrites is by passive means alone, whereas in others there is also active spread. Different conductance mechanisms (e.g., Na, Ca) with different time courses, fast or slow, may underlie the active properties. It is becoming apparent that it is part of the functional arsenal of dendrites that they may vary in this regard. It is important to realize that in all cases there is passive spread, and that analysis of dendritic electrotonus, as outlined in Chapter 5, is therefore necessary for understanding active properties.

In closing this section, it may be noted that there is a widely held assumption, deriving from the classical literature, that any process with the structure of an axon must generate action potentials. From this it has been only a short step to defining an axon as an impulse-generating process and any impulse-generating process as an axon. These definitions, however, do not have general validity, a point that has already been touched on in discussing synaptic arrangements in the previous chapter. We will encounter several examples of morphological dendrites that have impulse-generating properties (Chapters 7, 10, and 14), and we will encounter other cells with processes, classically defined as axonal, that do not generate action potentials (Chapter 9). In the previous chapter, we saw that, in many cases, the parts of the neuron do not admit of a simple distinction between axon and dendrite; it should, therefore, not be surprising that the relation between the structural parts of the neuron and their functional properties similarly do not admit of simple generalization. If we define structural parts of the neuron on the basis of structural criteria, and functional properties on the basis of physiological criteria, we will be taking a sound approach to the diversity that characterizes structure-function relations in the synaptic circuits of the brain.

NEUROTRANSMITTER
MECHANISMS

From the preceding account of synaptic actions one can draw the moral: control the conductance through the membrane and you control the potential across it. What then controls the conductance? At chemical synapses the control is by means of a chemical substance, a transmitter molecule, that is released by the presynaptic terminal and acts on the postsynaptic membrane. The mechanism is a complicated one, involving elements of ultrastructure, biophysics, and biochemistry. Certain features of the mechanism seem to be common to most synapses, at least those that have short-term actions. However, in other respects there may be many variations; for example, recent studies have suggested synaptic actions not associated with morphological junctions, and long-lasting actions that resemble hormonal effects. The uneasy feeling is growing that it will be difficult if not impossible to stretch the definition of synapse to cover all these cases. Our concern here is only with the best understood biochemical aspects of relatively short-acting transmitter mechanisms. We will be well-advised to remember, that "the more one finds out about properties at different synapses, the less grows one's inclination to make general statements about their mode of action!" (Katz, 1966).

MOLECULAR NATURE OF SYNAPTIC TRANSMISSION   The synapse that is best understood is the neuromuscular junction, due in large part to the brilliant investigations of Katz and co-workers (Katz, 1966, 1969). The junction, or end-plate, is formed by the axon terminals of a motoneuron on a muscle cell. As a chemical synapse it differs from its counterparts in the brain in several morphological respects: the presynaptic axon terminals are extremely extensive, covering an area of 2000 to 6000 μm^2

(compared with about 1 μm^2 for a simple synaptic terminal in the central nervous system); the synaptic cleft is relatively wide (500–600 Å) and contains a densely staining basal lamina; the postsynaptic membrane (of the muscle cell) forms a trough that receives the axon terminal, the walls of the trough being thrown into numerous folds. Some of these features are shown in Fig. 4.1 (A). This junctional complex is clearly a synapse, but it just as clearly falls at an extreme end of the morphological spectrum. In line with the comments in Chapter 2, it can be regarded as a specialized synapse of a giant terminal.

An impulse traveling in the motor axon invades the terminals and elicits a relatively large potential response in the muscle, as shown in Fig. 4.1 (B,1). This is the end-plate potential (EPP), and is equivalent to an EPSP, being due, as we have described in Chapter 3, to the ionic current that flows when the conductances to Na and K are transiently increased. It gives rise to the muscle action potential, which in turn activates the contractile machinery of the muscle.

Katz and his colleagues showed that the EPP is built up out of small unitary potentials with similar time courses, which are termed *miniature EPPs* (MEPPs). The summation of three MEPPs is shown in Fig. 4.1 (B,2). The unitary nature of the MEPP suggested that it is due to a packet, or *quantum*, of transmitter substance, and it has been calculated that the full EPP is due to the simultaneous release of a total of 100–200 quanta by the impulse in all the terminals. It has also been calculated that somewhere between 1000 and 10,000 acetylcholine (ACh) molecules are contained in each quantum. Traditionally, it has been tempting to equate one quantum to one vesicle, but recent studies suggest that a quantum may represent the simultaneous release of several vesicles (Wernig and Sterner, 1977; see also below).

The action of a single ACh molecule has been revealed by slowly passing ACh from a micropipette onto the end-plate, a technique known as microiontophoresis. Recordings from the end-plate show the expected slow depolarization, but in addition there are very small fluctuations in the baseline [Fig. 4.1 (B,3)]. Noise analysis has suggested that these are due to the opening and closing of the ionic channels by single ACh molecules as they interact with receptor molecules in the postsynaptic membrane (Katz and Miledi, 1972; Stevens, 1976). Further analysis has provided evidence for the brief membrane currents through the channels [Fig. 4.1 (B,4)].

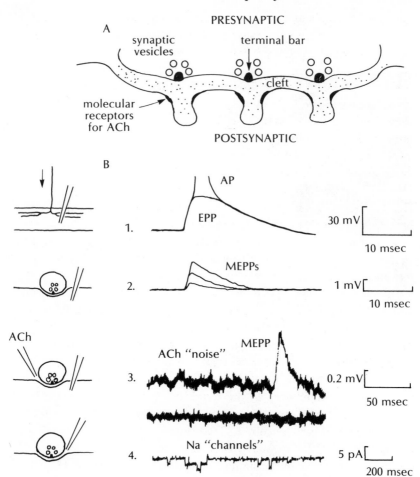

FIG. 4.1. Synaptic properties exemplified by the neuromuscular junction. (A) Schematic diagram of the junction. (B) Different types of recordings. (1) Intracellular recording of end-plate potential (EPP) giving rise to an action potential (AP) in the muscle cell: experimental set-up shown at left. (2) High-gain, showing summation of miniature end-plate potentials (MEPPs). (3) Very high gain recording, showing noise induced by iontophoresis of ACh (compare with control trace below). (4) Extracellular recording from junctional site, showing currents associated with Na "channels". [1–3 from Katz, Miledi and colleagues (see text); 4 from Neher and Steinbach, 1977]

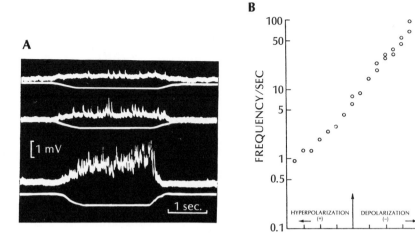

FIG. 4.2. Presynaptic control of the frequency of miniature end-plate potentials (MEPPs). (A) Recordings at three levels of depolarization of terminals (from del Castillo and Katz, in Katz, 1962). (B) Graph showing dependence of MEPP frequency on relative polarization of presynaptic terminals (From Liley, in Katz, 1962.)

Several lines of evidence suggest that the receptor for acetylcholine is a relatively large glycoprotein (MW = 20,000). By investigating the effects of toxins that bind to the receptor, it has been estimated that the receptor density is of the order of $10,000/\mu m^2$ (cf. Keynes, 1975). This implies that the receptors, and associated channels, are packed into the postsynaptic membrane extremely tightly, with only 100 Å or so between them. It may be recalled from Chapter 3 that this is similar to the density of Na channels in the node of Ranvier, but much higher than the channel densities in axons. This tight packing of the postsynaptic membrane with chemical receptors appears to be one of the defining characteristics of the synapse at the molecular level.

GRADED RELEASE OF TRANSMITTER QUANTA The release of transmitter molecules in quanta has been found at several types of synapses, and at present it is believed that such a mechanism may apply to all chemical synapses. We next inquire into the nature of the release. It is essentially controlled by the amount of depolarization of the presynaptic membrane; as shown in Fig. 4.2, the more the applied depolarization in the presynaptic terminal, the more the depolarizing response in the postsynaptic membrane. This is an expression of the generalization linking depolarization with transmitter release mentioned in the previous chapter. An important point is that the presynaptic depolarization increases the frequency (probability of occurrence) of the MEPPs; the individual amplitudes remain the same. The postsynaptic depolarization is therefore due to the summation of MEPPs overlapping in time.

The grading of postsynaptic responses with the amount of presynaptic depolarization is a crucial property for synapses in many central regions. A synapse from an incoming axon terminal is normally activated by an impulse invading the terminal, but a synapse from a dendrite may be activated by the graded depolarizations of synaptic potentials within that dendrite. This concept was first invoked in studies of the olfactory bulb, and appears to be applicable to the synaptic circuits in a number of regions, as we shall see in later chapters.

STEPS IN SYNAPTIC TRANSMISSION   The steps in the release process require time. At the neuromuscular junction there is a minimum *synaptic delay*, between the onset of a presynaptic depolarization and the postsynaptic response, of about 0.5 msec. Only about one-tenth of this (50 μsec) can be ascribed to the time for diffusion across the synaptic cleft. We may note in passing that this brief time for diffusion is an expression of an interesting aspect of dimensionality: processes that appear slow on a macroscopic scale are very fast on a microscopic scale. This is particularly relevant to the mechanisms at work at the microscopic level of synapses; we shall return to this point later (cf. Fig. 4.8).

What accounts for the rest of the synaptic delay? The answer has been sought by examining the junction between two giant nerve fibers which cross each other in the squid. The fibers are large enough to permit microelectrodes to be placed in both pre- and postsynaptic elements, an impossibility at most central synapses (and the reason our understanding leans so heavily on knowledge of peripheral junctions). The junctional area is enormous, 150,000 μm^2. Several steps, and the sequence of their timing, have been identified at this giant synapse, as shown in Fig. 4.3 (A). These studies have suggested that most of the overall synaptic delay is taken up by the opening of Ca^{2+} channels, and that the actual interval between the onset of inward Ca current in the presynaptic membrane and the onset of postsynaptic current flow is only some 200 μsec. Figure

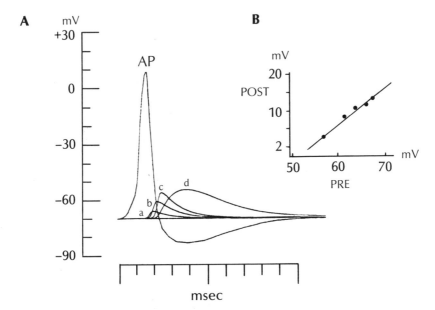

FIG. 4.3. Properties of giant synapse of the squid. (A) Model demonstrating sequence of events. (AP) Action potential in presynaptic terminal; (a) time course of calcium gate formation; (b) calcium current; (c) postsynaptic current; and (d) postsynaptic potential. (From Llinás, 1977.) (B) Graded relation between depolarization of pre- and postsynaptic terminals. (From Katz and Miledi, 1967.)

4.3 (B) shows that the amount of postsynaptic response at this junction varies with the amount of presynaptic depolarization, over a considerable part of the curve. It is thus a direct demonstration of the property of graded synaptic action discussed in the previous section.

The synaptic delay is a property that is frequently utilized in the analysis of synaptic circuits. By setting up synchronous volleys in input fibers and noting the times for neuronal responses, the electrophysiologist can determine the pathways for monosynaptic and polysynaptic connections within a local region. We shall encounter use of this technique in most of the regions of our study.

We may summarize the main steps in synaptic transmission thus far identified with the help of the series of diagrams in Fig. 4.4. In A, step 1 is a depolarization of the presynaptic terminal. In B, step 2 is an opening of the gates that permit Ca ions to flow inward (step 3) through their

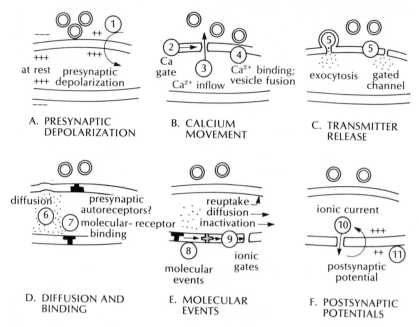

FIG. 4.4. Sequence of main events occurring at a synapse (see text for description).

conductance channels. The function of the Ca is believed to be promotion of fusion of synaptic vesicles with the plasma membrane (step 4).

The next step is release of transmitter (C, step 5). The nature of this release is keenly debated. Katz and his co-workers (see Katz, 1966, 1969) noted the possible relation between quanta and vesicles, and suggested that the quantal packets of transmitter are contained in the vesicles and extruded from them at release. Recent freeze-fracture studies have provided evidence for the attachment of vesicles to the plasmalemma (Akert et al., 1972), opening of vesicles into the cleft, and recycling of membrane to form new vesicles. The elegant experiments of Heuser and Reese (1973, 1977) have provided persuasive evidence for this sequence of events. The process is envisaged as similar to that of exocytosis, which is involved in the release of hormones (Douglas, 1977). On the other hand, it has been noted that transmitter is present in the cytoplasm of the terminal, and various lines of evidence have suggested that it may be released directly across the terminal membrane (albeit in quantal packets), with the vesicles playing a storage or otherwise complementary role.

The arguments for this view are presented in Cooper, Bloom, and Roth (1978).

After release, diffusion of the transmitter takes place across the cleft (D, step 6), followed by binding to the molecular receptors (step 7). One usually thinks of this as occurring on the postsynaptic terminal, but recent studies have suggested that in some cases a transmitter may also have an action on the presynaptic terminal (autoreceptors); we shall discuss this further in the chapter on the basal ganglia.

There then follow events at the molecular level (E, step 8) which range from the simple to the complex. The simplest event is a direct opening of ionic gates (step 9), such as occurs at the neuromuscular junction and the majority of central synapses that have been studied to date. However, in some cases a series of enzymatic reactions may occur. These have been demonstrated in the hormonal actions on target cells, and similar steps may be involved in some synaptic responses, as will be discussed in Chapter 6 on peripheral ganglia.

While these events are taking place in the postsynaptic membrane, the cleft is being cleared of transmitter by deactivation or hydrolysis, reuptake into the presynaptic terminal, diffusion, or uptake by glial cells.

The final steps, shown in F, are the current flows through ionic conductance channels (step 10) and the resulting synaptic potential (step 11). Of course, any of the steps can be refined to include substeps, or modified to account for other actions (e.g., a conductance decrease instead of increase in step 9).

METABOLIC PATHWAYS We have seen that morphologically synapses share certain fine-structural features, and physiologically they share certain steps and actions. This uniformity is remarkable when one considers the diversity of substances that can function as transmitters. We shall have occasion to assess the significance of this diversity as different neuronal systems are reviewed in later chapters. At this point it will be useful to obtain an overview of the metabolic pathways involved (see Cooper et al., 1978).

A summary of most of the substances that have been identified as transmitters in the mammalian nervous system, and the main metabolic pathways for their synthesis, is shown in the diagram of Fig. 4.5; their structure, synthesis, and inactivation are summarized in Fig. 4.6. The flow in Fig. 4.5 starts at the top, recognizing that metabolism begins with

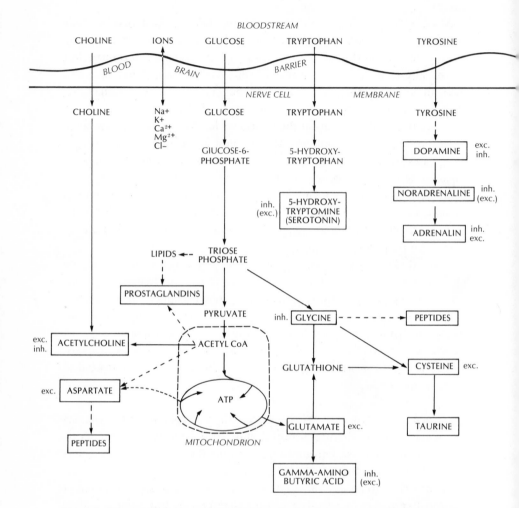

FIG. 4.5. Summary of neurotransmitters and related compounds, and some pathways involved in their transport from the bloodstream and their metabolism within the nerve cell. (Modified from Cooper et al., 1978.)

the substances provided from the bloodstream. This is a critical factor for nerve cells, because of the so-called *blood–brain barrier*. The barrier is formed by tight junctions between the capillary endothelial cells in the brain, which isolate the brain (with the exception of certain regions) from circulating substances in the bloodstream. The only substances to pass the barrier are ions, glucose, and essential amino acids and fatty acids. The central role of glucose in this regard, for energy metabolism and for synthesis of amino acids and proteins, is illustrated in the diagram. We shall recur to this point below, and later in the chapter.

The diagram indicates at the top the main transmitter categories: acetylcholine, catecholamines, amino acids, and peptides. The closed boxes indicate the different individual types of molecules. A few generalizations may be made at this point. The transmitter compounds are all low molecular weight, water soluble (polar) amines or amino acids and related substances. Acetylcholine and the catecholamines are synthesized from circulating precursors, whereas the amino acids and peptides are ultimately synthesized from circulating glucose.

The types of synaptic actions (excitatory or inhibitory) that have been correlated with particular compounds are also indicated in the diagram. Although it is commonly believed that a transmitter is associated with one or another specific action, it can be seen that this is not always correct. For example, acetylcholine has an inhibitory action on the heart, but at the neuromuscular junction we have seen that its action is excitatory. Both actions are therefore included beside the box for acetylcholine in the diagram. From this and other examples we recognize an important principle of synaptic organization, that *a specific transmitter substance cannot be identified with a specific postsynaptic action*. In more general terms, the nervous system can use the same substance for different purposes; obversely, the same function (i.e., excitation) can be mediated by different substances. This flexible relation between transmitter substance and physiological action may be regarded as a biochemical corollary to the flexible relation that exists between the structure and function of neuronal processes in different parts of the brain.

DALE'S PRINCIPLE Although the nervous system as a whole can use different substances at different synapses, this is not necessarily true for an individual neuron. The metabolic unity of the neuron would seem to require that it release the same transmitter substance at all its synapses. This is *Dale's Principle (Law)* and, since it can be easily misunderstood, it is well to quote the original formulation. In a review of synaptic transmission in the autonomic nervous system many years ago, Dale, one of the great pioneers in this field, wrote

COMPOUND	STRUCTURE	SYNTHESIS	INACTIVATION
ACETYLCHOLINE (ACh)	$H_3C-\overset{\overset{O}{\|\|}}{C}-O-(CH_2)_2\ \overset{+}{N}\ (CH_3)_3$	CAT	AChE
DOPAMINE (DA)	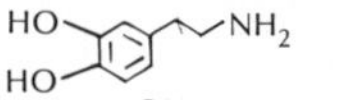 (catechol ring) HO–, HO– with –CH$_2$–NH$_2$	DDC	Reuptake MAO, COMT
NORADRENALINE (NA)	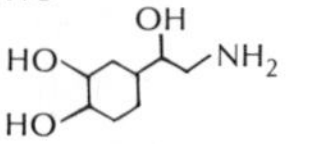 (catechol ring) HO–, HO– with –CH(OH)–CH$_2$–NH$_2$	DBH	Reuptake MAO, COMT
SEROTONIN (5HT)	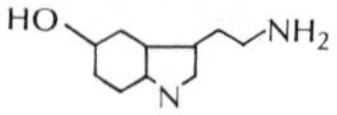 (indole ring) HO– with –CH$_2$–CH$_2$–NH$_2$	AADC	Reuptake MAO
GAMMA-AMINO BUTYRIC ACID (GABA)	$\overset{+}{H_2}N-(CH_2)_3-\overset{\overset{O}{\|\|}}{C}-OH$	GAD	Reuptake GABA-T
GLYCINE (GLY)	$\overset{+}{H_3}N-CH_2-\overset{\overset{O}{\|\|}}{C}-OH$	?	?
PEPTIDES THYROTROPHIC-RELEASING HORMONE (TRH)	(Pyro) Glu–His–Pro (NH$_2$)		
ENKEPHALIN	Tyr–Gly–Gly–Phe–Met–OH Tyr–Gly–Gly–Phe–Leu–OH		
OXYTOCIN	Cys – Tyr – Phe – Glu (NH$_2$) – Asp (NH2) – CyS – Pro – Lys – Gly (NH$_2$)		
SUBSTANCE P	Arg – Pro – Lys – Pro – Glu – Glu – Phe – Phe – Gly – Leu – Met (NH$_2$)		
SOMATOSTATIN (SOMATOTROPHIN RELEASE INHIBITING FACTOR)	Ala – Gly – Cys – Lys – Asn – Phe – Phe – Trp – Lys – Thr – Phe – Thr – Ser – Cys		
LIPID PROSTAGLANDINS (PGE)	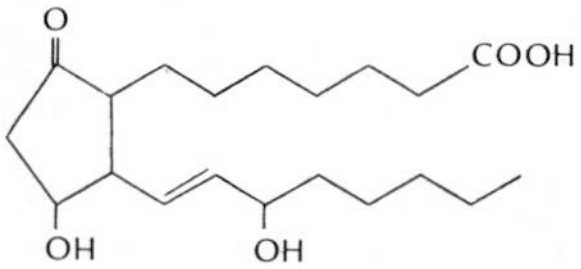 (prostaglandin structure with COOH, OH, OH)		

FIG. 4.6. Summary of molecular structures of neurotransmitters and neuromodulators, together with modes of synthesis and degradation of neurotransmitters. *Synthesis:* CAT, choline acetyltransferase; DDC, dopa decarboxylase; DBH, dopamine-B-hydroxylase; AADC, amino acid decarboxylase; GAD, glutamic acid decarboxylase. *Inactivation:* AChE, acetyl cholinesterase; MAO, monoamine oxidase; COMT, catechol-o-methyl transferase; GABA-T, GABA transaminase. (Modified from Mountcastle, 1974.)

... the phenomena of regeneration appear to indicate that the nature of the chemical function, whether cholinergic or adrenergic, is characteristic for each particular neurone, and unchangeable. When we are dealing with two different endings of the same sensory neurone, the one peripheral and concerned with vasodilatation and the other at a central synapse, can we suppose that the discovery and identification of a chemical transmitter of axon-reflex dilation would furnish a hint as to the nature of the transmission process at a central synapse? The possibility has at least some value as a stimulus to further experiment. (Dale, 1935)

This is the acorn from which the mighty oak has grown. The principle is profound, for it implies, as Iversen (1970) has pointed out, that during development some process of differentiation determines the particular secretory product a given neuron will manufacture, store, and release. The usefulness of the principle in the analysis of synaptic organization is explicit in Dale's statement, for, if a substance can be established as the transmitter at one synapse, it can be inferred to be the transmitter at all other synapses made by that neuron.

The point that is often misunderstood is that Dale's Law only applies to the presynaptic unity of the neuron; it does not apply to the postsynaptic actions the transmitter will have at the synapses made by the neuron onto different target neurons. These actions may be similar, or they may be different. We have already noted that the acetylcholine released at motoneuron nerve terminals has an excitatory action at the neuromuscular junction, whereas acetylcholine released from vagal nerve terminals has an inhibitory action in the heart. Similar possibilities for diversity of action exist for the transmitter released from a single neuron. Such neurons have been termed *multiaction cells*, and have been particularly well studied in invertebrates. Kandel (1976) has summarized the conclusions from this work as follows:

1. The sign of the synaptic action is not determined by the transmitter but by the properties of the receptors on the postsynaptic cell.
2. The receptors in the follower [postsynaptic] cells of a single presynaptic neuron can be pharmacologically distinct and can control different ionic channels.
3. A single follower cell may have more than one kind of receptor for a given transmitter, with each receptor controlling a different ionic conductance mechanism.
As a result of these three features, cells can mediate opposite synaptic actions to different follower cells or to a single follower cell.

These may be regarded as corollaries to Dale's Law. There is as yet limited evidence for multiaction cells in the vertebrate nervous system; an example will be discussed in the chapter on peripheral ganglia.

What of the possibility of cells with multiple transmitters? Recently, four putative transmitters have been identified in single neurons of

Aplysia (Brownstein et al., 1974). The fact that some synaptic terminals contain more than one type of synaptic vesicle is also suggestive in this regard. It has been thought uneconomical for a cell to synthesize, transport, and release different transmitters from different axonal terminals. However, this reservation need not apply to transmitter release from dendritic as compared with axonal terminals, or from different parts of a dendritic tree. We shall encounter evidence for this possibility in the olfactory bulb (Chapter 8).

IDENTIFICATION OF TRANSMITTERS   Thus far we have discussed transmitters as if it were known which substances function at different synapses. The identification of transmitters is in fact one of the most difficult, not to say vexatious, problems in all of neuroscience. Experimentally, certain criteria must be met; each involves a special methodology and, to a degree, indirect evidence, estimates, and inferences. The criteria may be summarized as follows (cf. Werman, 1966; Bullock, 1976):

> 1. *Anatomical:* presence of the substance in appropriate amounts in presynaptic processes.
> 2. *Biochemical:* presence and operation of enzymes that synthesize the substance in the presynaptic neuron and processes, and remove or inactivate the substance at the synapse.
> 3. *Physiological:* demonstration that physiological stimulation causes the presynaptic terminal to release the substance, and that iontophoretic application of the substance to the synapse in appropriate amounts mimics the natural response.
> 4. *Pharmacological:* drugs that affect the different enzymatic or biophysical steps have their expected effects on synthesis, storage, release, action, inactivation, and reuptake of the substance.

As Bullock has noted, "The value of these criteria is primarily that, if met, they can increase the probability of a substance being the natural transmitter. If not, they can rule out consideration of the compound." This touches on an interesting philosophical point, that proof in this endeavor is conditional; it grows by increment of evidence, building by as many independent methods as possible. This of course to a large extent is in the nature of biological research, and informs the strategy of a multidisciplinary approach to synaptic organization that is used in this book.

There is general agreement that the identification of acetylcholine as

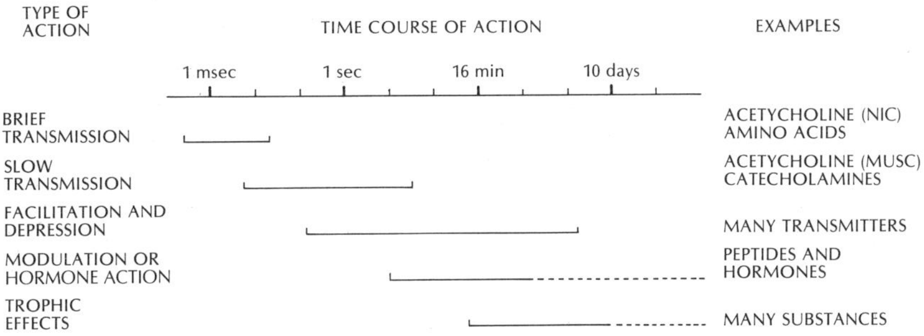

TYPE OF ACTION	TIME COURSE OF ACTION				EXAMPLES
	1 msec	1 sec	16 min	10 days	

BRIEF TRANSMISSION — ACETYCHOLINE (NIC) AMINO ACIDS

SLOW TRANSMISSION — ACETYCHOLINE (MUSC) CATECHOLAMINES

FACILITATION AND DEPRESSION — MANY TRANSMITTERS

MODULATION OR HORMONE ACTION — PEPTIDES AND HORMONES

TROPHIC EFFECTS — MANY SUBSTANCES

FIG. 4.7. Time course of action of neurotransmitters and related compounds.

the transmitter at the neuromuscular junction comes closest to fulfilling these criteria. There is also reasonable evidence regarding vertebrate autonomic ganglia (see Chapter 6) and several types of invertebrate neurons. For further discussion of these studies the reader is referred to Kuffler and Nichols (1976), Kandel (1976), and Cooper et al. (1978). In the vertebrate central nervous system our knowledge usually rests on one or two, or occasionally several, methodological approaches, carried out without benefit of direct observation. Although many of the results are intriguing, and indeed compelling, the evidence is nonetheless fragmentary. As we meet the members of the transmitter family in the various regions of the brain, we must remember that they all bear the same first name: putative.

NEUROTRANSMISSION AND NEUROMODULATION   An important development in recent years is the recognition of the wide range in the time course of action of different substances that mediate neuronal interactions. This is summarized schematically in Fig. 4.7. The time courses of action of the classical neurotransmitters, such as acetylcholine, represent the briefest types. The slower actions of neurotransmitters overlap with the periods of facilitation and depression that occur in the aftermath of activity, and with the effects mediated by peptides and hormones. These in turn overlap with trophic effects, and with the neuronal interactions that underlie such processes as development and plasticity.

We shall discuss later some aspects of the longer-lasting effects of synapses. For the present, Fig. 4.7 illustrates the problem that can arise in defining a neurotransmitter. Thus, to the traditional criteria mentioned previously, one must now add another dimension: the time course of action. At present, substances with brief actions are regarded as neurotransmitters, while those with long-term effects are often referred to as neuromodulators. The two may well represent extremes along a continuum. We must also recognize the differences in distances over which actions take place. The terminology will undoubtedly evolve as more substances are recognized and extrasynaptic interactions are identified.

TRANSPORT OF SUBSTANCES Closely related to synaptic transmission and its associated metabolic processes is the transport of substances within the nerve cell. Far from being the static structure visualized in microscopic sections, the neuron at the molecular level is in constant motion. As noted in the discussion of cell organelles in Chapter 2, there is ongoing synthesis of transmitter molecules, macromolecules, and vesicle membranes in the cell body; and movement out into the axon and dendrites (see Fig. 4.8 and Droz, 1975). Some of these substances pass out of axon terminals and are taken up by postsynaptic cells, as shown by trans-neuronal transport of labeled amino acids incorporated into protein. Proteins and small enzymes also are taken up by axon terminals and move in the axon toward the cell body; this is the basis of the mapping of axonal projections by the horseradish peroxidase technique (Kristensson, Olsson, and Sjöstrand, 1971). A similar movement of substances takes place in dendrites, involving transmitters, enzymes and even such molecules as nucleoside derivatives (Kreutzberg, Schubert, and Lux, 1975). Some of these substances are those taken up from neighboring terminals by trans-neuronal transport. Ions and small molecules move directly between cells through the channels of gap junctions. Thus, there is constant biochemical transport and communication between all parts of the neuron and between neighboring neurons.

These movements take place at different rates. Axoplasmic transport, in mammals, for example, ranges from slow (about 1 mm/day) to fast (100–400 mm/day). In line with an earlier comment, it is of interest to relate these rates to different levels of dimensionality. This can be done if we plot distance against time on logarithmic scales, as in Fig. 4.9. The fastest transport in axons thus translates to at rate of about 5 μm/sec. Surprisingly, this is similar to the rate that has been estimated for diffusion of the phospholipids in the cell membrane, as shown in the graph.

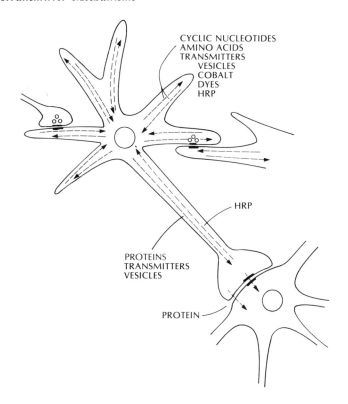

CYCLIC NUCLEOTIDES
AMINO ACIDS
TRANSMITTERS
VESICLES
COBALT
DYES
HRP

HRP

PROTEINS
TRANSMITTERS
VESICLES

PROTEIN

FIG. 4.8. Transport of substances within nerve cells.

Slow transport is at a rate of 0.01 μm (100 Å)/sec; this is even slower than the estimated rate of diffusion of proteins in the cell membrane. These values serve to emphasize that the membrane, as well as the internal cell substance, is in dynamic flux. Both slow and fast axoplasmic transport are dependent on the presence of Ca.

With regard to transport of synaptic transmitters and vesicular membrane, this would take many minutes even by fast transport in the shortest axons of a mm length, and would be a matter of hours in the longest axons. This helps to explain why axonal terminals contain some of their own metabolic machinery for transmitter synthesis and reuptake. In the case of output synapses from dendrites, however, the distances from the

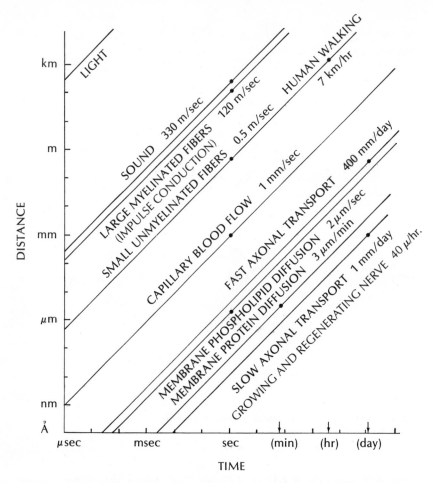

FIG. 4.9. Graph showing rates of movement of substances and conduction of activity for different dimensions of time and space. Small dots indicate common expression for rates (e.g., m/sec).

cell body are characteristically less than 1 mm, and the synapses would seem to be able to draw more directly on the metabolic resources of the cell body for sustaining their activity. For output synapses from the cell body itself, this of course becomes obvious.

Other rates are also shown in Fig. 4.9, for comparison. Note that the slowest rate of nerve conduction is more than 5 orders of magnitude faster than the fastest axonal transport; even the slowest impulses travel a micron in less than a microsecond. Synaptic transmitter diffusion through the cleft (see earlier in this chapter) works out to a rate of about one micron per millisecond, similar to the rate of capillary blood flow. The reader can insert other rates and relations as well. The general principle, that physiological processes at microscopic levels take place in incredibly short times, is readily apparent. It is also the reason why the time domain for microelectrode analysis of synaptic functions commonly falls into the range of milliseconds. The reader is referred to an interesting treatment of dimensionality in physiological processes by Adam and Delbruck (1964).

ENERGY METABOLISM AND 2–DEOXYGLUCOSE MAPPING   In discussing metabolic pathways we noted that the brain is virtually completely dependent on glucose for energy metabolism. Glucose is taken up by neurons and phosphorylated by hexokinase to glucose-6-phosphate. As in other cells of the body, it is then metabolized in the cytosol through the glycolytic chain to pyruvate, which enters the mitochondria and undergoes oxidative metabolism by the Krebs cycle to yield high-energy phosphates. The sequence is indicated in Fig. 4.5, and the initial steps in more detail in Fig. 4.10. The high-energy phosphate is incorporated into adenosine triphosphate (ATP) and made available for the on-going metabolism of the neuron and for the immediate demands related to nervous activity.

What types of activity require energy? We have seen that ions move passively through their conductance channels in the membrane; however, the concentration gradients are maintained by the metabolic pump, which requires energy. The squid giant axon can continue to generate action potentials for hours after metabolic poisoning, because the passive ion flows are small compared with the large amounts of available ions. However, the proportions increase in smaller fibers, with their larger surface-to-volume ratios; in the finest unmyelinated fibers, impulse activity places immediate demands on the metabolic pump. Similar factors are involved at synapses; the ion flows themselves are passive, but the restoration and maintenance of ion concentrations require energy, as does the synthesis of transmitters and the recycling of membrane. Also, higher rates of ion pumping may be expected at sites where the resting membrane potential is relatively low because of an increased permeability to Na (as at nodes of Ranvier, and in retinal receptors). The high

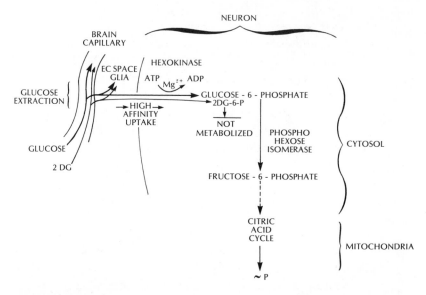

FIG. 4.10. Pathways involved in uptake and initial metabolism of glucose and 2-deoxyglucose (2DG) in nerve cells.

density of mitochondria in the small processes of axons and dendrites reflects to a large extent the energy demands of synapses at those sites.

These types of activity thus have immediate energy demands, and a new method makes use of this property to map the distribution of activity in the brain during different functional states. The method was introduced by Sokoloff and his colleagues (Kennedy et al., 1975; Plum, Gjedde, and Sampson, 1976) and makes use of an analogue of glucose, 2–deoxyglucose (2DG), which simply lacks an oxygen on the second carbon atom. As shown in Fig. 4.10, 2DG is taken up and phosphorylated by hexokinase like glucose. However, the resulting 2DG-6-P is not a substrate for phosphoglucose isomerase and cannot be metabolized further; it is trapped in the tissue. Sokoloff and his colleagues reasoned that if 2DG was labeled with radioactive carbon (14C) and injected in tracer amounts into an animal, the sites of increased 14C-2DG-6-P could be marked by exposing sections of the brain tissue to X-ray film. As many sections can be made as desired, so that the activity pattern associated with a particular functional state can be mapped throughout the entire brain.

The method has been applied to several systems. Among the most dramatic results are those that have been obtained in the visual system by Kennedy et al. (1976) and Hubel, Wiesel, and Stryker (1978). A monkey is injected a day after one eye has been removed. The autoradiograms of the visual cortex show alternating dark and light stripes, which represent the ocular dominance columns that had previously been demonstrated by electrophysiology and anatomical methods (see Chapter 15 for further discussion). These results are shown in Fig. 4.11 (A). The method has also been successfully applied to the olfactory system, (Sharp, Kauer, and Shepherd, 1975, 1977; Shepherd, 1976) where relatively little was known about spatial activity patterns. Surprisingly, after an injection into a rat breathing an odor, small intense foci of activity are found in the olfactory bulb over the glomerular layer, where the axons from the olfactory receptor cells terminate. These results are shown in Fig. 4.11 (B) (see Chapter 8 for further discussion of olfactory bulb organization).

These and other results indicate that the method holds considerable promise, not only for confirming and extending our previous knowledge about particular systems, but also for providing new insights into systems in which information about spatial activity patterns has not been obtainable by other methods. Because of the particular energy demands of synapses, the 2DG technique is well suited for identifying functional systems at the level of synaptic organization in different brain regions.

SYNAPTIC MODIFICATION The close link between metabolism and transmitter substances means that the intensity and duration of synaptic activity is an important variable in determining synaptic efficacy. Studies of the neuromuscular junction have delimited periods of facilitation and suppression that follow an initial period of high frequency stimulation (cf. Martin, 1967). Facilitation and depression have also been demonstrated at a number of central synapses. Internal calcium concentration at the terminal is becoming recognized as important in controlling these long-term dynamic properties. The calcium may originate from internal organelles such as mitochondria, sites on the internal surface of the membrane, and soluble molecules or macromolecules (cf. Erulkar and Rahamimoff, 1978).

The nervous systems of invertebrates are useful models for the study of these properties. In neurons of the leech, for example, a hyperpolarization occurs following impulse activity that appears to be due to an

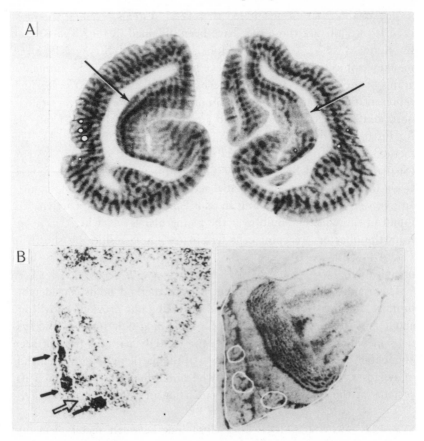

FIG. 4.11. Autoradiograms obtained using the 14C-2-deoxyglucose method. (A) Monkey visual cortex after removal of one eye (from Sokoloff et al., 1978). Arrows indicate blind spots. (B) Rat olfactory bulb after exposure to odor of amyl acetate. Left, autoradiogram showing three small dense foci (arrows) and intervening light region (open arrow). Right, outlines of dense foci fall precisely on small groups of glomeruli when superimposed on Nissl-stained section of bulb (From Stewart, Kauer and Shepherd, 1979.)

electrogenic sodium pump like that in fine axons (Baylor and Nicholls, 1971; also see above). It has been shown that this hyperpolarization has profound effects on synaptic transmission in the neuropil: increase in EPSP amplitude, decrease in IPSPs, conduction block in dendritic processes, and, probably, changes in amount of presynaptic transmitter release. Extracellular K accumulation due to repetitive activity not only may affect impulse conduction, it may also depress the release of transmitter at synapses by depolarizing the presynaptic terminal (Erulkar and Weight, 1977). In the snail, considerable evidence for conditioning of synaptic transmission and changes in reflex behavior has been provided by the elegant studies of Kandel (1976).

It is evident that the mechanism of synaptic transmission is not a simple, stereotyped, self-contained type of affair like that of an action potential. There are, as we have seen, many steps involved in a synaptic action, which encompass metabolic, biophysical, and electrical processes. For this reason, the synapse is the most vulnerable link in the neuronal circuits, the most sensitive site for modifying transmission, processing, and storage of information.

It is obvious that if modifications dependent on use or disuse occur at the central synapses of the vertebrate brain, they would provide a basis for changes underlying learning and memory. But because these changes can often be demonstrated only under extreme or artificial conditions, at peripheral and invertebrate junctions with no natural concomitant of learning or memory, caution is necessary in interpreting them.

Within the brain itself, synapses are, of course, modifiable during the differentiation and growth of neurons in embryonic and early life; the processes concerned are among the most profound problems of biology (Rakić, 1975, 1978; Lund, 1978). In the adult brain there is increasing experimental evidence of the modifiability of synapses. Rearrangements of synaptic inputs have been found following lesions of certain pathways (Raisman, 1970), and we will discuss the effect of de-afferentation on dendritic spines in the cerebral cortex in Chapter 15. There is also evidence that quite dramatic changes in synaptic potency occur during and after repetitive activation of the hippocampus and neocortex, similar to some of the effects elicited in neurons of the leech, as noted above. These effects, like those in invertebrate preparations, have been produced artificially, and the evidence for such changes as a basis for behavior must, thus, remain tentative. Nonetheless, it is widely accepted that synaptic changes do underlie learning and memory. The study of synaptic organization is, therefore, necessary for an understanding of all these aspects of vertebrate behavior.

5

DENDRITIC
ELECTROTONUS

Dendrites provide an elaboration of the surface area of a neuron, and synapses characteristically have different sites on this surface. The study of synaptic organization is, therefore, a study not only of action at a given synapse, but also of spatial relations between that synapse and the dendritic tree. These relations govern the effectiveness of a synaptic potential in generating a further output, whether that output be through a nearby dendrodendritic synapse or through an impulse-generating membrane within the dendritic tree or a soma or an axon hillock. These functional interactions are mediated by the flow of electrical currents set up by the synaptic potentials, and the task is to describe these current flows as rigorously as possible.

The analysis of current flows in neuronal processes has a long tradition in neurophysiology and biophysics. It began with the very earliest electrophysiological studies of activity in peripheral nerves in the 1840's. Much subsequent work in the 19th century was devoted to the problem of distinguishing the passive spread of current in peripheral nerves from the "action" currents associated with the action potential. From this work arose the concept of the nerve fiber as a core conductor, deriving from its high membrane resistance and relatively low internal resistance. Passive spread through the core conductor was termed *electrotonus*, and the changes in membrane potential caused by the passive spread were termed *electrotonic potentials*. These current flows and potential changes were described mathematically, and it was soon realized that the equations were essentially similar to those for the flow of current in an electrical cable, the flow of heat in a rod, and the diffusion of substances in a solute. The equations as applied to nerve cells are often referred to as the *cable equations*.

Application of the cable equations to experiments on the single nerve axon awaited the modern era, beginning with the analysis of the action potential mechanism and the development of the Hodgkin-Huxley model. The equations were adapted for use in studying conduction of the action potential in muscle fibers, and they were also important in Katz's analysis of the end-plate potential at the neuromuscular junction.

The application of the equations to these relatively simple cases (in a geometrical sense) was no easy task, and it therefore seemed that neuronal dendrites, with their limitless variety of shapes and branching patterns and their inaccessability to experimental approaches, were beyond the reach of rigorous analysis. Beginning in 1957, however, the systematic adaptation of the equations to dendrites has been carried out by Rall. Some of the key papers in this series are listed in the bibliography for the benefit of the biophysically minded student (Rall, 1957, 1959a,b, 1962, 1964, 1967, 1969, 1970, 1977). We will describe here only the essentials of the methods, in order to provide the student with the basic tools for understanding the spread of synaptic responses and the functional properties of dendrites. For further orientation to the mathematical methods, the reader is referred to the recent monograph of Noble, Jack, and Tsien, *Electric Current Flow in Excitable Cells* (1974), and to the lucid summary of Jack (1979).

STEADY-STATE ELECTROTONUS

The basic characteristics of electrotonic potentials are illustrated in Fig. 5.1. We consider a length of neuronal process (either axon or dendrite) as a series of membrane patches. A steady depolarization is imposed on the membrane of patch 1. This places a persisting excess of positive charge inside the membrane of patch 1. In this *steady-state* condition, the membrane capacitance acts as an open circuit, and we need only consider, therefore, the current flow through the resistance pathways of the neuron. Some of the current at point (a) will leak back through the membrane resistance of patch 1, but some will flow through the small internal resistance to point (b). At point (b), the current has two similar alternative paths: back through the membrane resistance of patch 2 or onward through the small internal resistance to point (c). The sequence repeats itself further along the neuronal process until all the current has leaked

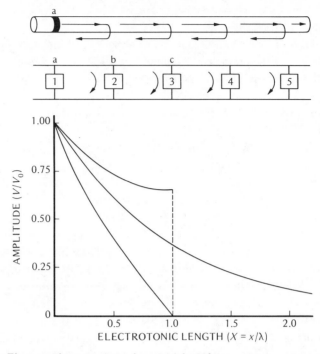

FIG. 5.1. Electrotonic currents and potentials. *Above*, a nerve process (axon or dendrite) with a steady depolarization imposed at (a); arrows, resultant current flows. *Middle*, current flows for a membrane patch model of nerve process. *Below*, distribution of electrotonic potential for the case of infinite length (continuous line); for termination of a process in an open (short-circuit) ending at $X = 1$ (lower line); for termination of a process in a closed ending at $X = 1$ (upper line). *Ordinate*, change in membrane potential (V) relative to its value at the site of current injection (V_0). (After Rall, 1959a.)

back across the membrane and returned to patch 1 to complete the circuit (cf. Fig. 3.7).

From the above, it can be seen that there will be a gradient of current flow along the fiber and a corresponding gradient of membrane potential. The difference between the membrane potential (V_m) and its resting value (E_r) at any point along the fiber is the *electrotonic potential* (V); $V = V_m - E_r$. For the idealized case of Fig. 5.1, we require that the electrical properties of a given patch do not change (as they do during action potentials and synaptic potentials). The properties are constant or, as we say, passive. Electrotonic potentials are, therefore, also called *passive potentials*.

If the electrical properties of the neuronal process are known, then, as the student familiar with Kirkhoff's elementary laws of electrical circuits knows, it is possible to describe the flow of current and the distribution of electrotonic potential exactly. The equation, as it applies to a neuronal process, is one of the so-called *cable equations*

$$V = \frac{d^2V}{dX^2} \qquad (5:1)$$

in which V = electrotonic potential, and X = length in electrotonic units, which we will define shortly.

One solution of this equation gives

$$V = V_0 e^{-x} \qquad (5:2)$$

in which $V_0 = V$ at $x = o$ (the starting point on the neuronal process), and λ = characteristic length. The significance of λ can be seen by setting $x = \lambda$; then $V = 1/e$ or, approximately, 0.37 of V_0. Thus, λ is the length over which the electrotonic potential falls to $1/e$ of its value at the origin. Like the notion of half-life, it is a way of characterizing and comparing electrotonic spread in different kinds of neuronal processes. It is a concept that is central to the analysis of dendritic organization.

A plot of Eq. (5:2) is shown in Fig. 5.1 (middle trace of bottom graph). The convention we will employ is to plot V relative to V_0 on the ordinate. On the abscissa is plotted the electrotonic length X, which is real length (x) relative to characteristic length λ, i.e., the exponent of Eq. (5:2).

To use Eq. (5:2) to describe the spread of synaptic potentials, we must take into account the geometry of the particular dendrites under study and their electrical properties. The basic geometrical variables whose numerical values we must determine are the *length*, the *diameter*, and the *branching* of the dendritic processes. Let us now consider these three aspects.

DENDRITIC LENGTH One of the assumptions underlying Eq. (5:2) is that the cable is of infinite length. For long axons, this assumption is acceptable, for virtually all the current has leaked back over several characteristic lengths (for example, V/V_0 is less than 0.02 at $X = 3$). Dendrites are relatively short, however, and the equation must obviously take this into account. This requires not only knowledge of the length of a dendrite, but also of its mode of termination, a "boundary condition" in mathematical terminology.

An intuitive grasp of the importance of these factors is provided in two cases illustrated by the different gradients in Fig. 5.1. We assume a dendrite of electrotonic length $X = 1$. In one case, the dendrite is assumed to have an open ending (i.e., $V_m = E_r$ at $X = 1$). At that point, therefore, the electrotonic potential must be 0, and associated with this is a much steeper gradient of electrotonic potential along the dendrite, as is shown by the lower line in Fig. 5.1. This case is relevant to situations in which a synaptic potential spreads toward a site of high conductance, as, for example, a strong inhibitory synaptic site, or a confluence of many branches. In such situations, the electrotonic gradient is steeper, and the spread of electrotonic potential is less (although usually not to the extent produced by the complete short circuit used for this illustration).

On the other hand, the dendrite may be assumed to terminate in a normal patch of membrane. This case will obviously cause the electrotonic potential to be greater at this point than it would be if the fiber extended to infinity. It can be shown that this is closely approximated by the assumption of a patch of infinite resistance across the end of the fiber, an assumption that is easier to work with mathematically. The electrotonic potentials along the dendrite, for this case, are shown by the upper line in Fig. 5.1. This case has general applicability to situations in which a synaptic potential spreads through a dendritic branch, as well as through an entire dendritic tree. In these situations, the electrotonic gradient is less, and the spread of electrotonic potential greater, than for an infinite cable.

DENDRITIC DIAMETER   All neuronal processes, including dendrites, vary in diameter as well as length. Intuitively, it is obvious that electrotonic spread will depend on diameter. Spread of current will be enhanced by a larger diameter, since the effective resistance inside a neuronal process (r_i) decreases as the diameter of the process increases. Similarly, spread will be enhanced by a relatively high membrane resistance (r_m), so that the current tends to spread internally through the process rather than across the membrane. These same factors indeed underlie the greater velocity of the action potential in larger fibers.

The dependence of electrotonic spread on diameter is incorporated in the equation for the *characteristic length* (λ). When the resistances are expressed in terms of unit area, the equation is

$$\lambda = \sqrt{\frac{r_m}{r_i}} = \sqrt{\frac{R_m}{R_i} \cdot \frac{d}{4}} \qquad (5{:}3)$$

where $r_m = R_m/2 \pi a$ = membrane resistance for unit length of cylinder (Ω cm), $r_i = R_i/\pi \alpha^2$ = internal resistance for unit length of cylinder (Ω/cm), R_m = specific resistance of unit area of membrane (Ω cm^2), R_i = specific resistance of unit volume of internal medium (Ω cm), a = radius of cylinder (cm), and Ω = resistance in ohms. In other words, the characteristic length (λ) varies as the square root of the diameter, given fixed values for R_m and R_i.

The variation of the characteristic length with the square root of the diameter is another key concept in the study of synaptic organization and the properties of dendrites. This relationship is illustrated in Fig. 5.2. In the construction of this nomogram, assumptions about the values of the electric properties R_i and R_m were required; R_i is relatively constant, and has been estimated at approximately 50 Ωcm for mammalian nerve, but R_m is more variable, and three values have, therefore, been used to cover most of the range found in mammalian nerve membrane.

Estimation of the specific membrane resistance (R_m) is by no means a simple procedure. One begins by passing current through an intracellular electrode and simultaneously recording the change in potential this produces. The current-voltage relation yields a value for the *whole neuron resistance* (R_N), also called the *input resistance*. The question arises: How much of the resistance (or, inversely, conductance) is due to the current that flows across the soma membrane and how much to that flowing out through the dnedrites? This requires an assessment of the branching pattern of the dendritic tree (see below), from which the relative contributions of *dendritic* and *somatic input conductance* are obtained, and expressed as the ratio (ρ). Since the ratio is usually greater than 1, it expresses *dendritic dominance*, in an electrotonic sense, just as measurements of surface area express dendritic dominance, in a spatial sense. An expression that includes ρ and various other factors is then used to obtain an estimate for R_m. These methods are explained by Rall (1959b, 1960, 1977), and the procedure, as it applies to the analysis of the motoneuron, is succinctly described by Lux, Schubert, and Kreutzberg (1970).

For general orientation, Fig. 5.2 provides the student with a starting point in assessing the range of possibilities for spread of currents in dendrites of different diameters. We will have occasion to refer frequently to this graph in our studies of the dendritic properties of differ-

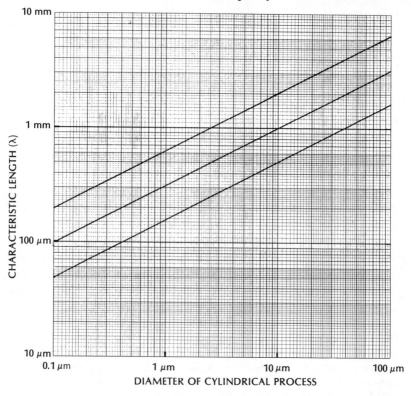

FIG. 5.2. Dependence of the characteristic length (λ) on the diameter and electrical parameters of a nerve process. *Ordinate*, characteristic length. *Abscissa*, diameter of a nerve process. The lines plot for three values of the ratio R_m/R_i: 10, 40, and 160 (e.g., R_i = 50 Ωcm; R_m = 500, 2000, and 8000 Ωcm²).

ent neurons. By way of general comment, it may be noted here that λ has a relatively high value even in very fine processes. Thus, the finest dendritic branches in the brain are of the order of 0.1 μm in diameter; as can be seen in Fig. 5.2, one might expect a λ of the order of 100 μm for them. Such branches are, in fact, rarely this long, which indicates that current spread may well be rather effective in small dendritic trees. On the other hand, the largest dendritic trunks (as, for example, in motoneurons and cortical pyramidal cells) are 10–15 μm in diameter. From Fig. 5.2 we might expect a dendrite of 10 μm in diameter to have a λ of the order of 1000 μm (1 mm). This is rather longer than the length of most large dendrites (but see the neocortex, Chapter 16), which again indicates

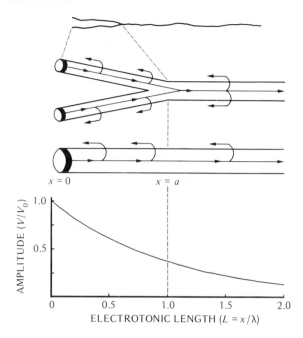

FIG. 5.3. Derivation of an equivalent cylinder for electrotonic current flow in a nerve process with two branches. *Steps from top to bottom,* branching process, cable model, equivalent cylinder. Steady depolarization imposed at $X = 0$; branch point is at (a); arrows, current flows. *Below,* continuous decrement of electrotonic potential, assuming a 3/2 power constraint at branch point, as defined in the text.

that the spread of synaptic current through them may be relatively effective. In contrast, the large axons of principal neurons are many times longer than their characteristic lengths; the longest motoneuron axons to the lower limb, for example, are over a meter (1000 mm) in length. Communication through these axons must be by action potentials rather than by passive potentials alone.

DENDRITIC BRANCHING The third basic characteristic of dendritic geometry is branching. Dendrites display a fantastic variety of branching patterns. How do the methods of Rall deal with this fact?

The basic approach is illustrated in Fig. 5.3. We consider, as usual, the simplest case first, that of a dendrite that divides into two branches. A steady depolarization is set up in the terminal patch of each branch, as might be due, for example, to steady excitatory synaptic potentials at those sites. In each branch, there is an electrotonic current flow, as depicted in Fig. 5.3. At the branch point, the currents summate and spread into the stem dendrite.

Now if both branches have the same diameter, length, and electrical properties, the gradient of electrotonic potential will be the same in them, and the gradient in one branch will be representative for both. We may then combine the branches into a single cylinder that represents the electrical properties, current flow, and potential spread for both branches. Thus, we obtain an *equivalent cylinder* for these branches: the length of the cylinder in Fig. 5.3 from $x = o$ to $x = a$.

What will be the gradient of electrotonic potential in the equivalent cylinder? This depends on the diameters of the branches, of course, but it also depends on the relations of the branches to the stem fiber. In other words, there is a boundary condition at the branch point. Let us imagine the simplest case, in which there would be continuity of the gradient through the branches and into the stem fiber. This is plotted in Fig. 5.3. Rall has shown that there is continuity if the branch diameters, taken to their 3/2 power and added, equal the 3/2 power of the diameter of the stem fiber.[1] This fulfills the requirement that the combined conductance for a given electrotonic length of the branches equals the conductance for the same electrotonic length of the stem fiber. Using this assumption, we can fit the equivalent cylinder for the branches to the cylinder for the trunk, as in Fig. 5.3, and obtain, thereby, a single cylinder for the entire dendritic system.

As a step in the construction of the equivalent cylinder, we have to generalize *electrotonic length* (X) in order to apply it to the combined branches; thus, $L = x/\lambda$ applies to both single dendrites and to parallel

---

[1]The dependence of dendritic input conductance (G_D) on the 3/2 power of the diameter of a dendrite of semi-infinite extension was derived by Rall (1959b) as follows

$$G_D = \frac{I}{V} \quad \text{(Ohm's Law)}$$

$$= (\lambda r_i)^{-1}$$

$$= \left(\frac{\pi}{2}\right)\left(\frac{1}{R_m R_i}\right)^{1/2}(d)^{3/2} \qquad (5:4)$$

branches, and L will be the designation we will use for electrotonic length hereafter.

Let us take a practical example. Assume that the branches in Fig. 5.3 are each 1 μm in diameter. This value raised to the 3/2 power is also 1; the sum for the two branches is, therefore, 2. The value for the stem dendrite which, raised to the 3/2 power, equals 2, is approximately 1.6. Thus, if the diameter of the stem dendrite is 1.6 μm, there will be electrotonic continuity at the branch point. If we make some reasonable assumptions about the electrical properties (taking, for example, the middle value for R_m in the graph of Fig. 5.2), we can then derive the characteristic lengths for the stem fiber and the branches and, finally, estimate the gradient of electrotonic potential through the system, as shown in Fig. 5.3. Note that, as a reflection of its larger diameter, the stem dendrite has a λ of about 400 μm, in comparison with 300 μm for the branches. This means that there is a continuity of the electrotonic gradient with respect to the electrotonic length (L) but not with respect to the actual length (χ); the gradient is less steep in the stem dendrite with respect to the real length. The student should be sure he understands this difference.

Just as the characteristic length provides a means for comparing spread of synaptic potentials in single dendrites of different size, so does the concept of equivalent cylinder provide the means for comparing spread in branching dendritic trees of different size. In subsequent chapters, we will derive equivalent cylinders, where possible, for dendritic branching systems by the steps outlined above.

It may be asked whether the 3/2 power relationship between a dendritic process and its branches has a general validity in the brain. This turns out to be, in fact, a reasonable first approximation for a number of dendritic trees. The equations are simple under this constraint (because the cylinder has a uniform radius throughout its length), but any branching relationship can be incorporated into the equivalent cylinder model with suitable assumptions. To emphasize the general applications, one may refer to it simply as an *electrotonic model* for whatever dendritic system one is interested in.

TRANSIENT ELECTROTONUS

Thus far we have described the spread of electrotonic current under steady-state conditions, that is, assuming a steady synaptic input. This is a necessary starting point for characterizing the electrotonic properties of dendrites. There are, indeed, cases in local brain regions of background depolarizations (as in the visual receptors of the retina) that are essentially steady states. There are also many types of slow synaptic potentials for which the assumption of a steady state is reasonable.

There are, however, many cases in which the essence of synaptic action is rapid transmission between neurons, an immediate triggering of an impulse within the same neuron, or both. The synaptic potentials for these functions have a rapid onset and decay; the description of these rapid transients requires an elaboration of the cable equations that is the biophysical foundation for the study of *transient electrotonus*.

Conceptually, the analysis of transient electrotonus is simple enough; it involves putting the capacitance of the membrane back into the picture. Rapid changes in electric charge across the membrane must first charge or discharge the membrane capacitance. This results in a time-dependent storage of electrical energy that delays, distorts, and attenuates the imposed signal. This is seen clearly in experiments in which a step of current is introduced through an intracellular electrode, and the voltage change is recorded through the same electrode. The voltage rises more slowly; we call it a *charging transient*. The time to reach a value ($1/e$) of the final level is called a *charging time constant* or, alternatively, the *whole neuron time constant* (τ_N). As in the case of the whole neuron resistance described above, it is necessary to take into account the electrotonic properties of the dendritic tree before an estimate of the membrane time constant (τ_m) can be made. These methods are described in Rall (1969, 1970).

SYNAPTIC POTENTIALS IN DENDRITIC TREES The membrane time constant, together with the electrotonic properties of the dendritic tree, determines the time course of a charging transient or a synaptic potential. Mathematically the description of these relationships is quite complicated. The essence of the methods, as they apply to the analysis of synaptic potentials, may be illustrated with respect to the diagram of Fig. 5.4. Consider a cell with an extensively branched dendritic tree, in which we wish to compare the synaptic potentials recorded in the cell body when the synaptic inputs are at three different sites: the cell body itself, midway in the dendritic tree, and at the far end of the tree. What will be the effect of the electrotonic properties of the dendrites on the characteristics of the synaptic potentials as they reach the cell body?

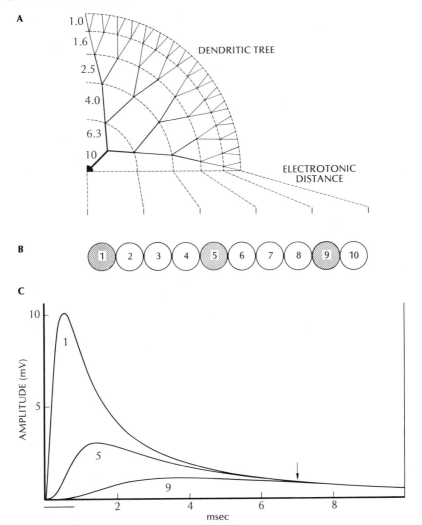

FIG. 5.4. Transient electrotonus in a dendrite tree. *Above*, diagrammatic representation of an extensively branched dendritic tree, in which a 3/2 power constraint applies to all branch points. *Middle*, equivalent cylinder for a dendritic tree, modeled as a chain of compartments (patches). *Below*, transient electrotonic potentials that would be recorded from the cell body (1) for the cases of brief synaptic conductance change (bar) in compartments (1), (5), and (9). *Ordinate*, amplitude (mV). *Abscissa*, time (msec). (Above and middle diagrams after Rall, 1964; bottom tracings calculated from the Rall model on a PDP-10 computer by K.L. Marton.)

To make this case tractable, it is assumed that each dendrite gives rise to two daughter branches that meet the 3/2 power constraint previously described. By suitable assumptions for the branch lengths, an equivalent cylinder is obtained in which increments of electrotonic length (ΔL) correspond to successive levels of branching. This modeling of an extensively branched system illustrates the power of the equivalent cylinder concept more vividly than the previous simple case.

For computational purposes the equivalent cylinder is put into the form of a chain of compartments, as shown in Fig. 5.4 (B). Each compartment represents a patch of membrane containing the simple electrical circuit of Fig. 5.1. Each patch is joined to its neighbor by transfer constants that incorporate the electrotonic properties of the dendrites. It can be seen that this approach is essentially similar to the compartmental analyses that are widely used in the study of metabolic turnover in many systems of the body.

To model a synapse in this system, we assume a brief conductance change, which places an excess positive charge inside the synaptic membrane. This depolarizes the membrane, giving rise to an EPSP, as in our previous simple model (Fig. 3.5). We assume the three different sites of synaptic input shown in Fig. 5.4 and ask the computer to compute the resulting voltage transients in the cell body due to electrotonic spread from these sites.

The results are shown in Fig. 5.4 (C). When the synaptic locus is in the soma, the EPSP at that site has an immediate and sharp rise and a rapid decay. For the middle dendritic input, the soma transient is reduced in amplitude and has a slower time course. This effect becomes more extreme with the peripheral input site. In these respects, the results agree with our intuitive expectations. The computer, however, allows precise measurements of these different EPSP's to be made and compared. For example, Rall has shown that certain kinds of *shape index*, such as the time-to-peak and the half-width, are sensitive indicators of the sites of input. This has been a valuable tool in the analysis of synaptic loci in motoneurons.

The model also permits one to be quite precise in describing synaptic current flows. For the soma input, for example, we can say that the decay of the EPSP is more rapid than would be the case for a single RC element (i.e., membrane patch) because, in addition to leakage of the charge locally across the membrane, there is a rapid electrotonic spread of the charge from that patch to the rest of the cylinder. Rall conceives of this as *equalizing spread*, for which *equalizing time constants* can be obtained through standard techniques of peeling exponentials from semilogarithmic plots of the decays (Rall, 1969, 1970b, 1977). As time goes by the charge gets evenly distributed throughout the cylinder, as is shown by the fact that the final decays of all the transients, regardless of their initial input locus, become similar [beginning at the arrow in Fig. 5.4 (C)].

Consider now the soma EPSP generated by the distant dendritic input. Not only is this transient slow and attenuated, but it has a very slow onset (i.e., a long time-to-peak). In fact, during the time of the synaptic conductance change in the periphery, no change in soma membrane potential is observed at all! This, of course, is a property of dendritic electrotonus, in that it takes time for the charge to spread along the capacitance of the equivalent cylinder.

The general conclusion from this type of analysis is that local inputs provide for rapid responses, whereas distant inputs provide for slower and more sustained activity. The rapid responses may have the function, in some neurons, of triggering impulses (as in the motoneuron of the spinal cord). In other neurons, their function may be the activation of local synaptic output from the same dendritic region (as in olfactory bulb neurons). Any local input will also contribute to the slow modulation of the background excitability of distant sites within its dendritic tree. It is important to realize that, because of the dendrodendritic synapses present in many brain regions, synapses onto small dendritic branches, although distant with respect to the site of impulse initiation in the soma, may be local with respect to postsynaptic interactions and to dendrodendritic synaptic output.

SYNAPTIC POTENTIALS IN DENDRITIC SPINES The smallest type of dendritic branch is the spine. These are found in many neurons, and provide targets for specific synaptic inputs and, in some cases, outputs as well. The spread of potentials into and out of the spine has been an intriguing question, particularly in view of the very thin spine neck in many cases. The small size of the spine has put this question out of reach of direct electrophysiological analysis. The general problem has been investigated computationally by Rall and Rinzel (1973), and a specific model for olfactory bulb dendrites has recently been developed (Shep-

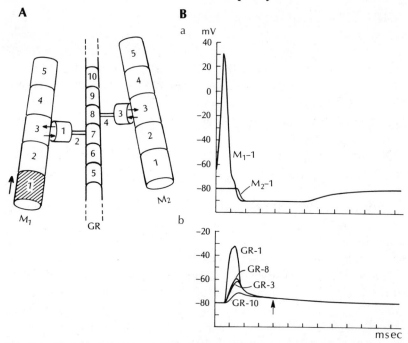

FIG. 5.5. Model of spread of potentials in dendrites and dendritic spines. (A) Compartmental model of two mitral cell dendrites (M_1 and M_2) and granule cell dendrite (GR) with two spines. Impulse is generated in compartment 1 of M_1 (shaded). (B) Potentials recorded in model: (a) Potentials in mitral cells; (b) Potentials in granule cell. (From Shepherd and Brayton, 1978.)

herd and Brayton, 1978) which illustrates some basic properties of spine input–output functions.

We consider in Fig. 5.5 (A) a compartmental model of a length of dendrite from which arise two spines. This represents a part of a granule cell dendritic tree, with each spine attached by reciprocal synapses to a neighboring mitral-cell dendrite. These particular dendrodendritic connections, and their physiological properties, will be discussed further in Chapter 8. For the present it is sufficient to note that an impulse spreading in mitral cell dendrite (M_1) activates an excitatory synapse onto spine (1). The EPSP in the spine in turn activates the inhibitory synapse of the reciprocal pair back onto the mitral cell dendrite (feedback inhibition). In addition, the EPSP spreads electrotonically into the dendrite and spine (3), activating its inhibitory synapse onto mitral cell dendrite (M_2) (lateral inhibition). This sequence of activity in the mitral cells is shown in Fig. 5.5 (B,1).

The electrotonic properties of the granule cell can be assessed by examining the potentials in different compartments. As shown in Fig. 5.5 (B,2) the EPSP in spine (GR-1) consists of a depolarization which rises and decays rapidly. The EPSP spreads from the spine head into the dendritic branch, where the potential amplitude is reduced to about half (GR-8). However, there is little further reduction in spreading from there into the second spine head (GR-3). This reflects the fact that the spine neck, although thin (only 0.2 μm in diameter) is extremely short (a very small fraction of a λ); also, there is a boundary condition in the spine head. Thus, most of the attenuation of the signal from the first spine is due to the conductance load of the dendritic branch and attached dendritic tree, rather than to decrement in passing through the spine necks. The bottom trace (GR-10) shows the potential in the end compartment representing the rest of the granule dendritic tree. Note that the transients all quickly equalize, and from the time indicated by the arrow all compartments are equipotential and decay together (compare Fig. 5.4 above).

The conclusions from this evidence are that (1) synaptic potentials in dendritic spines tend to be of large amplitude (2) there is spatial localization because of conductance loading, but also (3) significant electrotonic spread to neighboring spines. A spine can thus reach substantial levels of depolarization either by direct synaptic input or by summation of electrotonic potentials from many active neighboring spines. These factors are involved in integration and transfer of postsynaptic responses to the cell body, and they also govern input–output relations when the spines are presynaptic, as in the example above.

SYNAPTIC INTERACTIONS We previously discussed the interaction between an EPSP and an IPSP at the same site on a dendrite (Fig. 3.7), and we now must consider the effect different sites have on synaptic interactions. An example studied by Rall (1964) is illustrated in Fig. 5.6. We assume a dendritic cylinder divided into five compartments. The recording site is at 1. An excitatory input (e) occurs in the middle of the dendrite, and the resulting EPSP recorded at 1 is shown by the control tracing in the diagram. Note that the EPSP peak occurs well after the excitatory input occurs. This, of course, reflects the time required for electrotonic spread from the input site to the recording site.

Relative to this excitatory input, we have three basic possibilities for

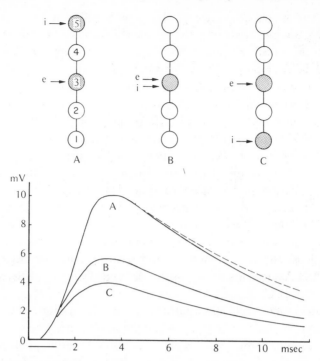

FIG. 5.6. Dependence of synaptic integration on the electrotonic relation between input sites. In all cases an excitatory synapse (e) is located in the middle of an equivalent cylinder (position 3). An inhibitory synapse (i) is located at one of three possible sites: peripherally (A), same site (B), or proximally (C). *Below*, resulting synaptic potentials recorded proximally (at 1) for these three cases. Dotted line, control response to an excitatory synapse alone. (After Rall, 1964.)

the site of the inhibitory input (i). One site is distal, further out on the dendrite (example A). Another is midway, at the same site as the excitatory input (example B). The third is proximal, at the recording site (example C). What is the effect on the recorded EPSP of a continuous inhibitory input at these three sites?

The computed results are shown in Fig. 5.6. The distal IPSP (A) has practically no effect on the peak of the EPSP but does cause it to decline more rapidly. The middle IPSP (B) cuts the EPSP peak to 57% of the control value. The proximal IPSP (C) is even more effective; it cuts the EPSP peak to 40%. We may remind ourselves that these interactions do not reflect an algebraic summation of the excitatory and inhibitory potentials. They are the outcome, rather, of the interactions of current flows induced by the synaptic conductance changes and then modified by the electrotonic relations between the sites.

This simple example will serve as a useful model for many of the cases of synaptic integration that we will encounter in local brain regions. It will apply, for instance, to the case of synaptic interactions within a single branch of a dendrite. For such a case the recording site might be located near a dendrodendritic synaptic output from this dendrite, and the synaptic potentials spreading to that site might determine, in a graded manner, the output from that synapse. On the other hand, the simple chain of compartments depicted in Fig. 5.6 could be used to represent, with suitable assumptions, the equivalent cylinder of Fig. 5.4, to illustrate the effect of inhibitory sites within an entire dendritic tree on the control of the generation of an impulse by an EPSP spreading to the soma.

A general conclusion from this latter type of analysis is that inhibitory sites become increasingly effective vis-à-vis control over the cell body as they are placed closer to the cell body. But this conclusion is subject to many qualifications. Timing, for example, is a crucial factor. In the model of Fig. 5.6, a steady IPSP was postulated for the sake of simplicity, but if we assume instead a brief IPSP, then, obviously, a well-timed IPSP at the middle dendrite will be more effective than an inappropriately timed IPSP at the soma. Also, Rall has made computations for more complicated branching systems and has shown that an inhibitory location that is identical with a peripheral excitatory location can produce more effective inhibition than an equal amount of inhibition applied at the soma.

This should be sufficient to indicate that many factors enter into the relative siting of excitatory and inhibitory synapses vis-à-vis the cell body and axon hillock. The nervous system provides examples of virtually every possible variation on this theme. In the stretch receptor cell of the crayfish, for example, inhibitory input has a peripheral location, near the site of excitatory input from the receptor terminals. Motoneurons provide examples of overlapping excitatory and inhibitory inputs throughout the dendritic tree. Hippocampal pyramidal neurons have inhibitory input directed to their cell bodies; olfactory and neocortical cells also have inhibitory synapses on the initial segments of their axons. These differences are obviously important to an understanding of the synaptic organization of different regions of the brain.

In addition to passive spread, a synaptic response may lead to the generation of an impulse. There are several possible relations between synaptic sites and active sites. There may be a patch of active membrane near the input site in the dendrites, which, in effect, serves as a booster for further electrotonic spread through the dendritic tree. There may be active membrane in the intervening dendrites, through which an impulse can propagate. And there may be active membrane only at a distance, with passive spread thereto. We will encounter examples of all these situations. For this reason, the study of dendritic electrotonus is a part of the larger study of *dendritic properties*, and this will, therefore, be our larger focus in the study of the neurons of each region.

In conclusion, it may be admitted that an understanding of dendritic electrotonus requires an effort that goes beyond the descriptions of dendritic branching patterns and the observations of physiological responses. But the extent to which these mathematical methods can be applied to the interpretation of the anatomical and physiological results is perhaps a direct measure of our progress toward building the foundations for a science of synaptic organization. Toward this end, an intuitive grasp of the methods is far better than none. The need has been succinctly expressed by Katz (1966):

> It can fairly be said that the cable properties of the neuron are the physical basis for all integrative processes at central nervous synapses. For example, spatial summation (or subtraction) of synaptic effects that interact within an effector cell depend upon the spread of subthreshold electric signals along the cell membrane. And as the synapses are clustered closely together within a fraction of a millimeter of the cell body, local integration of such signals can be handled by the subthreshold cable properties of the membrane. . . . It seems that the core conductor, or cable mechanism, is not involved in the transmission of signals *across* most synapses, although it undoubtedly is the basis of the *integration* of local messages, once these have been transferred to the common effector cell.

Part 2

ORGANIZATION OF NEURONAL SYSTEMS

6

PERIPHERAL GANGLIA

Peripheral ganglia are clusters of nerve cells wrapped in connective tissue capsules to form small nodules. They lie outside the central nervous system, in various places in the body. From an organizational point of view, the simplest of these, in fact probably the simplest collection of nerve cells anywhere in the nervous system, is the dorsal root ganglion attached to the spinal cord. It contains the cell bodies of the dorsal root ganglion cells (DRG cells) which transmit impulses from sensory organs in the periphery to relay stations in the spinal cord (cf. Figs. 1.1 and 6.1). As far as is known, there are no input fibers to the ganglion, and little integrative activity takes place within it.

More complicated are the ganglia found in the autonomic nervous system. As is commonly known, this system comprises the motor inner-vation of the internal organs of the body, and is divided into two subsys-tems. The parasympathetic system consists of fibers which arise from motoneurons in the brainstem as well as the most caudal part of the spinal cord, and have a generally inhibitory action on the viscera: slow-ing of heart rate, decreasing motility of the intestine, etc. In contrast, the sympathetic system, arising from motoneurons in the intervening part of the spinal cord, has a generally activating action: faster heart rate, in-creased gut motility, etc. There is a ganglion interposed in the motor pathway in each of these systems, located within the target organ itself in the parasympathetic pathway, and in a chain of separate ganglia in the sympathetic pathway (see Fig. 6.1).

The autonomic ganglia have long been studied with respect to their neurotransmitters, and indeed much of our knowledge about these sub-stances and their biochemistry and pharmacology is based on classical work dating back to Langley and Dale in the early years of this century

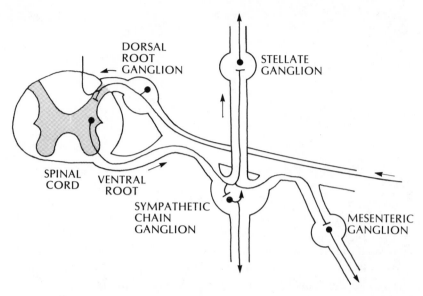

FIG. 6.1. Diagram of major types of ganglia in the sympathetic nervous system and their relation to the spinal cord and dorsal root ganglion.

(see discussion of Dale's Principle above, Chapter 4). For these purposes the ganglia have been considered merely as relay stations in the dullest sense of that term: little more than telegraph keys that click off and on. It is only with recent electron-microscopic and microelectrode studies that the nature of these ganglia as integrative systems in their own right has been realized.

We shall focus our description of synaptic organization on sympathetic ganglia, and make comparisons with parasympathetic ganglia and also with a sensory ganglion, the carotid body. We shall see that these have all served as accessible systems for the application of the methodologies described in the introductory chapters of this book, and that the results illustrate many of the principles that apply to the more complicated regions of the brain.

NEURONAL ELEMENTS

As noted in Chapter 1, there are three neural constituents in most regions of the nervous system: input axons, principal neurons, and intrinsic neurons. These elements are also the building blocks of peripheral ganglia, and we shall consider them in the same sequence used for other regions in our study. The description is based on classical material (Cajal, 1911; de Castro, 1932) and more recent studies (e.g., Elfvin, 1963, 1971; Williams and Palay, 1969; Matthews and Raisman, 1969). The reader should be warned that there are wide differences between different ganglia and different species.

INPUTS   The main input to a sympathetic ganglion is by way of thinly myelinated axons, approximately 3 μm in diameter, which arise from motoneurons in the lateral motor column of the spinal cord (Fig. 6.2). They are referred to as *preganglionic fibers*. Each ramifies sparingly, with numerous varicosities along the branches. There are also thin unmyelinated preganglionic fibers to some ganglia. In the classification of peripheral nerves, the myelinated fibers are B fibers and the unmyelinated are C fibers.

PRINCIPAL NEURON   There is one type of principal neuron, the *ganglion cell*. It is a relatively large cell, ranging in diameter from 15 to 60 μm. As shown in Fig. 6.2, it gives rise to two types of dendrite which, compared with those of other neurons, may be described as short and ultra-short! The short dendrites number 6–12, and are thin, only 1–3 μm in diameter; they branch sparingly and terminate after only 50–150 μm. The ultra-short processes are even thinner (a few tenths of microns) and only 1–3 μm in length; in fact, they appear as a kind of irregular spine (also termed accessory dendrite).

The axon arises from the cell body or, more commonly, from a dendritic trunk. The axon is thin (0.3–1.3 μm) and unmyelinated, and thus falls into the C category of peripheral nerve. It is called a *postganglionic fiber*. A thin axon arising from a large nerve cell is worth noting, there being usually a positive correlation between the sizes of cell bodies and their axons in the nervous system. Also remarkable is the fact that the axon does not give off any axon collaterals within the ganglion. This is an important point for the organization of intrinsic circuits. Axon collaterals are common in principal neurons elsewhere in the nervous system (though they are also lacking in the retinal ganglion cell).

INTRINSIC NEURON   Classical studies with the light microscope did not provide clear evidence for any other cell types in sympathetic ganglia.

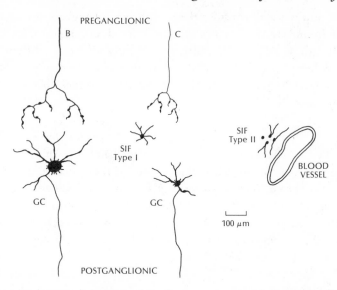

FIG. 6.2. Neuronal elements of the mammalian sympathetic ganglion.
Inputs: preganglionic B and C fibers.
Principal neuron: ganglion cell (GC).
Intrinsic neuron: small intensely flourescing (SIF) cell, types I and II.

There were isolated reports of small groups of cells giving a chromaffin reaction for catecholamines, like that of cells in the adrenal medulla. We now know that most of the catecholamines are lost in this method.

A much more sensitive test was provided by histofluorescence techniques, in which tissue is treated with formaldehyde (Eränkö, 1955) or formaldehyde vapors (Falck, et al., 1962). In the central nervous system this test has revealed several catecholamine-containing cell groups and fiber systems (cf. Basal Ganglia, Chapter 12). In sympathetic ganglia, the ganglion cells and their dendrites fluoresce lightly, because of their content of noradrenaline, and there are in addition "small, intensely fluorescing" cells, first described by Eränkö and Härkönen (1965), and known since then as SIF cells. Shortly thereafter, electronmicroscopists described a type of small cell containing an abundance of dense-core vesicles, and dubbed them "small, granule-containing" cells, or SGC cells. It was suspected, and recently proven (Grillo, Jacobs, and Comroe, 1974) that SIF and SGC cells are one and the same.

In the electronmicroscope these cells have a soma diameter of 6–12 μm. Two types have been distinguished (Fig. 6.2). Type I cells occur singly, near ganglion cells; they are rather amorphous in shape, and give off a number of short processes which vary from 0.2 to 1.5 μm in diameter and up to 100 μm in length. Type II cells occur in clusters of 3–12 cells. Within the clusters the cell bodies have apposed membranes, a not uncommon occurrence in the nervous system (cf. olfactory granule cells; dentate fascia granule cells). The clusters are commonly found near small fenestrated capillaries (i.e., capillaries in which the endothelial membranes have punctate fusions which permits easy passage of substances across the capillary wall; contrast with blood-brain barrier described previously). Satellite cells loosely envelope the clusters with sheet-like processes, except at the capillary appositions. Wide extracellular spaces are occasionally seen within the ganglion.

Because the processes of these cells remain within the ganglion, they are classified as intrinsic neurons. Neither of the two types has an axon. In this respect they resemble the anaxonal granule cells of the olfactory bulb and amacrine cells of the retina.

The internal fine structure of these cells and the other elements will be described in the section on Synaptic Connections below.

NEURONAL POPULATIONS   The elements just described vary widely in different ganglia in different species, with respect to their absolute and relative numbers. For example, in mammalian ganglia, preganglionic input fibers branch to contact a number of ganglion cells, whereas in the frog the ganglion cells of the V sympathetic ganglion are innervated by a single fiber (Blackman, Ginsborg, and Ray, 1963). Also, in the frog, the ganglion cells are described as being without dendrites.

Perhaps the greatest variation occurs in the intrinsic neurons. They are reported to be almost completely absent in the superior cervical ganglion of the cat (Elfvin, 1963; Williams et al., 1976), and those that are present are of the type II variety. In contrast, they are present in large numbers in the same ganglion in the rabbit, where they are mostly type I cells. Other species fall between these two extremes. Similar variations occur in the other types of sympathetic ganglia. We shall see that the ratio of intrinsic to principal neurons is correlated with the complexity of integrative activity in many regions of the nervous system. If that correlation applies to peripheral ganglia it would appear that the amount of processing can vary widely in different ganglia and in different species, though a

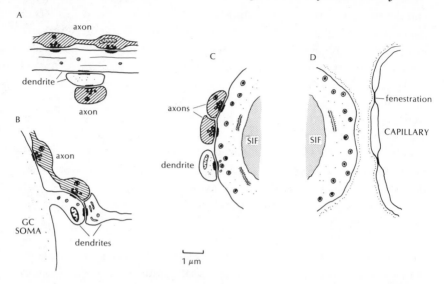

FIG. 6.3. Synaptic connections and neuronal relations in the mammalian sympathetic ganglion. (A) Synapses onto ganglion cell dendrites. (B) Synapses onto ganglion cell spines. (C) Synaptic connections of type I SIF cell. (D) Relation of type II SIF cell to fenestrated capillary. (A,B after Elfvin, 1971; C,D after Williams and Palay, 1969, Matthews and Raisman, 1969, Williams et al., 1976.)

degree of processing can be carried out by interactions between the principal neurons, as we shall see.

SYNAPTIC CONNECTIONS

The synapses in the sympathetic ganglion may be conveniently described in the sequence of those involving the principal neurons and those involving the intrinsic neurons.

The synapses involving the principal neurons have been seen most clearly in cat mesenteric ganglia, which lack intrinsic cells (Elfvin, 1971). As shown in Fig. 6.3 (A), the input (preganglionic) fibers make synapses onto the dendrites (A) and cell bodies and spiny processes (B) of the ganglion cells. These synapses are characteristically *en passant*, rather than by terminal boutons. The synapses have asymmetrical membrane densities and round vesicles, 300–500 Å in diameter; it is difficult to classify them as either type I or II (cf. Chapter 2). The terminals also have scattered larger vesicles, 500–1000 Å in diameter, containing moderately dense granules. We recognize here the point made in Chapters 2 and 4, that a process may contain more than one type of vesicle. The dense-core vesicles are never in contact with the synaptic region, however; the specific synaptic vesicles are thus the smaller, clear vesicles, clustered at the synaptic membrane, as previously defined.

Ganglion cells are also connected to each other by synapses. These occur between dendrites Fig. 6.3 (A) and between accessory dendrites (B). In the former case the membrane densities appear to have little asymmetry, and no synaptic vesicles are evident. In the latter case, small dense-core vesicles, 200–500 Å in diameter, are present in the processes near, though not actually in contact with, the junction. The membrane densities may show slight polarity.

The studies of synapses involving intrinsic cells are summarized in Fig. 6.3 (C) (Williams and Palay, 1969; Matthews and Raisman, 1969; Williams et al., 1976). Preganglionic fibers make synapses, often seen in pairs, onto the cell soma and processes. The synapses are similar to those made on ganglion cells (cf. A, B). The postsynaptic cells contain numerous large, dense-core vesicles, 500–1200 Å in diameter, which tend to be dispersed around the outer rim of the cytoplasm. The vesicles are thus of the same size as those scattered in the presynaptic terminals, but their cores are more electron-dense.

If the intrinsic cells receive synaptic input, yet have no axon, what kind of output do they have? It was first shown (cf. Williams and Palay, 1969) that there are output synapses from the soma and dendritic processes of these cells. As illustrated in Fig. 6.3 (C), this type has a distinct asymmetric membrane density; a few of the large-core vesicles are gathered near it. These synapses are made onto the cell bodies and processes of the ganglion cells. They are thus termed somasomatic, somadendritic, etc.

The intrinsic cells grouped in clusters have another possible output, by secretion of substances into the bloodstream. As shown in Fig. 6.3 (D), the plasma membrane of these cells is often next to a capillary, separated from it only by a space containing the two basement membranes. Note the fenestrations of the capillary endothelial cells, through which substances may pass between the cell and the bloodstream, in either direction.

BASIC CIRCUIT

It will be convenient to summarize the main patterns of synaptic connections for each of the local regions we study in a diagram, which will be

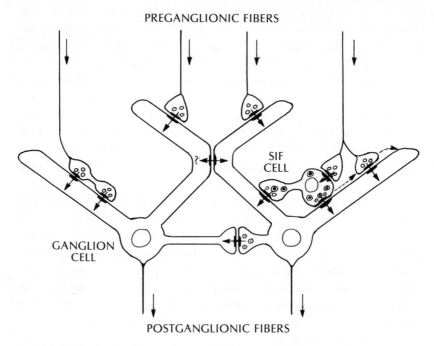

FIG. 6.4. Basic circuit diagram for the mammalian sympathetic ganglion.

referred to as a *basic circuit*. This will be useful in several respects: for identifying the principles of organization of that region; for describing synaptic actions and dendritic properties; and for making comparisons with the organization of other regions.

The basic circuit of the sympathetic ganglion is summarized in the diagram of Fig. 6.4. It draws on the anatomical evidence just considered, and looks forward to the analysis of physiological properties in the next section. It can be seen that the preganglionic fibers make synaptic connection onto the ganglion cells and, when they are present, the intrinsic neurons (SIF cells). The ganglion cells are interconnected through dendrodendritic contacts that take at least two forms: those between the longer dendrites and those between the accessory dendrites. The SIF cells have synapses through their soma and dendrites onto the ganglion cells.

The three elements that make up the synaptic triad are all present, and we can note some of the particular ways they are, or are not, interrelated. An input fiber sends separate terminals to the principal and intrinsic elements (cf. the large terminal with synapses on both types of element in cerebellum and thalamus). The connection onto the principal neuron provides a straight-through pathway for effecting output in the postganglionic fiber. The connection onto intrinsic cells provides an indirect pathway for more complex processing. The interactions between principal neurons contribute additional degrees of complexity. Note that there are no synapses from the principal to the intrinsic neuron, through either axon collaterals or dendritic synapses.

These kinds of arrangements will all become familiar as different regions of the brain are reviewed in later chapters. The form of the synaptic terminals and the geometry of the neurons will appear infinitely various, and the types of synaptic actions and neurotransmitters will show every conceivable permutation. However, whatever the medley, the changes will all be rung on three chimes, the triad of neuronal elements.

Given this basic circuit, we may note some of the aspects that are special for the sympathetic ganglion. First, compared with regions of the brain, the input is extremely simple. Many regions of the brain receive and integrate information from several inputs, often of different modalities; here, there is only one input, the preganglionic B fiber from the motoneurons in the spinal cord (sometimes also C fibers); hence, complex integration of different inputs is not involved. Second, spatial information is not conveyed in this input; this greatly simplifies the nature of the information processing. Third, the sympathetic system tends to function by mass action. On the other hand, the system exerts a variety of actions on postsynaptic targets, with varying time courses; these cover several of the ranges indicated in the diagram of Fig. 4.7.

It may be noted that the preponderance of interactions through dendritic pathways may seem a special aspect of this ganglion, but we shall encounter this type of organization in many regions of the nervous system (see later sections on other types of ganglia, and later chapters on olfactory bulb, retina, and thalamus).

It should be stressed that the basic circuit is not a static concept, but rather a flexible tool for dealing with variations and added details. For example, the variations in presence and numbers of SIF cells give rise to appropriately modified basic circuits for the relevant ganglia. Presynaptic and extrasynaptic actions can also be incorporated (see dotted lines in the diagram) as well as secretory activity of the SIF cells; these possibilities are considered further below in connection with synaptic actions and neurotransmitters.

SYNAPTIC ACTIONS

The electrophysiologist begins by setting up a volley of impulses in an input pathway and proceeds to examine the sequence of synaptic actions that takes place in the region under study. This requires an input that can be selectively activated, and a region that is accessible for recordings. The sympathetic ganglion was early recognized as a suitable, indeed advantageous, preparation for this purpose. Faced with the many variations among ganglia and species, we will focus here on the mammalian superior cervical ganglion (especially rabbit), and will base our description on only a few essential results from the many studies that have been reported.

The most direct information about the synaptic actions is obtained from intracellular recordings. A characteristic response of a ganglion cell to an orthodromic volley is illustrated in Fig. 6.5 (A). The impulses in the preganglionic fiber invade the terminals and, after a brief synaptic delay of 0.5 msec or so, give rise to a low-amplitude, slow, graded potential, the EPSP. When it reaches threshold the EPSP gives rise to one or two action potentials. The cell can be identified as a ganglion cell because a volley of impulses in the postganglionic fiber invades the cells directly, without a synaptic potential or delay (not shown). Antidromic impulse invasion of ganglion cell bodies often fails, however, presumably because of the low safety factor (high conductance load) in going from a thin axon to a large cell body (Erulkar and Woodward, 1968). This is a caution that antidromic identification is not always a reliable horse in the electrophysiologist's stable.

Intracellular recordings during several manipulations of neurotransmitters are also illustrated in Fig. 6.5 (A). Bathing the ganglion in d-tubocurarine reduces or abolishes the EPSP, a property of synapses with a nicotinic acetylcholine receptor. Appropriately, iontophoresis of acetylcholine by a brief pulse produces a potential resembling the EPSP, Fig. 6.5 (A,a). Perfusion of the ganglion with catecholamines also reduces the EPSP, as well as causing a slight hyperpolarization of the resting membrane. The effect of dopamine on miniature EPSPs is to lower their frequency but not their amplitude, Fig. 6.5 (A: b,c); in other words, it

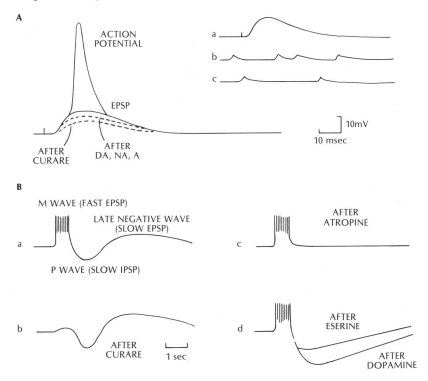

FIG. 6.5. Synaptic actions in sympathetic ganglia. (A) Intracellular recordings from ganglion cells, showing generation of action potential from EPSP elicited by a preganglionic volley, and reduction of EPSP by dopamine (DA), noradrenaline (NA), adrenaline (A), and curare. *Inset:* (a) iontophoresis of ACh elicits wave resembling an EPSP; (b) MEPPs (control recording); (c) MEPPs (after DA) (after Eccles, 1955; Erulkar and Woodward, 1968; Dun and Nishi, 1974). (B) Extracellular recordings in normal ganglion (a), and after various procedures (b–d); see text (After Libet, 1970, 1976).

reduces quantal content but not quantal size (cf. Chapter 4). The significance of dopamine as an interneuronal transmitter will be considered further below.

Intracellular recordings from mammalian ganglion cells are difficult to obtain; from SIF cells they have thus far been impossible. A more popular method has therefore been to record from extracellular electrodes on the surface of the postganglionic fibers. In the latter position the electrodes record the electrotonic potentials spreading into the axon due to the changes in the membrane potential of the cells.

This technique has been particularly employed in studies of slow potential changes induced by brief repetitive activation of preganglionic fibers, first reported by Laporte and Lorente de Nó (1950). As shown in Fig. 6.5 (B,a), the response of the normal ganglion consists of an initial extracellular negativity (N) during the stimulus train, due to the fast EPSPs and action potentials [compare with Fig. 6.5-(A)]. This is followed by a relatively slow positivity (P), lasting several hundred msec. Finally, a late negativity (LN) may be present. If the ganglion is curarized [Fig. 6.5 (B,b)], the early N potential is reduced (as expected from the intracellular recordings in A) while the P and LN potentials are enhanced.

The slow potentials have been of great interest in recent years, and the consensus is that the P wave represents a slow IPSP and the LN wave represents an even slower EPSP in the ganglion cell. There is also general agreement that the synapses of the input fibers mediating these actions have muscarinic cholinergic receptors: atropine blocks both of the potentials without affecting the fast N wave [Fig. 6.5 (B,c)]. Also, eserine, an anticholinesterase agent, prolongs the P wave; it has been suggested that this is due to prolongation of muscarinic excitation of an inhibitory interneuron.

The identity of the interneuron and its transmitter has been controversial. There is, of course, ample evidence for an interneuron, in the form of the SIF cell, receiving synapses as it does from input fibers and making synapses with the ganglion cells (cf. Figs. 6.2–6.4). The SIF cells contain catecholamines, the administration of which has the effect of enhancing the P wave in an eserinized ganglion [Fig. 6.5 (B,d)]. From this and other evidence Libet (1970) proposed that the SIF cell is a dopamine-releasing interneuron, mediating the slow inhibition of ganglion cells. Various lines of evidence have supported this hypothesis in those ganglia in which SIF cells contain dopamine. However, slow inhibitory potentials are also seen in ganglia with SIF cells that contain catecholamines other than dopamine (e.g., norepinephrine and epinephrine); in ganglia with SIF cells that lack efferent synapses; and in ganglia that have few SIF cells or lack them altogether. Thus it appears that the slow inhibition can be mediated by several different circuits, and several different transmitters (see review by Libet, 1976). This reflects the principle mentioned in Chapter 4, that there is a flexible relation between structure, function, and transmitters in the organization of synaptic systems.

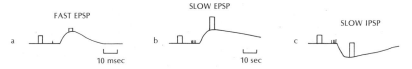

FIG. 6.6. Conductance changes during different types of synaptic potentials in sympathetic ganglion cells. (After Weight, 1974.)

The mechanisms of the slow synaptic potentials have been of interest. It was recognized from intracellular recordings that the slow potentials are not associated with conductance increases, as is the case with the fast EPSP [see Fig. 6.6 (a)] and most other rapid synaptic potentials in the nervous system (see Chapter 3). Weight and Votava (1970) first showed that in frog sympathetic ganglion cells a decrease in conductance occurs during the slow EPSP [see Fig. 6.6 (b)]. They demonstrated that the reversal potential for this response is near the equilibrium potential for potassium, and hypothesized that the slow EPSP is generated by a decrease in the resting potassium conductance of the membrane. Subsequently, Weight and Padjen (1973) showed that a decrease in conductance also occurs during the slow IPSP [Fig. 6.6 (c)], and that the reversal potential for this response is near the equilibrium potential for sodium. They hypothesized accordingly that the slow IPSP is due to a decrease of resting sodium conductance in the membrane (cf. Weight, 1974).

The experimental method of demonstrating the reversal potentials for these types of synaptic actions has been discussed earlier (Chapter 3). It may be noted that the electrogenic sodium pump may also contribute to the slow IPSP; the administration of ouabain reduces the slow IPSP (Nishi and Koketsu, 1967), presumably by inhibiting the electrogenic sodium pump and causing an accumulation of intracellular sodium (but see Smith and Weight, 1979). We shall see that conductance decreases underlie the synaptic actions of cells in other parts of the nervous system.

NEUROTRANSMITTERS

The evidence for neurotransmitters discussed above is summarized in the modified basic circuit diagram of Fig. 6.7. The input fibers release acetylcholine which elicits fast EPSPs by a nicotinic action and slow EPSPs by a muscarinic action in the ganglion cells; in addition, there is a muscarinic action on the SIF cells. The SIF cells release a catechola-

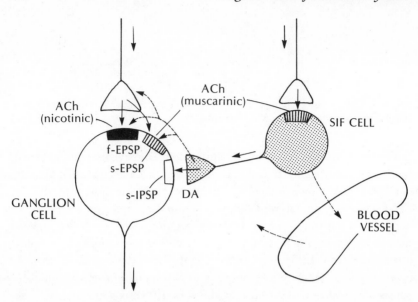

FIG. 6.7. Summary of putative neurotransmitters and their actions in sympathetic ganglion. (Modified from Libet, 1976.)

mine, in some cases dopamine, to elicit slow IPSPs in the ganglion cells. The catecholamines may also have modulatory effects (especially very slow inhibitory effects) on postsynaptic cholinergic sites on the ganglion cells, and perhaps also presynaptic sites on the input terminals [cf. Fig. 6.5 (A,a)]. The SIF cells may also secrete catecholamines directly into the bloodstream and exert effects within the ganglia (including some of the modulatory actions just described) or elsewhere in the body (Williams et al., 1976). These several modulatory actions are indicated by the dotted lines in Fig. 6.7. They should be kept in mind as possible types of actions in other regions of the nervous system (see especially the basal ganglia).

What of the mechanisms in the postsynaptic membranes, mediating the actions of the transmitter molecules and the changes in membrane conductance that underlie the synaptic potentials? In Chapter 4 we noted that there may be a direct relation between the receptor and the conductance change, or there may be several intermediary reactions (Fig. 4.4, step 8). The work of Greengard and his colleagues on the slow IPSP has been particularly illuminating in this regard. It was first shown that

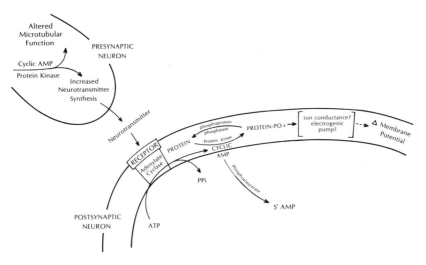

FIG. 6.8. Summary of proposed steps at synapse in which cyclic AMP and protein phosphorylation are involved. (From Greengard, 1976.)

preganglionic stimulation produces a several-fold increase in the content of adenosine $3',5'$-monophosphate (cyclic AMP) in the rabbit superior cervical ganglion (McAfee, Shorderet, and Greengard, 1971). Several lines of evidence suggested that the cyclic AMP activates a protein kinase (for example, theophylline, a phosphodiesterase inhibitor, causes an accumulation of cyclic AMP). The protein kinase in turn is believed to phosphorylate a protein constituent of the membrane, which causes the change in ionic conductance at the synapse.

This sequence of actions is summarized in the diagram of Fig. 6.8. Kebabian, Petzold, and Greengard (1971) showed that the administration of dopamine to a ganglion not only enhances the slow IPSP, as described above, but also stimulates adenylate cyclase activity, leading to increased cyclic AMP. This and other evidence suggests that the action of dopamine is mediated through activation of adenylate cyclase, either directly or through an associated receptor, as shown in Fig. 6.8. A thorough discussion may be found in the reviews by Greengard (1976; 1978). Some of the other possibilities for the actions of cyclic AMP in the cell are considered by Busis, Weight, and Smith (1978). The hypothesis of Fig. 6.8 has served as an important model for investigating the role of cyclic nucleotides as intracellular second messengers in nerve cells. It is believed to apply to several other systems, particularly to the dopaminergic cells of the substantia nigra (see Chapter 12).

DENDRITIC PROPERTIES

In most regions of the brain the majority of synapses are located on the dendrites of the principal and intrinsic neurons, and the properties of the dendrites are therefore of central importance for understanding how signals are integrated. In the mammalian sympathetic ganglion, the ganglion cells also have many synaptic inputs onto their dendrites. The short lengths mean that synaptic potential spread to the soma will be relatively effective, although different branches will be somewhat isolated electrotonically from each other.

In the frog, the ganglion cells have few if any dendrites; synaptic responses are therefore integrated with no weighting or isolation by electrotonic considerations, and there is a maximum opportunity for shunting effects between synaptic conductances acting simultaneously. This might be part of the explanation for the presence of synapses operating by conductance decreases, which have the effect of increasing rather than decreasing the effectiveness of synapses acting simultaneously. It may be noted that, in the frog, B and C inputs are segregated onto B and C ganglion cells; integration of the two inputs, for some unknown reason, is not permitted in a single cell.

The mammalian ganglion cell is of further interest for the interactions that can occur between its dendrites. We have seen that this involves specialized contacts between the long, slender dendrites and the short, accessory dendrites. Unfortunately, the significance of these contacts and these two types of dendrite is not understood. It is possible that the contacts could mediate the slow IPSPs onto neighboring ganglion cells in those ganglia that lack SIF cells (cf. Elfvin, 1971). Dale's Law (Chapter 4) would suggest that the transmitter in such a case would be norepinephrine, which is contained in the ganglion cells and liberated at their axonal terminals in the periphery.

The SIF cells lack an axon, and therefore their functions depend on soma and dendritic properties. Since the cells are so small and the dendrites relatively short, spread of potentials through them would be expected to be effective by passive electrotonus alone. This suggests that these cells may mediate their input-output functions without generating impulses. This is however still untested. There is evidence for impulse generation in similar cells in parasympathetic ganglia (see below), but not in chromaffin cells in the adrenal medulla. Either possibility—graded input-output functions, or impulse generation in an axonless cell—is interesting, and distinct from the classical model for neuronal function (cf. Chapter 1). We shall have occasion to consider these possibilities in other systems (olfactory bulb, retina, thalamus).

PARASYMPATHETIC GANGLIA

The parasympathetic nervous system has played a central role in the study of neurotransmitters, for it was Loewi's demonstration in 1921 that stimulation of the parasympathetic vagus nerve releases a substance that inhibits the heart, and the subsequent identification of the substance as acetylcholine, that marked the first persuasive evidence for chemical synaptic transmission. In contrast to the sympathetic system, in which the ganglia are situated along the nerves, parasympathetic ganglia are found within the organs which they innervate. Thus, it has been known that the inhibitory action of the vagus is mediated by a ganglion within the heart, but it is only very recently that the synaptic organization of the ganglion has been analyzed, thanks to a series of elegant studies by Kuffler and his colleagues.

As would be expected, the cardiac ganglion differs somewhat in different species; we shall consider briefly the ganglion in the mudpuppy. McMahan and Purves (1976) have investigated its structure, employing light microscopy of living and stained material as well as electron microscopy; the basic circuit summarizing their work is shown in Fig. 6.9. The vagus nerve terminates with chemical synapses on the principal (ganglion) cells. Most of the terminals are of the *en passant* type (site 1) on the cell body surface. The principal neurons are interconnected by electrical synapses (gap junctions) (site 2) and by axon collaterals with chemical synapses (site 3). There are also intrinsic neurons, which resemble the SIF cells of sympathetic ganglia. They are believed to receive input from the vagus, and are connected to the principal neurons by both chemical and electrical synapses (site 4). The output from the ganglion is by way of axons, sometimes double, from the ganglion cells to the cardiac muscle fibers (site 5). Note the lack of dendritic arborizations of ganglion cells. Each cell receives an average of only 22 vagal synapses.

In a companion study, Roper (1976) recorded from the cells in the ganglion, and some of the results are shown in Fig. 6.9 (B). A volley in

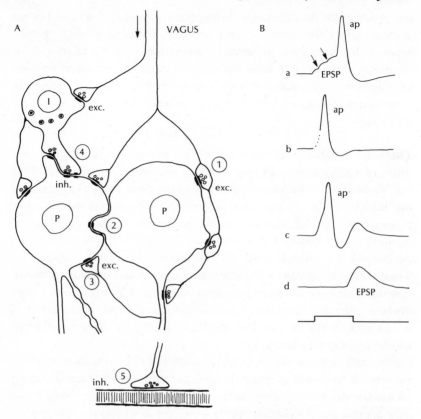

FIG. 6.9. Parasympathetic cardiac ganglion of the mudpuppy. (A) Basic circuit
diagram. P, principal cell; I, intrinsic cell; circled numbers indicate synaptic sites
(see text). (After McMahan and Purves, 1975.) (B) Synaptic actions revealed by
intracellular recordings (see text). (From Roper, 1975.)

the vagus gives rise to an EPSP in a ganglion cell and, at threshold, an
action potential (a). By adjusting the stimulus strength, steps can be seen
on the EPSP (arrows), indicating convergence of inputs from separate
vagal fibers onto this cell. Electrical coupling between cells can be demonstrated (not shown), but it is rather weak, especially for rapid transients such as the action potential (because most of the current goes to
charge the membrane capacitance of the postsynaptic cell). The SIF cells
are small and difficult to penetrate with an electrode; a few intracellular
recordings by Roper showed the ability of these cells to generate action
potentials (b). As discussed previously in relation to sympathetic ganglia,

the question of whether the axonless SIF cells generate action potentials is of some interest. Whether these cells in the cardiac ganglion generate action potentials in their normal function is not known; if they do, it would be an example in which the impulse mechanism is not used for long-distance communication.

The basic circuit of Fig. 6.9 (A) includes connections between the principal neurons by means of axon collaterals (site 3). Evidence for this connection was obtained by recording from two adjacent ganglion cells. When one cell was stimulated to produce an action potential [Fig. 6.9 (B,c)] an EPSP was evoked in the second cell (d). Several tests suggested that the EPSP was evoked through an axon collateral. These EPSPs are much smaller than those evoked by vagal stimulation, and the quantal content was found to be correspondingly smaller, a synaptic response comprising 1–5 quanta, in comparison with 22–23 quanta released by a single vagal stimulus.

Together these two studies provide a model analysis of structure-function relations at the level of synaptic organization. The triad of synaptic elements is evident, and it can be seen that the basic circuit established by the pattern of their connections shares many characteristics with the circuit for sympathetic ganglia. An interesting point is that the ganglion cells inhibit the cardiac muscle fibers but appear to excite each other, and both actions are mediated by acetylcholine. The ganglion cells are thus *multiaction cells,* and illustrate one of the corollaries of Dale's Law, as discussed in Chapter 4.

With regard to function one can speculate that the SIF cell might provide for inhibitory control over the ganglion cells; the ganglion cell collaterals in contrast might augment and prolong ganglion cell activity (cf. Roper, 1976). There is no direct insight into how these and other actions within this synaptic system are involved in the control of the heart, but one can safely surmise that the control is more complicated than previously suspected. One point does stand out clearly. The textbook statement that the vagus inhibits the heart can be seen to be, strictly speaking, incorrect. The synaptic action of the vagus itself is excitatory, by means of acetylcholine, on the cells of the ganglion; it is the ganglion cells, acting also through acetylcholine, that provide the fibers that actually inhibit the heart. This kind of transformation, or commutation, from one action to another, is a common function of synaptic connections in many systems.

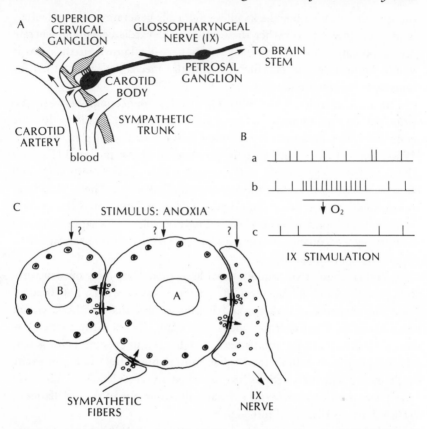

FIG. 6.10. Carotid body of the rat. (A) Diagram of vascular and nervous relations. (B) Representative recordings of impulses in glossopharyngeal nerve: (a) control; (b) during reduced oxygen tension in the blood; (c) during stimulation of the glossopharyngeal nerve. (C) Basic circuit diagram. Glomus cells are divided into A and B types, as shown. (Modified from McDonald and Mitchell, 1975.)

CAROTID BODY

We conclude our survey with brief consideration of the carotid body. As shown in Fig. 6.10 (A), this ganglion lies between the internal and external carotid arteries. It is a chemosensory organ; its function is to sense decreasing levels of oxygen in the blood by increasing the rate of discharge of impulses in the glossopharyngeal nerve supplying it [Fig. 6.10 (B)]. This information is integrated in the brainstem, where it contributes to pulmonary reflex systems for maintaining the oxygenation of the blood.

The afferent fibers carrying this information arise from cell bodies in the petrosal ganglion, a homologue of the dorsal root ganglion (cf. Fig. 6.1). Within the ganglion are two main constituents: the terminals of the nerve fibers, and glomus cells. The latter have relatively small cell bodies (8–15μm), few dendritic processes, and no axons. Also present are sympathetic preganglionic fibers passing through the nearby superior cervical ganglion, and a few sympathetic ganglion cells, which innervate the blood vessels within the carotid body.

The synaptic organization of the carotid body has been the subject of an elegant study by McDonald and Mitchell (1975), and Fig. 6.10 (C) is a basic circuit summarizing their work. The key findings are that the glomus cells are connected to each other and to the terminals of the glossopharyngeal nerve by synapses, and that these connections characteristically take the form of side-by-side pairs of synapses oriented in opposite directions. Therefore, these are reciprocal synapses, as described in Chapter 2 and discussed further in the chapters on the olfactory bulb and retina. The glomus cells contain many large dense-core vesicles. Two types of glomus cell, A and B, can be identified on the basis of the vesicle size, averaging 1160 Å and 910 Å, respectively [see Fig. 6.10 (C)]. Only type A cells take part in the reciprocal synapses with the nerve terminals. The terminals themselves are large and calyx-formed, and contain small, clear vesicles (average diameter 610 Å). Synapses from sympathetic fibers onto the glomus cells are also shown in Fig. 6.10 (C).

It may thus be seen that the organization of intrinsic synaptic circuits in the carotid body is almost exclusively based on local synaptic arrangements which are somatosomatic and somatodendritic in type, and reciprocal in pattern. McDonald and Mitchell noted the similarity of the glomus cells to SIF cells, on the one hand, and the similarity of the reciprocal synapses with those of inhibitory granule cells in the olfactory bulb. They postulate that the glomus cell may act as an inhibitory interneuron (possibly releasing dopamine), controlling the afferent discharge of impulses arising in the sensory nerve terminals. This of course does not exclude glomus cells from other functions; they may also be sensitive to anoxia and may act as secretory modulators within the ganglion, one of the functions postulated for SIF cells in sympathetic ganglion cells (see above). Thus, the glomus cell may be a *multifunction* intrinsic neuron.

The fact that a synaptic pathway is present from the afferent nerve terminals onto the glomus cells is also of interest in relation to the finding that stimulation of the glossopharyngeal nerve suppresses activity arising in the carotid body [Fig. 6.10 (B, C)] (Biscoe, Lall, and Sampson, 1970). One route for this effect, of course, could be via efferent nerves to the carotid body. However, McDonald and Mitchell postulate that the afferent nerves themselves mediate this effect, through the efferent synapses of their terminals onto the glomus cells. In this position they act, in effect, as presynaptic dendrites. The carotid body thus serves as an excellent example to illustrate that, unlike the classical doctrine, in which functional relations are strictly tied to particular nerve structures, our new concepts must recognize that a given structure may have several possible relations with neighboring structures, and mediate several possible functions.

7

SPINAL CORD:
VENTRAL HORN

The control of motor behavior is perhaps the most obvious and characteristic function of the central nervous system. Many parts of the brain are involved in this control; directly or indirectly, they all ultimately influence the brainstem and spinal cord, wherein lie the cells—the motoneurons—whose axons connect to the muscles. Within the cord, the motoneuron cell bodies are located in the ventral (anterior) horn, as is indicated in the diagram of Fig. 7.1. In Sherrington's felicitous phrase, the motoneuron is the "final common path" for the control of movement.

We have already seen that the motoneuron receives sensory inputs from the periphery through the dorsal root ganglion (DRG) cell. This was indicated in the diagram of Fig. 1.1. The fact that the DRG cell axons lie in the periphery has been of inestimable value to the experimenter; the axons can be stimulated by electrical shocks, or their receptors can be selectively activated by natural stimuli. If we add to this the fact that the axons of the motoneurons also lie in the periphery, and that they connect to muscles whose activity can be easily observed and measured, it can be readily appreciated that one has a near-ideal situation for an experimental analysis of input-output relations. This has afforded a shortcut, as it were, to the analysis of the spinal cord. From this approach, exploited so brilliantly by Sherrington, have developed the concepts of the reflex arc and the integrative organization of these arcs at the level of the spinal segment, concepts familiar to every student of biology, physiology, and psychology.

In recent years, there has been a growing realization that the spinal segmental apparatus must be viewed as part of its central, as well as its peripheral, connections. This realization has been abetted by improved techniques for studying activation of motoneurons through central pathways. From this work, it is possible, for the first time, to begin to gain a perspective on the integrative context of the motoneuron relative to internally generated behavior (which, after all, is what interests us most) as well as to reflex responses (see Burke, 1971; Evarts, 1971; Lundberg, 1975; Grillner, 1975). Our reconstruction of the synaptic organization of the ventral horn will reflect this new orientation.

NEURONAL ELEMENTS

The spinal cord is a complex structure. As is well known, the central gray matter is in the form of dorsal and ventral horns. A division of the gray matter into laminae was proposed by Rexed (1954); the inset in Fig. 7.1 provides a summary diagram. The region occupied by the motoneurons is lamina IX (actually, it is more in the form of a nucleus) and will be the focus of our interest.

The first step in understanding the organization of the ventral horn is to identify clearly the neuronal elements contained therein. We will proceed systematically in the sequence used for all regions of our study. First to be identified are the long-distance axons that bring input to the ventral horn. Next are the axons that carry output from the ventral horn; in identifying these, we at the same time specify and describe the principal neuron that gives rise to these axons. Last, we identify the intrinsic neurons whose processes and connections are contained entirely within this region.

INPUTS   The inputs to the ventral horn fall into two main categories, peripheral and central. The *peripheral* or *afferent* fibers are, as already indicated, the axons of the DRG cells. The diameters of these fibers cover a wide range, from 20 μm down to about 2 μm. Most of the smaller axons are unmyelinated.

A wide range of sensory modalities is carried in this array. The classical concept has been that different modalities are carried in different-sized axons; from muscle stretch receptors in the largest axons; from touch and pressure receptors in the large- and intermediate-sized axons; and from pain and temperature receptors in the finest axons. Many of these borders are becoming blurred, however, from the results of recent work; for example, pain and temperature, as well as some tactile, stimuli are carried in axons of different diameters.

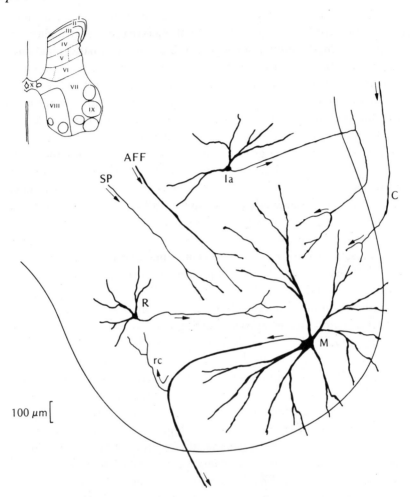

FIG. 7.1. Neuronal elements of the ventral horn of the mammalian spinal cord.
  Inputs: central (C) descending from brain; relays from other parts of spinal cord (SP); afferent sensory fibers from the periphery (AFF).
  Principal neuron: motoneuron (M) with recurrent collateral (rc).
  Intrinsic neurons: interneuron in Ia afferent pathway (Ia); interneuron in Renshaw pathway (R).
  Laminae of spinal cord grey matter according to Rexed (1954).

As Fig. 1.1 indicates very schematically, the afferent fibers, upon entering the spinal cord, join one of a number of tracts that ascend to higher centers in the brain. In addition, they give off branches within the spinal cord, the primary afferent collaterals. Some of these collaterals reach the ventral horn directly, as shown in Fig. 7.1. Here they bifurcate and run in a longitudinal direction for one to four segments, giving off collateral branches in their course. The collaterals of the largest, Ia fibers from muscle receptors have been effectively visualized by cobalt injections (Iles, 1976) and HRP transport (Brown and Fyffe, 1978). By virtue of these branches, there is *divergence* of the peripheral input; by virtue of the overlap of branches from different axons, there is *convergence* of the peripheral input. These are fundamental features in characterizing the inputs to all local regions in the brain.

An interesting point is that some afferents to the spinal cord arrive in the ventral, not the dorsal, root. These are central processes of small DRG cells, which enter the ventral root as fine unmyelinated fibers (15–30% of all ventral root fibers), and project to the spinal cord (Coggeshall, Coulter, and Willis, 1974; Maynard et al., 1977). As Coggeshall and his colleagues point out, the law of separation of functions (sensory in dorsal roots and motor in ventral roots), dating back to Magendie and Bell in the early nineteenth century, is no longer completely accurate.

Central inputs are classified not by their fiber diameter or their "modality" but by their site of origin within the brain. The most distant site is the cerebral cortex. As indicated in Fig. 1.1, there is, in many mammals, a direct connection from the cortex to the spinal cord. These fibers form the *corticospinal tract*. As shown in Fig. 7.1, these fibers (labeled C) distribute directly, in primates, in the ventral horn and indirectly, through connections in the intermediate gray (labeled SP). This pathway from the cortex is called *suprasegmental*, to distinguish it from the pathways within and between the spinal cord segments themselves. There are other suprasegmental pathways descending from other parts of the brain, for example, the *red nucleus*, the *reticular nucleus*, and the *vestibular nucleus*. These are not shown in Fig. 7.1 for the sake of simplicity. Like the peripheral input axons, these central input fibers characteristically distribute longitudinally over several spinal segments.

There are also many pathways within the spinal cord itself, connecting one segment with another (*intersegmental*) and one side with the other (*commissural*). Although these pathways are essential to the mechanisms of the spinal cord, we will concentrate on the other connections.

PRINCIPAL NEURON The output of the ventral horn is to the muscles, and the principal neuron whose axon carries this output is the *motoneuron*. There are two types of motoneurons, depending on the muscle fibers innervated. The *alpha motoneuron* sends its axon to skeletal (extrafusal) muscles; it is the main type of principal neuron. The *gamma motoneuron* sends its axon to the intrafusal fibers of muscle spindles. These fibers make a negligible contribution to the work done by the skeletal musculature, but their contractile state (controlled by the activity of the gamma motoneurons) sets the sensitivity of the spindle as it monitors the extrafusal muscle contractions. In mammals, the gamma motoneurons are specialized for this particular function. Such a clearcut division among principal neurons is unusual for local regions in the brain.

The alpha motoneurons have cell bodies that range in size from 25–100 μm in diameter; they are among the largest neurons in the vertebrate brain, as well as among the most variable in size. Each cell body gives rise to several large dendritic trunks, 10–15 μm in diameter at their origin. These are among the largest dendrites in the brain. The dendrites branch relatively modestly and reach considerable lengths, up to 1000 μm (1 mm) distance from the cell body. The dendritic surface is generally smooth; there are occasional spiny protuberances, and varicosities may be present near the terminations.

The gamma motoneurons are, on average, smaller than the alpha motoneurons, with cell bodies ranging from 15–40 μm in diameter. Their dendritic trees are, by and large, smaller versions of those of the alpha motoneurons. The size difference applies also to the axons, the alpha axons being 12–20 μm in diameter, the gamma axons 2–9 μm. The designations alpha and gamma derive from the classical terminology for the size ranges of the peripheral axons.

Within the ventral horn, the motoneurons have a definite topographical arrangement. The motoneurons that supply the muscles of the trunk and neck are located medially, whereas those that supply the muscles of the limbs are located laterally. The motoneurons for the limbs are further localized to the cervical and lumbar enlargements of the cord, which supply the upper and lower limbs, respectively. The motoneurons that supply the more distal limb muscles, particularly those of the primate hand that are under the finest control, are located more dorsally and more caudally than those that supply the proximal muscles. These aspects are admirably described by Brodal (1969).

We say, then, that there is a *somatotopical organization* of the ventral horn, reflecting, to some extent, the spatial relations of the muscles innervated. The groupings of motoneurons take the form, not of rounded nuclei, but, rather, of longitudinal columns within the ventral horn, a fact not adequately brought out by the cross-sectional diagram of Fig. 7.1. The motoneuron dendrites, like the input axons mentioned above, also reflect this by their predominantly longitudinal orientation; there is considerable overlap of the dendritic trees of the motoneurons within these longitudinal columns. Because the ventral horn is spread out over a considerable longitudinal extent in this way (40 cm, i.e. 400,000 μm, in the adult human), it is much more difficult to define "local region" here than in most other parts of the brain.

Near its origin from the cell body, the motoneuron axon gives off one or several collateral branches. Like the dendrites, these have a generally longitudinal orientation. They attain lengths of 1–2 mm and are believed to terminate in the ventral horn of the same spinal segments (Ryall, Piercey, and Polosa, 1971). Some motoneurons do not have axon collaterals, at least none that are impregnated by the Golgi method. We will see that axon collaterals are characteristic of the principal neurons in most (but not all) of the regions of the brain. Motoneuron axon collaterals are considered to be intrinsic processes, confined within the region from which they arise. They are termed *recurrent collaterals*, to distinguish them from collateral branches that only extend laterally, and from collateral branches that distribute to different regions (as, for example, the primary afferent collaterals of the DRG axon).

In the periphery the axons of motoneurons branch and terminate on the muscles to form there the presynaptic processes of the neuromuscular junctions. A single alpha motoneuron, together with all the muscle fibers it innervates, was termed a *motor unit* by Sherrington. The size of a motor unit (i.e., the number of axonal branches to different muscle fibers, or divergence ratio) is a measure of the fineness of motor control; the smaller the unit, the finer the control. The variation in motor unit size is quite considerable, from about 100 for the smallest muscles of the hand to 1900 for the large muscles of the leg. If we consider the different kinds of muscles in the body—the extraocular muscles that control the eye, the muscles in the larynx, and the muscles in the face, as well as those in the hands, limbs, and trunk—it should be evident that we are dealing with systems that may be quite different in many respects. This is a necessary caution in drawing inferences about general principles of motor organization that apply to all these systems.

INTRINSIC NEURONS There has never been any doubt that the ventral horn contains neurons other than motoneurons; they are usually termed *propriospinal neurons* by anatomists and *interneurons* by electrophysiologists. Their functional identity, however, has been very difficult to establish. Only recently has it been possible to stain cells subjected to electrophysiological analysis (Jankowska and Lindström, 1971, 1972) and identify thereby the types of intrinsic neurons that are involved in particular pathways.

The cell bodies of intrinsic neurons are scattered throughout the ventral horn, but, from recent studies, it appears that there are two main regions of concentration. One is situated just dorsal to lamina IX (see Fig. 7.1). The cell bodies here have diameters of 20–30 μm. Each cell body gives rise to several dendritic trunks, 3–5 μm in diameter. The dendrites have generally smooth surfaces, they branch sparingly, and they terminate some 200–500 μm from the cell body. They thus resemble the smaller motoneurons in size and dendritic pattern. It is noteworthy that the dendrites have a dorsal-ventral orientation, in contrast to the longitudinal orientation of motoneuron dendrites. These cells have been identified as the interneurons in the Ia inhibitory pathway to the motoneurons (Jankowska and Lindström, 1971; see Fig. 7.3 and later).

The other area of concentration of intrinsic neurons is near the site where the motoneuron axons gather to leave the ventral horn. The cells stained in this region by Jankowska and Lindström (1972) are, in general, similar in size and shape to those just described. The evidence that these cells may be the interneurons in the Renshaw pathway for recurrent inhibition of the motoneurons will be discussed later in the section on Synaptic Actions.

These two types of intrinsic neuron fall into the category of propriospinal neuron. The general similarity in form between intrinsic neurons and motoneurons is a notable feature of the ventral horn. In most of the regions of the brain in our study, the intrinsic neurons can be sharply differentiated from the principal neurons in size and shape. In many regions we will find intrinsic cells of the *short-axon* type, the axon of which is very limited in its extent and distribution. Although definite short-axon cells are present in other parts of the spinal cord, they appear to be scarce or absent in the ventral horn (Scheibel and Scheibel, 1966; Jankowska and Lindström, 1971, 1972).

The term propriospinal denotes the fact that the axon distributes within the ventral horn itself. This is the basis upon which we designate it as an intrinsic neuron. The extent of the axon varies considerably, however; some axons distribute within one or two segments of their cell of origin, while others distribute many segments away. The axon characteristically enters a tract (see Fig. 7.1) through which it runs to the distant sites. It, therefore, becomes a matter of definition whether these propriospinal axons are to be regarded as intrinsic neurons, or as another type of principal neuron; this is yet another example of the problem of determining what constitutes a local region within the spinal cord. A similar problem is encountered with regard to the types of neurons in the cerebral cortex that give rise to association fibers.

NEURONAL POPULATIONS An analysis of synaptic organization must ultimately include quantitative data about the number of neuronal elements involved. We will, therefore, note such data as are available. They are, unfortunately, very difficult to obtain, and they almost invariably represent rough estimates, so rough, in some cases, as to be misleading. An additional problem is that populations vary greatly in different species. This is dramatically shown for the spinal cord by the comparative study summarized in Table 7.1. The great increase in numbers in this series reflects both an increase in size and an increase in complexity of motor control as one ascends the vertebrate series. One moral of this example is that quantitative data have little meaning unless the species from which they were obtained is identified. The student may well ponder the implications of this fact in considering general models of ventral horn organization.

In the human spinal cord, the total number of motoneurons on one side has been estimated at about 200,000, as shown in Table 7.1. The ratio of alpha to gamma motoneurons is about 3:1, and one obtains, therefore, a total of some 150,000 alpha motoneurons and 50,000 gamma motoneurons. These totals are quite modest compared to the numbers of principal neurons in other regions of the brain; compare, for example, the 7,000,000 Purkinje cells in one side of the human cerebellum. The average number of motoneurons per spinal segment

Table 7.1

Quantitative estimates of numbers of peripheral afferent input fibers (in dorsal root) and of output axons from motoneurons (in ventral root) for spinal cords of different species

	DORSAL ROOT (*afferent axons*)	VENTRAL ROOT (*motoneurons*)	RATIO
Toad	8,000	5,700	1.4:1
Mouse	45,000	23,000	1.9:1
Dog	300,000	150,000	2:1
man	1,000,000	200,000	5:1

From Agduhr (1934).

works out to be about 5500 alpha motoneurons; this is so small as to raise the question of whether a single segment can be considered an independent local region.

Two quantitative ratios are important in the study of synaptic organization. One is the convergence ratio of input fibers to principal neurons. The data in Table 7.1 can only indicate an upper limit for this ratio as it applies to the ventral horn, since many of the dorsal root fibers go elsewhere in the cord. The ratios, at any rate, can be seen to vary from 1.4 in the toad to about 5 in the human. Thus, this ratio increases to a much smaller degree than the numbers of neuronal elements. This ratio for the spinal cord is very low compared to that for many other regions of the brain; in the retina, for example, the over-all ratio may be as high as 1000:1. Individual afferent fibers, however, diverge through multiple branches and terminals, as has been described above. This increases the overall convergence ratio, although at the expense of spatial discreteness in the input-output relations.

The other ratio of importance concerns the relative number of intrinsic and principal neurons. In anatomical studies, the ratio of small neurons (presumably intrinsic neurons) to motoneurons, in the ventral horn of the cat, has been estimated to be about 7:1 (see Brodal, 1969). This is greater than in some other regions (e.g., the thalamus) but much smaller than in others (e.g., the olfactory bulb). In most of the regions of the brain, the number of intrinsic neurons reflects their relative contribution to the processing of information in the input pathways and in the pathways for lateral and recurrent control. As we shall see, this is not so obvious in the ventral horn.

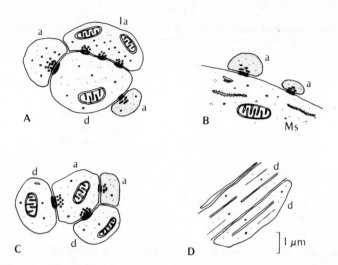

FIG. 7.2. Synaptic connections in the mammalian ventral horn. (A) Axodendritic synapses from axon terminals (a) to a motoneuron dendrite (d). Note the multiple contacts made by the Ia axon terminal. (B) Axosomatic synapses onto a motoneuron cell body (Ms). (C) Synaptic cluster with serial synapses (axoaxodendritic). (D) Dendrodendritic membrane juxtaposition.

(After Bodian, 1966, 1972; Charlton and Gray, 1966; Uchizono, 1966; Conradi, 1969; McLaughlin, 1972a, b; Matthews, Willis, and Williams, 1971.)

SYNAPTIC CONNECTIONS

Although the ventral horn has certain topographical patterns of organization, as described above, it lacks the rigid separation of neuronal elements into laminae that is so characteristic of other parts of the brain in our study. Because of this, identification of the synaptic connections between the neuronal elements is a much more difficult task than in other regions. The following account draws on a variety of studies (see Fig. 7.2).

There are two major morphological types of synaptic terminals in the ventral horn of mammals. As is illustrated in Fig. 7.2 (A), one type, the larger, is 1–4 μm in diameter. The synapse consists of a presynaptic cluster of spheroidal vesicles and a prominent densification of the postsynaptic membrane. These are, therefore, type I chemical synapses, as described in Chapter 2. These synapses are found at all levels of the motoneuron—the cell body and the proximal, intermediate, and distal dendrites—although the distribution tends to favor the distal dendrites.

The other major kind of synaptic terminal is somewhat smaller, being 0.5–3 μm in diameter [Fig. 7.2 (B)]. The vesicles tend to be flattened or variable in shape, and the synaptic membranes are more equally dense. These, therefore, tend to fall into the category of type II chemical synapses. They, too, are found at all levels of the motoneuron, but their distribution tends to be skewed toward the cell body. Each of these types accounts for approximately 40% of the total population of terminals in the ventral horn, so together they provide most of the input to the motoneurons.

Among the other much less frequent types of synaptic terminals, one is of particular interest. This is the largest type in the ventral horn, with a diameter 4–7 μm. The contacts made by these terminals are type I chemical synapses. One of these single terminals may have as many as five to eight synapses onto a single postsynaptic profile (McLaughlin, 1972b). Multiple contacts from one terminal to another are unusual in the nervous system, although we will encounter an even more striking example of this type of arrangement in the retina.

The identification of the sources of the different types of terminals is a forbidding task, and there is relatively little evidence with regard to most of the type I and type II synapses described above. The best evidence relates to the large terminals. After dorsal root section, these terminals degenerate, and it is inferred that they are the monosynaptic terminals from the largest fibers in the dorsal root, the IA afferent axons from the muscle spindles. There is general agreement that these terminals constitute less than 1% of the total number onto motoneurons.

From the preceding description, it can be seen that most of the connections in the mammalian ventral horn are made by simple terminals with simple synapses, as defined in Chapter 2. The main orientation of the synapses is axosomatic and axodendritic. In these respects, the synaptic repertoire of the ventral horn is rather limited; lacking are the specialized terminals and the rich variety of interconnections, particularly between dendrites, that are found in such other regions as the olfactory bulb, retina, and thalamus. Nor is there the grouping of terminals into synaptic complexes and glomeruli, as is seen in the cerebellum and thalamus.

Irregular small groups of terminals are sometimes seen, however, and of interest in this respect is the occasional serial sequence of synapses, as is illustrated in Fig. 7.2 (C). A large terminal can be seen making a synapse onto two presumed dendritic branches; in addition, the terminal is postsynaptic to another terminal. It has been postulated (Gray, 1962) that such sequences provide the morphological basis for presynaptic inhibition of motoneurons. It is not clear, however, whether such sequences are present within the lamina IX (McLaughlin, 1972b) or whether they are in nearby parts of the spinal cord. Similar sequences have been reported in the dorsal horn (see Ralston, 1968; 1979), where it is possible that some of these sequences are dendrodendritic rather than axoaxonal.

It may finally be noted that there are membrane-to-membrane appositions between motoneuron dendrites in some species [see Fig. 7.2 (D)]. These appositions may provide an opportunity for the spread of current between the motoneurons (Gogan et al., 1977). No tight or gap junctions have been reported in mammals, although they have been found in the frog (Sotelo and Taxi, 1970).

The number of synapses on a single motoneuron has been estimated to be as high as 20,000 (Gelfan, 1963). This is one of the largest numbers for any neuron in the brain, exceeded only by cortical pyramidal cells and cerebellar Purkinje cells. The total surface area of cell body and dendrites of a large motoneuron can be calculated to be as high as 100,000 μm^2, so it appears that there is room for this many synapses. Most of the motoneuronal surface area (estimated 80%) and most of the synapses are on the dendrites (Aitken and Bridger, 1961).

BASIC CIRCUIT

In the ventral horn, the lack of distinct cell types and lamination makes the task of identifying the main synaptic pathways on the basis of available anatomical evidence alone very difficult. For that reason, the basic circuit depends to a great extent on the results of the electrophysiological analyses of synaptic transmission. We anticipate that evidence in the diagram of Fig. 7.3.

A prominent feature of the ventral horn is the large number of different functional pathways that feed into it. Figure 7.3 is a very schematic diagram that summarizes only some of the simplest of these functional pathways. Particular emphasis is given to the central connections of the motoneurons and to the organization of the interneurons. The orientation is somewhat different from that of the usual diagrams of spinal cord organization in that the central pathways (1–4) are here considered as the main inputs to the ventral horn and arrive from the top of the diagram. The peripheral afferents (5 and 6) are considered as feedback inputs from

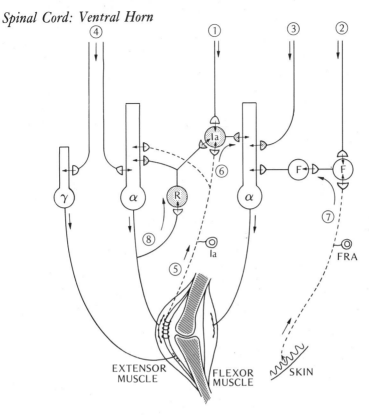

FIG. 7.3. Basic circuit diagram for the mammalian ventral horn. *Input pathways:* central descending pathways for the brain (1–4) (see text); the Ia afferent excitatory pathway from muscle spindles (5); the Ia afferent inhibitory pathway (6); the flexor afferent pathway (FRA) from the skin (7); the Renshaw recurrent inhibitory pathway (8). *Principal neurons:* alpha (α) motoneurons to flexor and extensor muscles; gamma (γ) motoneurons to intrafusal muscle fibers of muscle spindles. *Intrinsic neurons:* Ia interneuron in the Ia afferent pathway; F interneuron in the flexor reflex pathway; R, Renshaw cell in the recurrent inhibitory pathway. Neurons and terminals with presumed excitatory actions are in open profiles; those with presumed inhibitory actions are shaded in this and corresponding diagrams in other chapters.

the sites of ventral horn output and arrive, therefore, from the bottom of the diagram.

Let us first consider the central input pathways. Most central motor control in vertebrates is effected through fibers descending from the brain that relay through interneurons in the spinal cord. These relays may be through either inhibitory (pathway 1) or excitatory (pathway 2) interneurons. Depending on the number of synaptic relays, these pathways are either *disynaptic* or *polysynaptic*. The interneurons in these pathways may be the ones located within the ventral horn itself (i.e., the Ia interneuron in pathway 1), or they may be located in other parts of the spinal cord (i.e., the intermediate nucleus of Cajal and the dorsal horn).

Monosynaptic pathways from the brainstem and cerebral cortex provide direct central control of some motoneurons in the primate. These pathways play onto both flexor (pathway 3) and extensor (pathway 4) motoneurons. The central monosynaptic pathways are especially directed to motoneurons that supply such distal muscles as those of the hand (see Phillips, 1971). Pathway 4 in Fig. 7.3 indicates that central activation of the alpha motoneurons to the hand muscles is frequently linked to activation of the gamma motoneurons that supply the spindles in the hand muscles. Thus, at the same time that the alpha motoneurons cause the muscle (an extensor muscle, in the example of Fig. 7.3) to contract and shorten, the gamma motoneurons cause the spindles of that muscle to contract and shorten also. This was called *alpha-gamma linkage* by Granit (1955) and is considered to be the mechanism whereby the length of the muscle spindle is adjusted according to the length of the surrounding muscle, so that the spindle continues to be sensitive to changes in length or tension as movements are carried out.

The orientation of the diagram in Fig. 7.3 emphasizes this role of the muscle spindle in providing feedback information to the motoneuron from the site of motoneuron output. This information travels, as an impulse discharge, in the large Ia axons of DRG cells (pathway 5), and it has two destinations within the ventral horn. One destination is an excitatory monosynaptic connection onto motoneurons that supply that muscle and its synergists. The other destination (pathway 6) is a disynaptic connection through an inhibitory interneuron (the Ia interneuron in Fig. 7.3) onto motoneurons that supply antagonist muscles. This is an expression of the Sherringtonian principle of *reciprocal inhibition*, which is considered to be basic to the reciprocal relation of muscle movements about a joint. Note that these Ia inhibitory interneurons are the same ones that are under central control from descending pathways, i.e., the reciprocal organization is built into the central as well as the peripheral connections. This important new concept is discussed more fully by Lundberg (1970, 1975), Burke (1971), and Grillner (1975).

Muscle spindles, thus, have a role to play within the whole context of centrally generated movements, in addition to their more local role in reflex behavior at the spinal level. As is well known, this latter role revolves around the *stretch reflex*. Traditionally, this has been regarded as the basic spinal mechanism for the maintenance of muscle tone and the activation of extensor muscles that oppose gravity and thereby maintain upright posture.

In addition to the Ia afferents from muscle spindles, there are also Ib afferents from Golgi tendon organs and II afferents from the spindles. These afferents have their own spinal connections that contribute to centrally generated movements and to particular types of reflex behavior. For simplicity, they are omitted from Fig. 7.3. Muscle receptors and their central actions are fully described by Matthews (1972) and Phillips and Porter (1977).

In addition to muscle afferents, there are many other types of peripheral inputs. For the most part, they make polysynaptic excitatory connections, particularly onto flexor motoneurons (pathway 7), and are, therefore, often referred to collectively as *flexor reflex afferents* (FRA). As is well known, they provide the basic mechanism for reflex withdrawal of a limb from a noxious or painful stimulus. The FRA interneurons are located in other laminae of the spinal cord; like the Ia interneurons, they are also part of central descending pathways.

In addition to the long feedback loops through the periphery, there are also short feedback loops within the ventral horn due to the presence of motoneuron axon collaterals. As indicated in pathway 8, the axon collaterals connect to an interneuron, the so-called Renshaw cell, that makes inhibitory connections onto motoneurons as well as interneurons. This is the pathway for recurrent inhibition in the ventral horn. Note that the Renshaw cell also connects to Ia interneurons, which, themselves, are inhibitory to motoneurons. Through this connection, the recurrent inhibitory pathway can bring about a decrease of the feedforward inhibition through the Ia pathway, an action that is termed *disinhibition*. There are many permutations of these kinds of effects within the local circuits of the ventral horn (see Lundberg, 1975).

In later chapters, we will have frequent occasion to compare aspects of the organization of other brain regions with those of the ventral horn. For the present, it will suffice to note certain of the most important aspects. First, the pathways in the ventral horn are mainly from axons to cell bodies and dendrites; there are limited interactions between dendrites. In this respect, the ventral horn resembles the cerebellum and differs from the olfactory bulb, retina, and thalamus. Second, the triad of input, output, and intrinsic elements is loosely, or diffusely, arranged; this is similar to most parts of the cerebral cortex and differs from the tightly organized triadic relations between these elements in the olfactory bulb, retina, cerebellum, and thalamus. Third and finally, most of the input pathways onto the motoneurons are polysynaptic, through interneurons in the ventral horn and elsewhere in the spinal cord. The excitatory interneurons provide for a preliminary integration and processing of inputs to the motoneurons; we will see examples of this kind of relay in the granule cells of the cerebellum, the granule cells of the dentate fascia, and, possibly, the stellate (granule) cells of the neocortex as well. Inhibitory interneurons also provide for a functional inversion, or commutation, of excitatory to inhibitory inputs; among the other regions of our study, the neocortex offers possible examples of this type of relay. The spinal gray thus provides a polysynaptic substrate wherein diverse afferents act together in different combinations to effect an extremely flexible and infinitely variable control of the movements of the body (Lundberg, Malmgren, and Schomburg, 1977).

SYNAPTIC ACTIONS

Analysis of synaptic actions within the ventral horn must begin with the simplest and most accessible input to the motoneurons. This is through the largest Ia fibers from the muscle spindles (pathway 5 in the basic circuit diagram of Fig. 7.3). The electro-physiologist proceeds by delivering a single shock to a dorsal root or muscle nerve in order to set up a synchronous volley of impulses in these fibers. The impulses invade the axon terminals and activate the synapses onto the motoneurons. The pioneering experiments of Eccles and his co-workers (Eccles, 1953) showed that an intracellular electrode within a motoneuron records a depolarizing response, such as that in Fig. 7.4 (A). The latency of onset of the response is brief but sufficient to allow for a 0.5 msec synaptic delay, as is characteristic of chemical synapses. This is, therefore, a monosynaptic EPSP, mediated by a type I chemical synapse. It has a relatively brief time course: a rapid rise of several milliseconds and a longer decay of 10–20 msec.

The threshold for generation of an action potential is about 15 mV. Electrophysiological analysis has shown that the impulse initiation site is

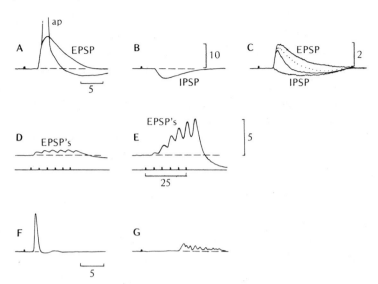

FIG. 7.4. Main types of synaptic actions in the ventral horn, as recorded intracellularly from the motoneuron. (A) EPSP at threshold for generating an action potential (ap) (After Eccles, 1953.) (B) IPSP. (After Eccles, 1957.) (C) Integration of EPSP and IPSP gives the result shown in the middle trace, which differs from a simple algebraic summation (dotted line). (After Rall et al., 1967.) (D) Reproducible EPSPs elicited over the Ia monosynaptic pathway. (E) Rapid buildup of EPSPs elicited over the monosynaptic corticospinal pathway. (From Phillips and Porter, 1964.) (F) Extracellular recording of a brief discharge in motoneuron axons (ventral root) in response to a single Ia volley (pathway 5 in Fig. 7.2). (G) Prolonged response to a single volley in flexor reflex afferents (pathway 7 in Fig. 7.2). (After Lloyd, 1943.) Vertical bars, millivolt calibration; horizontal bars, milliseconds.

in the axon hillock and initial segment. The spread of the synaptic potential to the impulse initiation site is governed by the electrotonic properties of the motoneuron dendrites. This will be explained further in the next section.

The volley in the Ia spindle afferents also activates the interneurons that connect to antagonist motoneurons (pathway 6 in Fig. 7.3). From such a motoneuron, the hyperpolarizing response shown in Fig. 7.4 (B) is recorded. This is an IPSP, presumably mediated by the type II chemical synapses in the ventral horn. These IPSPs have simple brief rise times and decays, the time course being somewhat longer than that for the monosynaptic EPSPs.

The interaction of an EPSP and an IPSP serves as a paradigm for synaptic integration as discussed in Chapter 3. Figure 7.4 (C) shows recordings from an experiment in a motoneuron, in which an EPSP (upper trace) and an IPSP (lower trace) were timed to occur simultaneously. The middle trace shows the result of this interaction; it is significantly different from the dotted line which indicates the transient that would have occurred if the interaction had been an algebraic summation of the two. In some cases, the interactions are, in fact, linear, but in other cases, as in this example, the interaction is nonlinear. This illustrates the point made in Chapter 3 that the interactions between EPSPs and IPSPs depend on the interactions of the synaptic conductances and the point made in Chapter 5 that they also depend on the relative positions of the synapses and their electrotonic relations within the dendritic tree.

The response of a motoneuron to a sequence of six Ia volleys is shown in Fig. 7.4 (D). The later responses resemble the first; there is a deadbeat quality to the sequence. But synapses do not all have this simple action, as has been shown in experiments on the central monosynaptic inputs to the motoneurons. One such input comes through the pyramidal tract fibers that originate in the cerebral cortex (cf. Fig. 1.1). Figure 7.4 (E) shows that, when this pathway is repetitively stimulated, there is a dramatic increase in amplitude of the synaptic potentials (Phillips and Porter, 1964). This increase is due to an overlap of the synaptic potentials (*temporal summation*) as well as to the increased amplitudes of successive responses (*facilitation*).

These findings are significant for several reasons, as Phillips and Porter have pointed out. They show that central synapses differ in their potency. They also show that the high frequency discharges of which pyramidal neurons are known to be capable would be especially effective in activating the motoneurons over the monosynaptic pathway. This pathway appears to provide for the fractionation of movement that underlies the exquisite control of the hand in primates. The directness of this pathway should increase the accessibility of hand motor units to the complex intracortical neuronal systems that control the cortical pyramidal output. Last, the increased synaptic potency is what is needed for the cerebral cortex to override other inputs to the motoneuron in its role of initiating and controlling sudden or precise movements. We will later discuss the even more dramatic changes in synaptic potency in the hippocampus and neocortex.

These monosynaptic responses may be compared with the responses of motoneurons to inputs arriving over polysynaptic pathways. As shown in Fig. 7.4 (F, G), the response to even a single volley in the flexor afferent pathway (FRA, pathway 7, in Fig. 7.3) consists of a response that builds up slowly and long outlasts the initial volley. Many factors may be involved in this type of response: delayed transmission through the synaptic relays in the spinal interneurons; prolonged transmitter action and prolonged EPSPs; prolonged spike discharges aroused by the EPSPs; and reverberating activity due to re-excitation loops among the circuits of the spinal cord. Similar activity can be induced by stimulation of central pathways. It is clear that much of the ongoing control of motoneurons is mediated by this type of activity, but it is equally clear that analysis of these pathways is one of the most difficult challenges facing the electrophysiologist.

RECURRENT INHIBITION Among the local circuits of the ventral horn, the recurrent inhibitory pathway has been the most intensively studied and has been of the greatest interest as a model for similar pathways in other regions of the brain. It has already been shown in Fig. 7.3 (pathway 8). The inhibitory action of this pathway is best revealed by setting up a single volley in a ventral root that invades the motoneurons antidromically. The response in a motoneuron consists of the antidromic impulse followed by a prolonged hyperpolarization, as shown in Fig. 7.5 (A). By using a shock that excites only the axons of neighboring motoneurons, it can be shown that the hyperpolarization is not the afterpolarization of the impulse but, rather, is due to an IPSP. The latency of the IPSP is sufficient for two synaptic relays, and it is concluded that the pathway is from the motoneuron axons through their collaterals onto an interneuron that has inhibitory synapses onto the motoneurons.

The name proposed by Eccles, Fatt, and Koketsu (1954) for this interneuron is the Renshaw cell, in honor of Birdsey Renshaw, who obtained the first physiological evidence for its existence in 1946. The cells respond to the ventral root volley with a prolonged discharge of impulses, as shown in Fig. 7.5 (B). The frequency is extremely high, starting at 1500/sec (i.e., an interspike interval of only about 0.6 msec); the spikes are, correspondingly, extremely brief in time course and refractory period. The cells are difficult to record from, apparently being rather small. The intracellular recordings show that the spikes arise from an

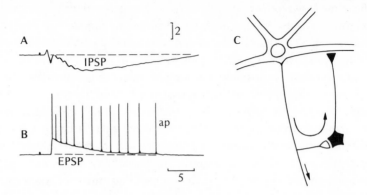

FIG. 7.5. Recurrent inhibition in the ventral horn. (A) Intracellular recording of a prolonged IPSP in a motoneuron elicited by a volley in motoneuron axons (ventral root). (B) Intracellular recording of a high frequency discharge of a Renshaw unit. Postulated pathway for activation of the Renshaw cell and inhibition of the motoneuron. (After Eccles, 1969 and Willis, 1970.)

EPSP with an unusually sharp initial peak and a very long tail; the latency of onset is about one synaptic delay before the onset of the motoneuron EPSP. The frequency of the discharge is similar to the frequency of the ripples that are sometimes discerned on the IPSP in the motoneuron; see Fig. 7.5 (A).

These various lines of evidence have indicated that the single volley of impulses in motoneuron axon collaterals sets up a prolonged EPSP and spike discharge in these interneurons, which, in turn, set up the prolonged IPSP in motoneurons through inhibitory synapses from their axon terminals [Fig. 7.5 (C)]. This is the Renshaw pathway in the spinal cord. It was the only model for recurrent inhibitory pathways in the central nervous system until the discovery of the dendrodendritic pathway in the olfactory bulb, to be described in the next chapter. A nagging problem was the histological identification of the Renshaw cell itself. It was early supposed that it was a type of short-axon cell, but, as we have seen, this type is rare in the ventral horn. The possibility that Renshaw discharges are recorded from the terminal boutons of the motoneuron recurrent collaterals themselves was suggested by Weight (1968) (see also Erulkar, Nichols, Popp, and Koelle, 1968). The recent experiments of Jankowska and Lindström (1971) support the anatomical evidence that the Renshaw cell is a type of propriospinal neuron. Because of these uncertainties, many observers have used the noncommittal term "Renshaw element" (see Csillik, Toth, and Karesu, 1973).

In addition to the question of identification, the role of recurrent inhibition in the ventral horn has been by no means clear. An analogy with surround or contrast inhibition in sensory systems has seemed obvious, but the evidence for such a function 'has not been compelling. Renshaw cells may be involved in complex disinhibitory interactions with each other (Wilson and Burgess, 1962) and with the interneurons in the Ia inhibitory pathway onto the motoneurons (Hultborn, Jankowska, and Lindström, 1968). The unusual properties of these elements—their abruptly rising and long-lasting EPSPs and their extremely high discharge rates—are not understood. All these unanswered questions indicate that there is still much work to be done on the significance of recurrent inhibitory pathways in the ventral horn (see Willis, 1971, for a comprehensive review).

TYPES OF INHIBITION   Many different types of inhibition are involved in mechanisms of synaptic integration, and it is appropriate at this point to distinguish between them as they affect the motoneuron. Inhibition directed predominantly to control of impulse output is indicated at the *soma* and *axon hillock* in Fig. 7.6. In motoneurons of lower vertebrates (e.g., Mauthner cells in the goldfish), the control is quite specific, through highly differentiated terminals that surround the hillock region. This type of inhibition tends to prevent impulse initiation without spatial discrimination of the sources of excitatory inputs. We will see examples of this type in the cerebellum and hippocampus.

Most synaptic inputs to mammalian motoneurons are directed to the dendrites; *proximal* and *distal* synapses are indicated in Fig. 7.6. Because their action may not be evident in intracellular recordings taken from the cell body, the latter is referred to as *remote inhibition* (Frank and Fuortes, 1957). Its significance lies mainly in its local interactions with other dendritic inputs (see under Dendritic Properties).

A final type is *presynaptic inhibition*, in which inhibition is exerted over an excitatory terminal. The pathway is indicated in Fig. 7.6, and the electrophysiological evidence for the mechanism is shown schematically in Fig. 7.7. An impulse is set up in an input axon (1); the impulse invades the presynaptic terminal (PT) and elicits an EPSP in a motoneuron. The intracellular recordings of the PT impulse and the motoneuro-

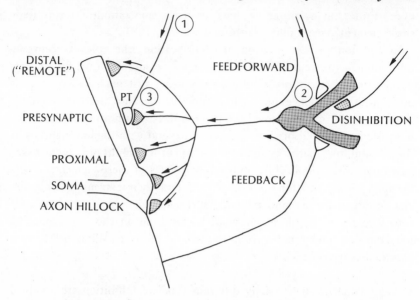

FIG. 7.6. Types of local inhibitory connections and pathways onto motoneurons.

nal EPSP are shown in Fig. 7.7. Repetitive activation of an inhibitory interneuron (2) causes a long-lasting *depolarization* of the PT by the action of the inhibitory neuron terminals (3), but no detectable response in the motoneuron itself. When (1) occurs during the response to (2), the EPSP in the motoneuron is reduced. This is ascribed to the fact that, in the PT, the action potential amplitude is reduced by the amount of the underlying depolarization, and hence the number of transmitter quanta released by the PT is reduced to q' compared with the normal q. Associated increases in potassium conductance and sodium inactivation contribute to the effect. Through presynaptic inhibition this type of excitatory input can be effectively opposed without affecting the excitability of the motoneuron itself; (see B-2 in Fig. 7.7). It is therefore, hard to distinguish this type experimentally from remote inhibition. Much evidence has been obtained in electrophysiological experiments (cf. Eccles, 1964), and there is electron-microscopic evidence for synaptic sequences between axon terminals [see Fig. 7.2 (C)], but the role during natural activity has not yet been determined.

The foregoing types of inhibition are defined in relation to the motoneuron itself; indeed, their significance cannot be assessed without refer-

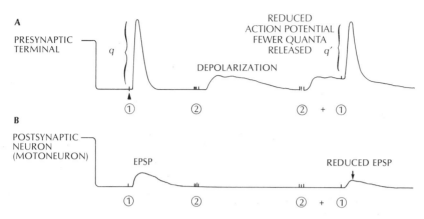

FIG. 7.7. Diagrams illustrating the principle of presynaptic inhibition. (A) Representative intracellular recordings from presynaptic terminal. (B) Recordings from postsynaptic neuron (see text).

ence to the electrotonic properties of the motoneuron. In addition, there are inhibitory actions that are defined in relation to intrinsic pathways. The two main types are depicted in Fig. 7.6. *Feedback inhibition* has already been discussed in relation to the Renshaw pathway. *Feedforward inhibition*, on the other hand, is exemplified by an interneuron in an input pathway, as shown in Fig. 7.6. There has been much interest recently in the role of feedforward circuits, both excitatory and inhibitory, in the central control of movement (see Evarts, 1971). Finally, Fig. 7.6 shows an inhibitory connection to the inhibitory interneuron, a connection providing for *disinhibition* of the inhibitory input from the interneuron to the motoneuron.

All these types of pathways are found generally throughout the brain, and we will see many examples in the regions of our study.

NEUROTRANSMITTERS

In their investigation of Renshaw inhibition, Eccles et al. (1954) reasoned, from Dale's suggestion, that if acetylcholine is the neurotransmitter at the neuromuscular junction, one would expect it also to be the transmitter at the axon collateral synapses onto Renshaw cells. A variety of evidence has supported this postulate (Eccles, 1964). The action is excitatory, as at the neuromuscular junction. A nicotinic receptor appears to mediate the initial high frequency response (cf. Fig. 7.5) and a

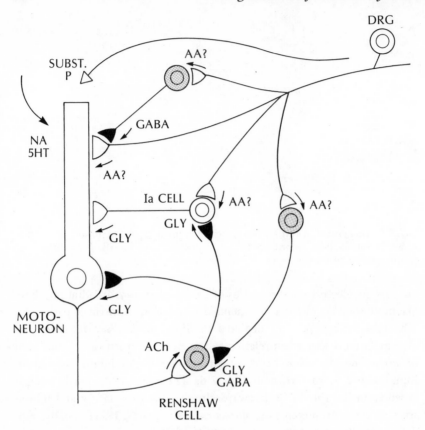

FIG. 7.8. Summary of putative neurotransmitters and their actions in the ventral horn of the spinal cord. AA, amino acids (e.g., glutamate, aspartate).

muscarinic receptor the later slower discharge (Curtis and Ryall, 1964). The similar presence of both types of cholinergic receptors on sympathetic ganglion cells may be recalled. This was the first central synapse, and for many years the only one, at which a neurotransmitter could be identified with some certainty. It is indicated diagramatically in Fig. 7.8.

The inhibitory action of Renshaw cells on motoneurons appears to be mediated by glycine. Iontophoresis of this substance hyperpolarizes and inhibits spinal neurons, by increasing membrane conductance to Cl⁻ (Werman, Davidoff, and Aprison, 1968). This action, and Renshaw inhibition, is reduced by administration of strychnine, an antagonist of glycine-mediated synaptic inhibition.

Renshaw cells, identified by their responses to ventral root volleys, have been further studied with respect to their responses to dorsal root volleys, which cause both polysynaptic excitation and inhibition. The excitation appears to involve an amino acid, possibly aspartate; early brief periods of inhibition are mediated by glycine, the later phases by GABA. Strychnine administration reduces the former, whereas picrotoxin and bicuculline, antagonists of GABA-mediated inhibition, reduce the latter (but see below). Some of the synapses and transmitters postulated by Curtis et al. (1976) on the basis of these results are indicated in Fig. 7.8. A great deal of further evidence—regarding local concentrations and enzyme activities, and high affinity uptake in synaptosomes—is consistent in general with this scheme, but will not be detailed here.

It may be noted that, despite the usefulness of strychnine, picrotoxin, and bicuculline as tools in transmitter identification, their mechanism of action is not yet understood. A fundamental problem is whether these antagonists act specifically on receptor molecules or nonspecifically on the ionophores controlled by the receptors (steps 8 and 10 in Fig. 4.5). The nonspecific actions of these drugs have come increasingly into question (see Roberts, 1975; Cooper et al., 1978), which has the effect of shifting the burden of proof to other methods, such as immunocytochemistry. Glutamate decarboxylase (GAD), the enzyme that synthesizes GABA from glutamate, has been localized by immunocytochemical methods to some of the terminals making synapses on motoneurons (McLaughlin, et al., 1975).

GABA is also believed to be the transmitter of the interneurons that mediate presynaptic inhibition of motoneurons (Schmidt, 1971). It will be recalled that presynaptic inhibition is due to a depolarization of the afferent terminals onto motoneurons (cf. Fig. 7.7) rather than a hyperpolarization which characterizes the action of GABA elsewhere in the spinal cord and at inhibitory synapses in many other regions. Some of the evidence for this action is indirect, such as the observation that GABA increases primary afferent depolarization, and that this is antagonized by picrotoxin but not by strychnine. Dorsal root ganglion cells are depolarized by direct iontophoresis of GABA onto their cell bodies (Feltz and Rasminsky, 1974; Gallagher, Higashi, and Nishi, 1978), which is consistent with the postulate of a similar action at their terminals. Immunocytochemical studies have demonstrated GAD-containing terminals that are presynaptic to large terminals (presumably the Ia afferents) that make synapses onto motoneurons, which supports the evidence that GABA may be the transmitter mediating presynaptic inhibition (McLaughlin et al., 1975). GAD-positive terminals take part in even more extensive axo-axonal synaptic arrangements in the dorsal horn (Barber et al., 1978).

Figure 7.8 also indicates several other transmitter pathways onto motoneurons. Iontophoresis of noradrenalin causes a hyperpolarizing inhibition of motoneurons, with no change or slight increase in membrane resistance (Engberg and Marshall, 1971). This is similar to the effect of noradrenalin on cerebellar Purkinje cells. A noradrenergic projection to the spinal cord from the locus coeruleus has been described (Nygren and Olson, 1977). Substance P has a slow excitatory effect on motoneurons (Takahashi et al., 1974; see also Belcher and Ryall, 1977). It is present in dorsal root fibers and thus could function as a neuromodulator in relation to sensory input. Its presence in small cells and unmyelinated afferents in the dorsal horn, and its overlap with the distribution of opiate receptors there, has suggested a possible role in pain mechanisms (Hökfelt et al., 1975).

DENDRITIC PROPERTIES

Like roads leading to Rome, the pathways in the ventral horn lead to the motoneuron. The terminals are mainly distributed over the dendrites, so the study of input-output mechanisms in the ventral horn comes down, largely, to a study of the properties of the motoneuronal dendrites. This was the original object of Rall's analysis, and modern studies of synaptic integration in the motoneuron are now firmly based on his methods. The motoneuron has thus come to serve as a model for the analysis of the dendritic properties of other neurons in the brain.

The basic approach involves the construction of an equivalent cylinder for the dendritic tree of the motoneuron. The steps in this procedure have been outlined in Chapter 5 and are summarized in the diagram of Fig. 7.9. The electrical properties used in constructing the cylinder are derived from experiments in which current is passed through an intracellular electrode, while the voltage change is simultaneously recorded. Such experiments have yielded values between 0.5 and 5 MΩ (average, 1.65 MΩ) for the whole neuron resistance (R_N) of the motoneuron (Frank and Fuortes, 1956) and a time constant for the charging transient of 2–3 msec. From such data, estimates of 4–7 msec for the membrane time

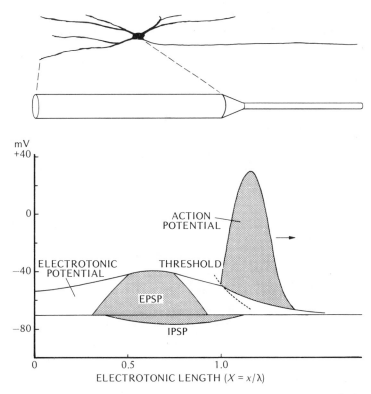

FIG. 7.9. An electrotonic model of a motoneuron, illustrating the spread of potentials in the dendritic tree. *Above*, derivation of an equivalent cylinder from the motoneuron. *Below*, types of potentials and their distribution (see text). *Ordinate*, intracellular potential (mV). *Abscissa*, electrotonic length.

constant (τ_m) and 2000–4000 Ωcm^2 for the specific membrane resistance (R_m) are obtained (Rall, 1959b, 1970; Lux et al., 1970). These experiments, combined with measurements of motoneuron dendritic geometry, have permitted estimates of the electrotonic length (L) of the equivalent cylinder. The best estimates appear to lie between 1 and 2 (Burke and ten Bruggencate, 1971; Jack and Redman, 1971); a value of 1 is used in the illustration in Fig. 7.9. In recent experiments, it has been possible to carry out these studies in single motoneurons identified with intracellular markers, by autoradiographic techniques (Lux et al., 1970), and with Procion dye (Barrett and Crill, 1974).

In our discussion of dendritic electrotonus, it was shown that the shape of a synaptic potential, as recorded from the cell body, varies according to its site in the dendritic tree because of the electrotonic properties of the dendrites (Chapter 5; see Fig. 5.4). This principle was early recognized in the frog motoneuron by Fadiga and Brookhart (1960). As developed by Rall, the shape indices of synaptic potentials have provided a useful tool for ascertaining the sites of some of the synaptic inputs to the motoneurons. The case of the Ia monosynaptic input is illustrated in Fig. 7.9. The moderately rapid rise time and decay of the EPSP indicate that the synapses are widely distributed over the motoneuron surface, with a predominance in the middle portion of the dendritic tree. This is indicated diagrammatically by the shaded area in Fig. 7.9; (see also Iansek and Redman, 1973).

The synaptic potential must spread to the site of impulse initiation in the initial segment, as previously mentioned, and Fig. 7.9 shows how this comes about. The motoneuron dendritic membrane is electrically passive, hence the spread of synaptic potentials is governed by the electrotonic properties of the dendrites. The significance of the electrotonic length calculated for the dendritic tree is that it is sufficiently short to allow for effective spread of passive current through the dendrites to the cell body. Thus, the synaptic potential in the dendrites is linked to the action potential in the initial segment by the electrotonic potential in between.

This is a common arrangement in neurons. For example, a model for the stretch receptor cell of the crayfish would be very similar to that shown in Fig. 7.9, except that the location of the excitatory input would be more distal in the dendrites. In that cell, too, the site of impulse initiation is well out in the initial segment, as first shown in the classical experiment of Edwards and Ottoson (1957). This illustrates an important principle, namely, that the location of the cell body has no necessary significance in the integrative organization of a neuron. In the motoneuron, it happens to be (usually, but not always) at the convergence point for current flow from dendrites to initial segment. We will see examples in other neurons in the brain in which the cell body is completely irrelevant for particular input-output relations.

Motoneurons of different size have been found to have similar electrotonic lengths for their equivalent cylinders; the values for L lie between 1 and 2 (Burke and ten Bruggencate, 1971). Thus, in the smaller motoneurons, the smaller diameters of the dendrites are balanced by their shorter lengths. This introduces a *scaling principle* in the electrotonic properties of dendritic trees of different size, which may have a general application to neurons in other parts of the brain (cf. Rall and Rinzel, 1973).

The electrotonic properties of the smaller motoneurons (and of smaller neurons, in general) have an important consequence: a given synaptic input gives rise to a larger synaptic potential in them. This is because the resistance (the *input resistance*) through which the synaptic current will have to flow in the smaller dendrites is higher. This may be related to the fact that smaller motoneurons tend to be more excitable and display more spontaneous activity. The alpha motoneurons have low levels of spontaneous activity (0–10 impulses/sec), whereas the smaller gamma motoneurons fire at rates of 30–50/sec. The functional significance of this difference is that the continual activity of the gamma motoneurons keeps the spindles slightly contracted, thereby providing continual Ia feedback excitation of the alpha motoneurons, whose resulting slow discharges are the basis for resting muscle tone. Such differences in spontaneous activity between different types of neurons are important factors in understanding the dynamics of synaptic organization, as we will also see in other regions of the brain.

Differences in excitability between alpha motoneurons of different size have been found; this has been termed a *size principle* by Henneman (1966). According to this principle, increasing activity over a given input pathway successively excites motoneurons according to their increasing size. The extent to which this principle, deduced from electrophysiological experiments, is operative in the normal ongoing control of the muscles is currently under investigation (cf. Phillips and Porter, 1977).

In the electrotonic model for the motoneuron, it is assumed that the spread of the synaptic potentials through the dendritic tree is by passive means alone. This appears to be generally true for the normal motoneuron. In motoneurons undergoing chromatolysis after sectioning of their axons, however, small amplitude spike-like activity can be recorded, and it has been concluded that this indicates the generation of impulses or impulse-like activity in restricted parts of the dendritic tree (Eccles, Libet, and Young, 1957). This is an important finding; it provides a model for active properties of dendrites in other parts of the brain (the cerebellar Purkinje cell and the hippocampal pyramidal cell), and it shows that the properties of dendritic membrane depend, to a certain extent, on the functional and metabolic state of the cell.

SYNAPTIC INTEGRATION   The locus for Renshaw recurrent inhibition is also shown in Fig. 7.9 (IPSP). It is mainly in the proximal dendrites, closer to the cell body than the Ia excitatory input. In the early experiments it was inferred that this reflected a general rule, that inhibitory synapses are placed close to the cell body in order to be most strategically placed to control impulse generation. As discussed in Chapter 5, this rule no longer has a general validity. In the crustacean stretch receptor cell, for example, the inhibitory synapses occur far out on the dendrites. The strategy of that placement appears to be to permit them to oppose directly the excitatory sensory input to the dendritic terminals. In the motoneuron there appears to be a mixture of the two cases: some inhibitory synapses directly oppose the excitatory synapses through the overlap in their distribution (in the distal dendrites, this results in remote inhibition; see below). Others tend to be closer to the cell body, the more effectively to control impulse initiation in the initial segment. These two kinds of inhibition are clearly seen in the cerebellar Purkinje cell.

The distributions of several of the other inputs to the motoneuron are shown in Fig. 7.10. Some of these distributions have been deduced by Rall's methods, others from such evidence as susceptibility to intracellular Cl⁻ and reversal by intracellular currents. In some cases, different parts of a motoneuron dendritic tree may receive different inputs; this was termed a "fractionation of dendritic field" by Sprague (1958). In general, however, there are relatively wide distributions and extensive degrees of overlap between the sites of central, afferent, and intrinsic connections. These are important features in the synaptic organization of motoneurons and are in contrast to the organization of many other principal neurons of the brain, in which there is a sharp localization of different inputs to different parts of the dendritic tree. The overlap of inputs provides the fullest means by which the many different inputs to the motoneuron can interact dynamically with each other.

To understand the nature of these interactions, it is necessary to know the input provided by a single synapse. The large amplitude EPSP, depicted in Fig. 7.9, represents the summated response to many individual synapses. For a single Ia afferent terminal, Kuno (1971) has obtained evidence that a single quantum causes a unit ("miniature") EPSP of about 100 μV and that there are, on average, only 1–2 quanta/terminal. Therefore, if the impulse threshold is about 10 mV, the synchronous

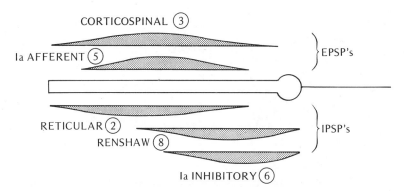

FIG. 7.10. Distribution of some synaptic inputs to the motoneuron. Numbers refer to pathways in Fig. 7.3. (After Porter and Hore, 1969; Burke et al., 1970; Kuno and Llinás, 1971; Jack, Miller, Porter, and Redman, 1971.)

input from about 50 Ia terminals is needed to initiate an impulse in the motoneuron. This may be compared with the relation between quanta and the end-plate potential at the neuromuscular junction (Chapter 4). It may be noted that the amplitude of a postsynaptic potential depends on input resistance and spatial distribution; depending on these variables, the amplitude of unit synaptic potentials elicited by other inputs may vary from 0.05 to 0.5 mV.

We can now see more fully the significance of the fractionation of inputs by means of the small contacts from small terminals, as discussed in Chapter 2. It means that a single input is rarely effective itself in initiating or controlling output from the motoneuron; it must always combine with many others. The summing of the inputs must depend on accurate timing and on appropriate siting vis-à-vis the electrotonic properties of the dendritic tree. Because each input is small, the summation will be finely graded. And because the impulse threshold is relatively high, a great amount of finely graded interaction occurs in the dendrites before output occurs in the axon. The ongoing control of the muscles is, therefore, the outcome of a complex process in the motoneuron, in which a multitude of local synaptic interactions precedes the final integration at the site of impulse initiation in the axon hillock.

8

OLFACTORY BULB

The olfactory bulb, protruding like an incandescent fixture from the forebrain, is the main relay station in the olfactory pathway. It occupies in this respect a position similar to that of the retina in the visual pathway. It is here, as is shown in the diagram of Fig. 8.1, that the axons of the olfactory receptor cells in the nose terminate. The output of the bulb is directed to several brain regions, and there are, in return, connections to the bulb from the brain. The main outlines of these connections are indicated in Fig. 8.1; they will be described in further detail below and in the later chapters on the olfactory cortex and hippocampus.

The classical histologists of the late nineteenth century took a keen interest in the olfactory bulb. This was by virtue of its very distinct laminations and its several sharply differentiated types of neurons. The deductions drawn by Cajal (1911, 1955) and his contemporaries about the organization of neurons in the olfactory bulb played a central role in the development of the functional concepts of the classical neuron doctrine. Following this period, however, interest waned, due in large part to the almost complete lack of progress in understanding the nature of the olfactory stimulus.

Interest in the olfactory bulb was revived by the anatomical studies of le Gros Clark and his co-workers (Clark, 1951; 1957; Allison, 1953) and the physiological studies of Adrian (1950; 1953). Knowledge of synaptic organization began in the early 1960's, with electrophysiological investigations using single unit recordings. These studies took advantage of the fact that the input and output pathways of the bulb are completely separated, the kind of situation that made the ventral horn of the spinal cord such an admirable subject for study. Electron-microscopic and biophysical studies followed, and more recently, studies of neurotransmitters, which together have put our knowledge on a sound basis.

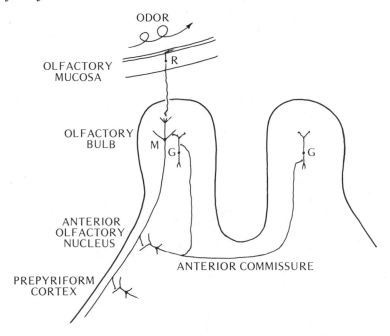

FIG. 8.1. Connections of the olfactory bulb. R, olfactory receptor cell; M, mitral cell; G, granule cell.

The results have shown that, in its functional organization, the olfactory bulb goes significantly beyond the framework of the classical neuron doctrine as formulated on the motoneuron model. It is appropriate, therefore, to consider the olfactory bulb at this point, in order to compare it with the ventral horn and with two other highly organized regions of the brain, the retina and cerebellum.

NEURONAL ELEMENTS

INPUTS The neuronal elements of the olfactory bulb are shown in Fig. 8.2. The *afferent* (peripheral) input is through the axons of the receptor cells in the olfactory mucosa in the nasal cavity. The axons are all unmyelinated and extremely thin, approximately 0.1–0.3 μm in diameter. The fact that the input fibers are all of the same modality (olfactory), and they all have small diameters and no myelin, stands in the sharpest possible contrast to the variety of input fibers to the ventral horn of the spinal cord.

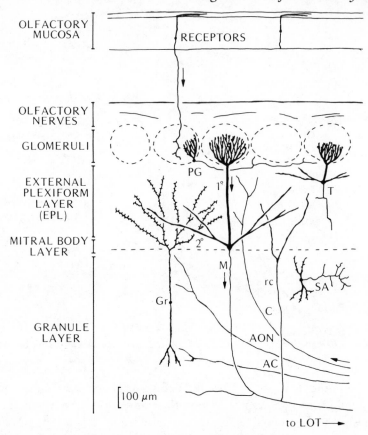

OLFACTORY
MUCOSA

RECEPTORS

OLFACTORY
NERVES

GLOMERULI

EXTERNAL
PLEXIFORM
LAYER
(EPL)

MITRAL BODY
LAYER

GRANULE
LAYER

PG

1°

T

2°

M

rc   SA

Gr   C

AON

AC

[100 μm

to LOT⟶

FIG. 8.2. Neuronal elements of the mammalian olfactory bulb.

Inputs: afferent fibers (above) from olfactory receptors; central fibers (below) from three sources; centrifugal fibers (C) from the nucleus of the horizontal limb of the diagonal band; ipsilateral fibers from the anterior olfactory nucleus (AON); contralateral fibers from the anterior commissure (AC).

Principal neurons: mitral cell (M), with primary (1°) and secondary dendrites (2°) and recurrent axon collaterals (rc); tufted cell (T).

Intrinsic neurons: periglomerular short-axon cell (PG); deep short-axon cell (SA); granule cell (Gr). LOT, lateral olfactory tract.

(Based on Cajal, 1911; Price and Powell, 1971; Pinching and Powell, 1972; Shepherd, 1972.

The olfactory axons enter at the bulb surface and terminate in a layer composed of spherical regions of neuropil, termed *glomeruli*. These structures are 100–200 μm in diameter; like the glomeruli ("barrels") in the cerebral cortex, they are at a macroscopic level of organization compared with the synaptic glomeruli of the cerebellum and thalamus. A general definition of the term glomerulus, as it applies to different levels of organization, is given in Chapter 10.

The olfactory axons do not branch on their way to the glomeruli, but once inside they ramify, to varying extents, and terminate. An essential feature of bulbar organization in all vertebrates is that all the olfactory input terminates within the glomeruli.

There are several *central* inputs to the bulb from the brain. Some sites of origin have been indicated in the diagram of Fig. 8.1. Axons that are relatively large (several microns in diameter) but few in number come the farthest distance, from a region at the base of the brain called the diagonal band (DB). Other axons, finer and much more numerous, come from the region just posterior to the bulb, the anterior olfactory nucleus (AON). Some of these come from the AON of the same side; others come from the contralateral side through the anterior commissure (AC). The central inputs are also referred to as *centrifugal* fibers to indicate their outward orientation from the brain.

These inputs have terminals at different though overlapping levels in the bulb, which is indicated very approximately in the diagram of Fig. 8.2 and will be further described later.

PRINCIPAL NEURON The output from the bulb is directed centrally (not peripherally, as in the case of the ventral horn) and is carried in the axons of *mitral cells*. As indicated in Fig. 8.2, the mitral cell bodies are arranged in a thin sheet about 400 μm below the glomerular layer. As principal neurons go, the mitral cell is small-to-medium sized, its cell body being 15–30 μm in diameter. Each cell sends an unbranched *primary dendrite* to a glomerulus, to terminate there in a tuft of branches. The tuft has an extent of 100–150 μm and, therefore, fills much of the glomerulus it lies within. The diameter of the primary dendrite ranges from 2–12 μm, and the length is 400–600 μm, depending on the angle of direction across the external plexiform layer (EPL). Each mitral cell also gives rise to several secondary dendrites, which branch sparingly and terminate in the EPL. Secondary dendrites are 1–8 μm in diameter and up to 600 μm or so in length.

The primary and secondary dendrites have generally smooth surfaces, like the dendrites of motoneurons. They are also similar to motoneuron dendrites in diameter and length. But the differentiation into primary and secondary types, the strict localization of afferent input to the terminal tuft of the primary dendrite, and the separation of intrinsic circuits in relation to the two types of dendrite, are specializations that have no counterparts in the motoneuron.

The mitral cell axons proceed to the depths of the bulb and then run posteriorly to emerge together to form the lateral olfactory tract (LOT). During their course within the bulb they give off two kinds of collaterals: *recurrent collaterals* that terminate in the EPL and *deep collaterals* that terminate in the granule layer (GRL). Smaller versions of the mitral cells, the so-called *tufted cells*, have cell bodies scattered throughout the EPL. Many of these appear to send axons to the LOT and, thus, carry part of the bulbar output. They are, therefore, a smaller type of principal neuron. Whether they are differentiated to perform some specific function, as are the smaller gamma motoneurons of the ventral horn, is not known. Their collaterals appear to be preferentially distributed within a thin layer just deep to the mitral cell bodies. The LOT axons range from 0.2 to 3.0 μm in diameter, and are all myelinated (Price and Sprich, 1976). They are among the thinnest myelinated axons in the nervous system.

The output axons in the LOT distribute collateral branches and terminals to several central regions; these are indicated in Fig. 8.1 and will be further discussed in Chapter 13. The distances over which this output is carried are rather short, not much more than a centimeter or so. Note that the principal neuron of the olfactory bulb terminates in several distinct types of distant region, each with different functions; this is in contrast to the motoneuron, whose output goes exclusively to one destination, the muscles. Thus, the two regions offer an interesting contrast in that the input is multimodal and the output is unimodal in the case of the motoneuron, but the reverse in the case of the mitral cell.

INTRINSIC NEURONS   In contrast to the difficulty in identifying interneurons in the spinal cord, we can recognize three distinct types of intrinsic neuron in the olfactory bulb.

Surrounding the glomeruli are the cell bodies of *periglomerular* (PG) *cells* (see Fig. 8.2). The cell body is small (6–8 μm in diameter), far smaller than any cell in the ventral horn, and among the smallest in the brain. Each cell has a short bushy dendritic tree that arborizes to an extent of 50–100 μm within one of the glomeruli. The axon distributes to neighboring glomeruli, reaching distances of 500 μm or so. Significantly, the axon does not distribute to the glomerulus containing the dendritic tree of its parent cell.

We have previously touched on the identification of *short-axon cells* in discussing the intrinsic neurons of the ventral horn, and we may now deal more fully with this question with regard to the PG cells. We will define a short-axon cell as *a cell whose axon distributes within the same histological region*. Note that this differs slightly from the oft-quoted classical definition, of a cell whose axon ramifies within the field of the dendritic tree of its parent cell. Thus, once we have characterized a region in terms of its characteristic nuclear or laminar arrangements, any cell whose axon distributes within that region is a short-axon cell. A cell whose axon distributes outside the local region is consequently a long-axon cell and, by definition, a principal neuron.

In the case of "loosely organized" parts of the brain, such as the ventral horn and, as we shall see, the cerebral cortex, a clear distinction between the two neuronal types may sometimes not be possible. In the case of more rigidly organized regions, however, the distinction is usually clear. Within this general definition of a short-axon cell, we will encounter many varieties: axons that distribute within the dendritic field of the parent cell (e.g., some cells in the thalamus) and those that distribute outside it (e.g., the PG cell); those axons that distribute within the same histological lamina (e.g., the PG cell) and those that distribute within a different lamina (e.g., some cells in the cerebellum).

Deep to the layer of mitral cell bodies is a thick layer containing the cell bodies of *granule cells* (see Fig. 8.2). These cell bodies are also very small (6–8 μm in diameter); hence the name granule, a very general term applied by the early histologists to the "grains" they saw in their primitive microscopic preparations. Each granule cell has a superficial process that ramifies and terminates in the EPL. The branching tree has a lateral extent of 300–500 μm within the EPL. The shaft of the tree is up to 500 μm or more long, depending on the depth of the cell body from which it arises. In their branching pattern and their investiture with many small spines (gemmules), the superficial processes resemble the apical dendrites of cortical pyramidal cells. They contrast with the smooth appearance and infrequent branching of the dendrites of mitral cells and of motoneurons. Each granule cell also gives off an inner process that terminates deeper in the granule layer.

The outstanding feature of the granule cell is that it lacks a morphological axon; repeated Golgi studies and, more recently, electron-microscopic studies, have confirmed this fact. In this respect the granule cell resembles the amacrine cell of the retina. These cells have thus always stood out as exceptions to the classical model of the neuron based on the motoneuron. The lack of an axon has raised the question of the identity of the processes of the granule cell; some would call them "primitive" or "axon-like". One need not hesitate, however, in calling them dendrites on the grounds of their general fine structural features and close resemblance to cortical cell dendrites. The lack of an axon has posed a severe challenge to the interpretation of the functions of these cells, which has only been initiated in the studies of recent years.

There is also within the bulb a third type of intrinsic neuron, a *short-axon cell* found rarely in the glomerular layer but more frequently in the granule layer. The latter have cell bodies 8–15 μm in diameter and dendritic trees of variable extent (up to 200–300 μm across). Their axons ramify either in the EPL or the GRL (see Fig. 8.2).

CELL POPULATIONS   The numbers of receptor cells have been estimated at about 50,000,000 on one side of the nose in the rabbit; this is therefore the number of afferent axons entering one olfactory bulb. This number of afferent elements is exceeded only by the number in the visual pathway. The number of mitral cells is of the order of 50,000, so there is considerable convergence, on the order of 1000:1, onto the principal neurons. There are about 2000 glomeruli in a rabbit's bulb, so there are approximately 25,000 olfactory axons and 25 mitral cells per glomerulus (Allison and Warwick, 1949).

The ratios of intrinsic neurons to principal neurons are also high in the olfactory bulb. Approximate estimates are 20:1 for the PG cells:mitral cells, 200:1 for the granule cells:mitral cells, and perhaps 1:1 for the short-axon cells:mitral cells. These ratios by themselves strongly support the presumption that a considerble amount of information processing takes place within the intrinsic circuits of the olfactory bulb.

SYNAPTIC CONNECTIONS

The lamination of the olfactory bulb greatly simplifies the analysis of synaptic connections as seen under the electron microscope; in addition, identification has been put on a sound basis by the extensive use of serial

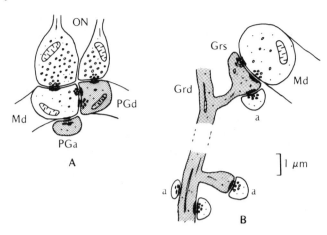

FIG. 8.3. Synaptic connections in the mammalian olfactory bulb. (A) Axodendritic and dendrodendritic connections in the olfactory glomerulus. ON, olfactory nerve; Md, mitral dendrite; PGd, periglomerular cell dendrite; PGa, periglomerular cell axon. Note the serial and reciprocal synaptic sequences. (After
Andres, 1964; Reese and Brightman, 1970; Pinching and Powell, 1971; White
1972.) (B) *Above,* dendrodendritic connections in the external plexiform layer
between a mitral secondary dendrite (Md) and a granule cell dendritic spine (Gr
s); note also the centrifugal axodendritic connection onto the spine. *Below,* axodendritic connections in the granule layer. (After Rall et al., 1966; Price and
Powell, 1970a.)

reconstructions. The analysis has been carried out at three main levels in
the bulb.

GLOMERULAR LAYER   Within the glomeruli the terminals of olfactory
axons make synaptic contacts onto the dendritic tufts of the principal
neurons, the mitral (and tufted) cells (Andres, 1970; Reese and Brightman, 1970). As shown diagrammatically in Fig. 8.3, the terminals are
moderately large (1.0–3.0 μm in diameter), particularly when viewed in
relation to the very thin axons from which they arise. The contacts are
type I chemical synapses. The axon terminals also make synapses onto the
dendrites of the intrinsic neurons, the PG cells, in most species that have
been studied. An exception is a particular strain of mouse (Balb/c), in
which these connections are missing. This finding has been well documented by White (1972, 1973) in serial reconstructions and points up a
very interesting genetic difference at the level of synaptic connectivity.

By the use of serial reconstructions and careful comparisons with

Golgi preparations, it has been established that there are numerous synaptic connections between the mitral and PG cell dendrites within the glomerulus (Pinching and Powell, 1971; White, 1972). The mitral-to-PG synapses are type I, whereas the PG-to-mitral synapses are type II [see Fig. 8.3 (A)]. These dendrodendritic synapses may be arranged in serial sequences or in reciprocal, side-by-side pairs (cf. Fig. 2.6, Chapter 2). About 25% of the synapses are involved in reciprocal pairs. A group of axonal and dendritic terminals is sometimes set apart to form a synaptic complex in a manner somewhat resembling the synaptic glomeruli in the cerebellum and thalamus. Synapses between two presumed PG cell dendrites have also been observed. At the borders of the glomeruli are axon terminals on the larger mitral dendritic branches; these terminals come from PG cell axons; a few also come from central inputs (DB).

EXTERNAL PLEXIFORM LAYER (EPL)   In the EPL, the dominant type of synaptic connection is a pair of reciprocal contacts (Hirata, 1964; Andres, 1965; Rall et al., 1966). Serial reconstructions (Rall et al., 1966) established that these contacts occur between the secondary dendrite of a mitral cell and the spine (gemmule) of a granule cell dendrite [see Fig. 8.3 (B)]. These were the first dendrodendritic synapses identified in the nervous system. The mitral-to-granule synapse is type I, whereas the granule-to-mitral synapse is type II (Price and Powell, 1970a). Over 80% of all synapses in the EPL are involved in such reciprocal pairs. If we consider that there are a hundred or more granule cells for each mitral cell, and that each granule cell has perhaps a hundred or more spines, it is obvious that these dendrodendritic connections provide for extremely powerful and specific interactions with the mitral cells. Indeed, electron micrographs show the EPL to be a neuropil composed almost entirely of mitral and granule cell dendrites and their synaptic interconnections (see Reese and Shepherd, 1972).

Recently, Ramon-Moliner (1977) pointed out that the granule-to-mitral synapse sometimes appears indistinct or missing in single sections, and suggested that the inhibitory action of granule cells might be mediated by a nonsynaptic mechanism. However, Lieberman and his colleagues have carefully re-investigated the question (Jackowski, Parnevalas, and Lieberman, 1978) using several EM techniques, and have confirmed that the granule-to-mitral synapses are approximately equal partners in the reciprocal pairs, as originally described. This of course does not rule out the possibility of additional nonsynaptic interactions.

GRANULE LAYER In the granule layer, axon terminals are found on the shafts and spines of the granule cell dendrites [see Fig. 8.3 (C)]. The studies of Price and Powell (1970b) have shown that these axon terminals derive from both intrinsic and extrinsic (central) inputs. The *intrinsic* sources include the axon collaterals of mitral and tufted cells and the axons of the deep short-axon cells. There is evidence that the synapses of these terminals are type II. The *extrinsic* sources have been shown to make connections at different levels of the granule dendritic tree. The AC distributes mainly to the deep processes. The AON distributes over the middle part of the dendrites, including the spines in the EPL. The DB axons distribute mainly to the spines in the EPL; some terminals are also found at the borders of the glomeruli. The synapses made by these inputs from the brain appear to be type I. In the EPL, the synapses made by these terminals are on the same spines that take part in the reciprocal connections with mitral dendrites, providing thereby a means for presynaptic control of the spines.

It should be noted that all the synaptic connections in which the granule cell takes part are oriented toward the granule cell, with the sole exception of the dendrodendritic synapses from the granule spines onto the mitral dendrites in the EPL. The latter are, therefore, the only output avenue from the granule cells.

It can be seen that there is a much richer variety of patterns of synaptic connections in the olfactory bulb than in the ventral horn. In the ventral horn, nearly all the connections are axodendritic or axosomatic, with the exception of some serial arrangements presumed to be axoaxonic. The olfactory bulb also contains many axodendritic synapses, but, in addition, there are dendrodendritic, somatodendritic, dendrosomatic, and axodendrodenritic synapses, as described above. The purely local circuits are, therefore, much more complex in the olfactory bulb than in the ventral horn.

GLIA The olfactory bulb has provided favorable opportunities for observing the relation of glial membranes to the neuronal elements and synapses. The incoming olfactory axons are gathered into bundles of

100–200 axons contained within one glial (Schwann) cell. Within the glomeruli, a synaptic complex, such as that shown in Fig. 8.3 (A), is often seen to be surrounded by one or more loose folds of glial membrane; this is similar to, though not nearly as distinct as, the synaptic glomeruli of the cerebellum and thalamus (Pinching and Powell, 1971). A similar relation is sometimes seen around the reciprocal synapses in the EPL.

Within the EPL, in most vertebrate species, several loose folds of glial membrane surround the primary dendrite of the mitral cell near the glomerular boundary. In primates, it has been found that the folds of membrane are packed down into typical myelin, which may surround not only the primary dendrite but even extend to the cell body in the case of tufted cells (Pinching, 1971). As already noted in Chapter 2, this finding shows that a dendrite may be myelinated and that myelin is not exclusively associated with axons.

BASIC CIRCUIT

The synaptic organization of the olfactory bulb may be summarized in a basic circuit diagram; see Fig. 8.4. Because of the clear cell types and laminae in the bulb, the diagram can be constructed largely on the basis of the foregoing anatomical evidence.

First, by way of brief summary: the olfactory axons make synapses within the glomeruli onto mitral (and tufted) cell dendrites, as well as onto PG cell dendrites in most species. Between the dendrites of mitral and PG cells are synaptic connections, both reciprocal and serial. The PG cell axons connect to mitral dendrites in neighboring glomeruli. In the EPL, the major type of connection is the reciprocal dendrodendritic synapse between mitral dendrites and granule dendritic spines. Finally, the input fibers from the brain have terminals at several levels on the granule cells: AC axons to the deep granule processes; AON axons to the middle portions; and DB axons to the peripheral dendritic spines.

With regard to the three main types of neuron, an outstanding feature is the fact that they all take part in dendrodendritic synaptic connections. The principal neuron (mitral cell) not only has synaptic *inputs* to all parts of its dendritic tree, it also has synaptic *outputs* from virtually every part of that dendritic tree. Much the same can be said of the PG cell dendrites. The granule cell also has synaptic inputs over all its dendritic tree, but its synaptic outputs are localized to the spines in the EPL.

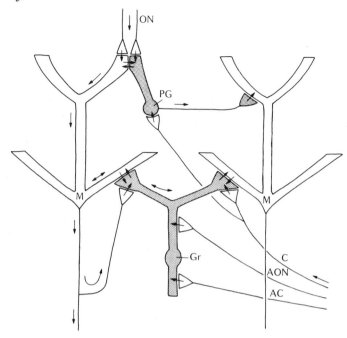

FIG. 8.4. Basic circuit diagram for the mammalian olfactory bulb. Abbreviations as for Fig. 8.3.

Thus, the granule cell differs from the other two types of bulbar neuron not in having synaptic output from its dendrites (all three types have that) but rather in having that output localized to only one part of the tree, and in lacking an additional axonal output pathway.

The diagram of Fig. 8.4 illustrates the principles upon which this variety of interconnections is organized. An obvious feature of the basic circuit is that there are vertical pathways for direct, "straight-through" activity and horizontal pathways for interactions between the vertical paths. The horizontal connections are organized in two distinct levels, or tiers. The first level is the glomerular layer, which is obviously concerned with reception of the olfactory input and the initial processing of that input. The second level is the EPL, which is obviously concerned with control of the bulbar output from the mitral cell bodies. The intrinsic neurons are specific to these levels and functions, the PG cells to input processing, the granule cells to output control.

In the general arrangement just described, there is an interesting simi-

larity to the basic circuit of the retina. This will be discussed further in
the following chapter. For now it may be noted that in both these
regions there is a framework of vertical and horizontal pathways such as
cannot be discerned in the ventral horn. Also, in both regions, there is
little ambiguity about the positions of the intrinsic neurons in the vertical
and horizontal pathways, so that the functional roles of the intrinsic
neurons are much clearer than in the case of the ventral horn.

Let us now look more closely at the synaptic organization within the
olfactory bulb, using Fig. 8.4.

The olfactory glomeruli are the most characteristic feature of the olfactory bulb in the vertebrate series. Within the glomeruli, three neuronal
elements come together: olfactory axon, mitral cell dendrite, and PG cell
dendrite. In more general terms, the three elements are input fiber,
principal neuron, and intrinsic neuron. These are the basic elements in
the synaptic organization of the local regions of the brain, and as noted
(Chapter 1) we refer to them as a *synaptic triad*. Within the triad, the
synapses between the input and principal elements provide the necessary
basis for input-output transmission, whereas synapses between the principal and intrinsic elements provide for modulation and control of the
input-output transfer.

The synaptic triad in the glomerulus involves synapses from the input
onto both the principal and (in most species) the intrinsic elements. This
is a common pattern in the brain; the same type of arrangement is found,
for example, in the retina, cerebellum, and thalamus. In the latter regions, as we shall see, the synapses onto the principal and intrinsic
elements arise from a single large input terminal, whereas, in the olfactory bulb, the synapses are made by separate terminals. The arrangement in the olfactory bulb appears to be more flexible and, possibly,
more precise. In order to assess its functional significance, however, one
needs to know if the separate terminals arise from separate olfactory
axons; if they do, does this mean that some olfactory receptors project
only to the principal neuron, whereas others project only to the intrinsic
neuron? Such questions are fundamental to understanding the nature of
information processing in this sensory pathway.

After the initial input to the principal and intrinsic elements in the
glomerulus, further processing takes place through the dendrodendritic
synaptic connections between them. In all regions of the brain, the principal and intrinsic elements stand in some kind of relation to each other. In

the olfactory glomerulus, the multitude of reciprocal and serial connections appears to maximize the possibilities for complex information processing. A similar variety of connections is present in the retina. In the thalamus, the dendrodendritic connections are mainly oriented from the intrinsic to the principal elements. In the cerebellum, there is a notable absence of connections between the dendrites of the two elements.

These different arrangements will be discussed in due course. Here it may simply be noted that almost every conceivable variation is rung on this triadic theme in the various local regions of the brain; in any given region, the variation is specific for the type of information processing carried out there. The basic patterns are easiest to identify in tightly organized regions, like those just mentioned. In more spread-out regions, like the ventral horn and cerebral cortex, the arrangements are diffuse and more difficult to identify. Even in these cases, however, the three basic elements still stand in some kind of relation to each other, be it in parallel or in sequence, and it is, therefore, useful to use the concept as the basis for understanding the synaptic framework of a region and comparing it with other regions.

If we turn now to the second level of organization in the olfactory bulb, we see that the mitral and granule cell dendrites form the principal and intrinsic elements, respectively. The input elements at this level are of two types. The afferent input comes by way of the mitral primary dendrite; there is therefore an exclusive input to the principal element of the triad by this route. The central input, on the other hand, makes synapses onto the granule cell, and this input therefore is directed exclusively to the intrinsic element.

As a consequence of the two-tier separation of connections within the bulb, the mitral and PG cell synapses within the glomeruli are concerned exclusively with olfactory processing, whereas, at the deeper level, the mitral and granule cell synapses are concerned both with olfactory processing and with integration of information passing forward from the brain through the granule cell, as described above. Some of the information from the brain may be in the form of feedback through long loops from the olfactory projection areas. Some of it, however, may be in the form of nonolfactory signals from hypothalamic and limbic structures. The granule-to-mitral synapse is, therefore, of interest as a specific site at which there is an overlap of distinct functions. One may characterize it in this regard as a *multifunctional*, or *multiplex*, synapse.

The lamination of central inputs to the granule cell is an important aspect of functional organization, which will be discussed further with respect to dendritic properties.

Two points relevant to the organization of the olfactory bulb as a cortical structure may be noted. There is a strong implication that a glomerulus may function to some extent as a functional unit. This has been long suspected on anatomical grounds (see Clark, 1957). Recent anatomical studies indicate that there may be several levels of organization within a single olfactory glomerulus (Land and Shepherd, 1974). There is physiological evidence for glomerular specificity for different olfactory stimuli (Leveteau and MacLeod, 1966), and the 2-deoxyglucose experiments indicate strongly that there are groups of glomeruli with similar specificities for a given odor (Sharp et al., 1977; see Chapter 4). It has been pointed out that if glomeruli have this functional specificity, then the group of mitral, tufted, and PG cells with dendrites connected to a particular glomerulus would all share this specificity. This would imply a horizontal constraint on the organization of functionally related neurons in the bulb, which may be analogous to the functional columns of the cerebral cortex (Shepherd, 1972a). We will return to this question when we discuss the glomeruli (barrels) and columns of the cortex.

One of the chief functions of the principal neuron is to provide the vertical conducting and integrating loci across the bulbar cortex, as shown in Fig. 8.4. The lamination of the bulb, therefore, reflects the sequence of interactions carried out in relation to the principal neuron. A key point is that this sequence is nonrepeating: at successive depths, the structures are different, the synaptic connections are different, and the functional interactions are different. There is, therefore, a *nonrepeating sequence of structure and function* in relation to the principal neuron at progressive depths in the cortex, and this expresses itself in the sequence of laminae; it is an *oriented multicellular system*. Such considerations as these may be said to touch on the essence of cortical organization, in contrast to the classical considerations of such points as the numbers of layers, granules, etc. We shall have occasion to amplify this theme in later chapters.

SYNAPTIC ACTIONS

It would be nice if synaptic actions in the olfactory bulb could be elucidated using natural stimuli, as can be done in the retina. But such things

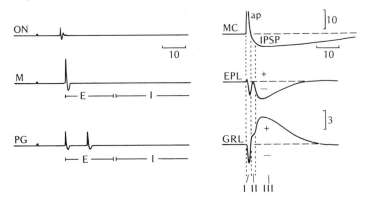

FIG. 8.5. The main types of synaptic actions in the olfactory bulb.

Left, ON, extracellular recording of an afferent volley in olfactory nerves; M, extracellular recording of the spike response of a mitral cell; PG, extracellular recording of the spike response of a periglomerular cell. Periods of excitatory and inhibitory action, as revealed by a second test volley, are indicated by E and I, respectively. (After Shepherd, 1963; Getchell and Shepherd, 1975a,b.)

Right, MC, intracellular recording from a mitral cell body, showing an anti-dromic impulse (ap) followed by an IPSP. (After Yamamoto et al., 1962; Phillips et al., 1963; Nicoll, 1969; Mori and Takagi, 1978a,b). EPL, summed evoked potentials in the external plexiform layer; GRL, summed potentials in the granule layer. Time periods of EPL and GRL response are indicated by dotted lines and I, II, and III below (see text). (After Phillips et al., 1963; Rall and Shepherd, 1968.)

are not yet possible, and analysis has had to rely on electrophysiological techniques. Fortunately, the bulb is admirably suited for this, for it shares with the ventral horn the advantage that its input and output pathways are quite separate and can, therefore, be activated independently. Since the intrinsic neurons are small, the analysis of their properties has had to be based on extracellular recordings of units and summed potentials.

A single volley set up by an electrical shock to the olfactory nerves gives rise to a sequence of actions depicted on the left of Fig. 8.5. The volley reaches the bulb after a long delay (ON in Fig. 8.5), due to the slow conduction velocity (0.3–0.5 m/sec) in the thin unmyelinated axons. The impulse volley depolarizes the axon terminals, activating excitatory synapses onto the dendrites in the glomeruli. The EPSP set up in a mitral cell dendritic tuft has two functions. One is to spread to the primary dendrite and through it generate impulses in the mitral cell (M in Fig. 8.5). The other function is to activate the local synapses of the dendritic tuft onto the dendritic terminals of the PG cells. This EPSP in the PG cell dendrites also has two functions: it spreads to the PG cell axon hillock to generate an impulse discharge (PG in Fig. 8.5), and, locally, it activates the dendritic synapses of the PG cell onto other dendrites, including the reciprocal synapse back onto the mitral cell dendrites. These pathways can be traced in the basic circuit diagram of Fig. 8.4. There is evidence that the output of the PG neuron is inhibitory at both its dendrodendritic and axodendritic synapses (Shepherd, 1971; Getchell and Shepherd, 1975b).

We turn next to the actions engendered by the impulse in the mitral cell body. These have been investigated most directly by backfiring the mitral cell antidromically from the LOT. An intracellular electrode in the cell body records the response shown in MC in Fig. 8.5, an impulse followed by a long-lasting hyperpolarization. This has been shown to have the characteristics of an IPSP (Yamamoto, Yamamoto, and Iwama, 1963; Phillips, Powell, and Shepherd, 1963; Nicoll, 1969; Mori and Takagi, 1978 a,b).

The synaptic pathway for this IPSP was deduced from an analysis of the summed extracellular potentials evoked by the antidromic volley. In the external plexiform layer (EPL), three successive time periods were identified in the evoked potential (Fig. 8.5). The first two are brief and are related to the invasion of the impulse into the cell body (period I) and the spread into the dendrites (period II); period III, on the other hand, is generated primarily by an EPSP in the granule cell arborization. The potentials in the granule layer (GRL in Fig. 8.5) can be divided into the same periods, but they have polarities that are generally the inverse of those in the EPL, and they differ in magnitude, according to a potential divider effect in the external recording circuit. By reconstructing the mitral and granule cell population responses with biophysical models (see below), and incorporating the external recording circuit, it was possible to reconstruct the physiological results. From this analysis it was postulated that the predominant pathway for the recurrent inhibition of mitral cells was by way of dendrodendritic connections through the granule cells. This was confirmed by the electron microscopic evidence, summarized in Fig. 8.3. The details of the analysis may be found in Rall and Shepherd (1968), Rall (1970), and Shepherd (1972). With regard to the extracellular potential analysis, perhaps the most important point for the general reader to grasp is that it was based on a division of the response into successive time periods, rather than into labeled components, as is the usual practice in studies in other parts of the brain. The stereotyped lamination of the bulb provided an important advantage for this approach.

Certain features of these synaptic actions in the olfactory bulb are of particular interest. One is that the major actions between principal and intrinsic neurons are through dendrodendritic synapses. The synapses are activated either by a graded presynaptic depolarization (in the case of the synapses in the glomerulus, and the granule-to-mitral synapse in the EPL) or by a presynaptic impulse (in the case of the mitral-to-granule synapse in the EPL). The properties of these synapses are in principle the same as those of the neuromuscular junction and the axodendritic synapses onto motoneurons; thus, there is nothing unusual in the mechanism of dendrodendritic synapses, as far as these properties are concerned.

The long-lasting nature of the synaptic actions in the olfactory bulb is notable. It may be recalled that the synaptic potentials in motoneurons are relatively brief; long-lasting responses, as in the case of the recurrent IPSP, are due to repetitive firing of interneurons. But in the olfactory bulb, a single volley gives rise to prolonged synaptic actions, as witness the prolonged excitatory period in the mitral tuft (M in Fig. 8.5) or the IPSP caused by the granule cell input to the mitral dendrites (MC). These persistent actions are not associated with impulse firing throughout; they must be due, rather, to prolonged release of transmitter, sequestration of transmitter, or persistent postsynaptic responses to the initial transmitter released. Similar long-lasting synaptic actions occur in other parts of the brain, as we shall see.

DENDRODENDRITIC RECURRENT INHIBITION   The postulated mechanism of the dendrodendritic pathway between mitral and granule cells is considered in more detail in Fig. 8.6. In (A) is shown the sequence of mitral depolarization (I), granule spine EPSP (II), and mitral IPSP (III). Note that the sequence is such that the IPSP in the mitral dendrite follows the initial brief impulse; it thus occurs in the repolarizing aftermath of the impulse. This sequence ensures that the impulse and the IPSP do not clash or in some way "short-circuit" each other; the IPSP always follows the impulse, and the repolarization, in fact, sums with the IPSP action.

The spatial aspects of the inhibition are illustrated in Fig. 8.6 (B). Here, it can be seen that the granule EPSP not only provides for self-

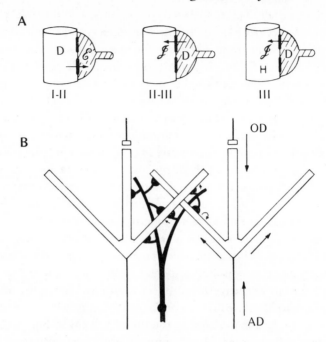

FIG. 8.6. (A) Postulated mechanisms of action of the dendrodendritic synaptic pathway between mitral (open) and granule (shaded) cells, during successive time periods I, II, and III following an antidromic volley. D, depolarization; H, hyperpolarization; E, excitation; I, inhibition. (B) Diagram of the pathways for self and lateral inhibition through dendrodendritic connections. OD, orthodromic (normal) activation; AD, antidromic activation. (From Rall and Shepherd, 1968.)

inhibition of an active mitral cell, but also lateral inhibition of neighboring mitral cells. This is by virtue of the spread of the EPSP to neighboring spines of the same granule tree, and of the numerous connections a single granule cell makes with different mitral cells. By this means the granule cells mediate both feedforward and feedback inhibitory control of the mitral cells.

The mechanism postulated in Fig. 8.6 has been supported by subsequent experimental studies (Nicholl, 1969; Getchell and Shepherd, 1975a; Mori and Takagi, 1978a,b), and recently has been tested by the computational model of Shepherd and Brayton (1978), as discussed in Chapter 5. The spread of activity within the granule tree will be considered further in the section on Dendritic Properties.

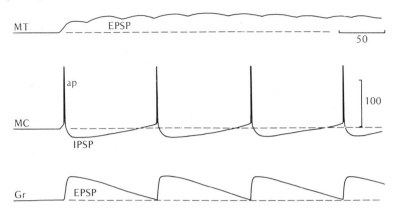

FIG. 8.7. Postulated mechanism whereby the dendrodendritic pathway may provide for rhythmic activity in the olfactory bulb. Postulated intracellular potentials are shown for the mitral dendritic tuft in the glomerulus (MT), mitral cell body (MC), and granule cell (Gr). See text.

The reciprocal dendrodendritic synapses can be seen as providing for recurrent inhibition by a pathway different from that for Renshaw inhibition. The essence of the difference is that the dendrodendritic pathway is local in character; the inhibitory actions of a given mitral cell are confined to the cell itself and to neighboring mitral cells. Even the additional Renshaw-like pathway through the mitral axon collaterals has a local character, in being directed to individual granule spines (see Fig. 8.4). Recurrent inhibition in the spinal cord, on the other hand, entails the activation of an impulse in the Renshaw interneuron that invades all the axonal branches; it, therefore, has a wide field of action. Because the granule cell has different input-output relations in different parts of the dendritic tree, there is a fractionation of these relations.

RHYTHMIC ACTIVITY   The sequence of dendrodendritic interactions described above is of additional interest in that it provides the basis for the generation of rhythmic activity in the neuronal populations of the bulb. The mechanism will be briefly described (Fig. 8.7).

As illustrated in Fig. 8.7, the sequence begins with a long-lasting EPSP in the mitral dendritic tufts (MT) in the glomeruli, due to the olfactory nerve input or the intrinsic activity at the glomerular level. The first mitral impulse generated by the EPSP (MC) synchronously activates all the granule cells with which that mitral cell has synaptic connections (GR). These deliver feedback inhibition of the activated mitral cell, and feedforward inhibition of neighboring inactive mitral cells, in the way already described relative to Fig. 8.6. As the mitral IPSP subsides, a point is reached at which the EPSP is again at threshold; an impulse is again initiated, and the cycle repeats itself. Through the extensive interconnections between the mitral and granule cells, a steady input in the glomeruli is converted into a rhythmic impulse output in the mitral cell population, locked to a rhythmic activation of the granule cell population.

The activity in these populations generates electric current, which flows through the cells according to the electrotonic properties to be described below. The current flows from the individual neurons summate in the extracellular spaces in and around the olfactory bulb and give rise, thereby, to summed extracellular potentials, which are recorded by an electroencephalograph (EEG). Such rhythmic EEG potentials are a prominent characteristic of the olfactory bulb in the resting state as well as during olfactory-induced activity (Adrian, 1950). Similar mechanisms, although not involving dendrodendritic synaptic connections, have been proposed for the generation of EEG waves in the prepyriform cortex, thalamus, and cerebral cortex. They will be described further in later chapters.

SENSORY PROCESSING   From the foregoing account it can be seen that enough is known about synaptic circuits to inquire into their role in olfactory processing. One approach to this question has been to develop methods for precise control of the stimulus, corresponding to the pulses of light, tone pips, etc., that have been employed so successfully in the analysis of other sensory systems. Using small jets of odor, Kauer and Moulton (1974) showed that single mitral cells in the salamander olfactory bulb are either excited, suppressed, or unaffected by any given odor. The excitation tends to be elicited from restricted areas on the olfactory mucosa, whereas the suppression is elicited from large areas. This was the first evidence for receptive field organization in the olfactory system, and correlates with anatomical evidence for topographically organized projections (cf. Shepherd, 1972a; Land and Shepherd, 1974). The large fields for suppression have been postulated to reflect the widespread dendrodendritic connections of the granule cells mediating inhibition of the mitral cells.

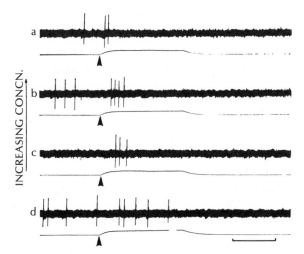

FIG. 8.8. Mitral cell responses to odor stimulation at increasing concentrations. Extracellular unit recordings in salamander; amyl acetate odor. Note prolonged impulse discharge in response to odor stimulation at lowest concentration (d), changing to brief bursts followed by supression at higher concentrations. Lower traces show stimulus monitor; arrow heads show time of stimulus onset. bar: 2 sec. (From Kauer and Shepherd, 1977.)

Analysis of temporal aspects of responses, using brief step pulses of odor, has shown that excitatory responses consist of a prolonged impulse discharge at weak, threshold, odor concentrations, changing to a brief, high frequency burst followed by prolonged suppression as concentration is raised (Kauer, 1974; Kauer and Shepherd, 1977). A typical result is illustrated in Fig. 8.8. Suppressive responses, by comparison, are similar throughout the concentration range. These results indicate that inhibition plays a powerful role in shaping excitatory response patterns, as well as suppressing many mitral cells completely. There is the impression from these experiments of a broad curtain of inhibition drawn across the olfactory bulb, through which excitation pierces, carrying specific information about the stimulating molecules. The inhibition contributing to these effects may be mediated through both glomerular and granule cell circuits.

Another approach to the analysis of sensory olfactory processing has been to analyze the patterns of activity in the olfactory bulb during natural stimulation with odors in awake, behaving animals. The

2-deoxyglucose method has provided a means for achieving this (Sharp et al., 1975; 1977), and the patterns revealed by this method have been illustrated in Fig. 4.10 (Chapter 4). The patterns suggest that the primary excitatory drive is provided by groups of receptors whose axons converge onto glomeruli within topographically confined regions of the olfactory bulb.

These recent studies thus provide clear evidence for the interplay of excitatory and inhibitory mechanisms in olfactory processing in both spatial and temporal domains. The results are consistent with the postulate that these mechanisms are to be found in the synaptic organization of the glomerular and granule cell levels, as summarized in the basic circuit of Fig. 8.4. They provide an interesting comparison with the mechanisms for sensory processing revealed in studies of the retina and the sensory cortex, as discussed in later chapters.

NEUROTRANSMITTERS

Adding to its interest as a model system is the fact that the olfactory bulb contains many of the major types of transmitters. Figure 8.9 summarizes our present information.

The best evidence relates to GABA and the granule-to-mitral inhibitory synapses. The granule cells take up GABA (Halasz, Llungdahl, and Hökfelt, 1978b), and GAD has been localized in the granule cells and the granule cell spines by EM immunocytochemistry (Ribak et al., 1977; see Fig. 2.3). Microiontophoresis of GABA causes a depression of mitral cell firing; bicuculline counteracts this effect, and also reduces the inhibition of test responses after conditioning LOT volleys (McLennan, 1971; Nicoll, 1971).

Studies of the mitral-to-granule excitatory synapse have emphasized the importance of knowledge of synaptic organization in interpreting neuropharmacological results. Microiontophoresis of amino acids, particularly aspartate and DL-homocysteate, tends to inhibit mitral cell activity. This appeared at first to be rather confusing, in view of the usual excitatory effects of these amino acids on other neurons. However, closer consideration suggested that the action of these substances was to excite the granule cell spines, which then inhibit the mitral cells (McLennan, 1971; Nicoll, 1971). This serves as a model for the local interactions that must be taken into account in interpreting microiontophoresis studies.

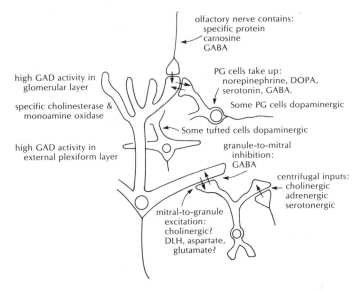

FIG. 8.9. Summary of putative transmitters in the mammalian olfactory bulb. (Modified from Shepherd, 1977.)

The case for aspartate as the transmitter at all the output synapses made by the mitral cell dendrites in the olfactory bulb is strengthened by the evidence for aspartate as the transmitter at the axon terminals of the mitral cells in the olfactory cortex (see Chapter 13); this would be an example of the workings of Dale's Law. However, there are other candidates. Recently, alpha-bungarotoxin binding has been localized to the external plexiform layer and the glomerular neuropil, consistent with an interpretation that the mitral cells might be cholinergic at their dendritic output synapses (Hunt and Schmidt, 1978).

In the glomerular layer, histofluorescence studies show that some periglomerular cells are positive for dopamine-synthesizing enzymes (Halasz et al., 1977). In addition, some cells and their dendrites contain GAD, and take up GABA (see Ribak et al., 1977). These results show that a single morphological type of neuron—the PG cell—can be fractionated biochemically into two types with regard to possible transmitters. And this is not all; some external tufted cells also appear to be dopaminergic (Halasz et al., 1977). This offers yet a third transmitter candidate for at least some of the mitral and tufted cell dendritic synapses. The evidence for inhibitory actions of PG cells (Getchell and Shepherd, 1975b) is consistent with either GABA or dopamine at PG cell synapses.

The olfactory nerves have received considerable attention in studies of axonal transport and biochemical composition. They have been found to contain high concentrations of the dipeptide, carnosine, as well as a specific olfactory protein (MW = 20,000) (Margolis, 1978). However, there is as yet no direct evidence regarding transmitters at the olfactory nerve terminals in the glomeruli.

The central inputs to the olfactory bulb include noradrenergic fibers from the locus coeruleus, and serotonergic fibers from the raphe nucleus (see Halasz et al., 1978b; Broadwell, 1978). It is of interest that the olfactory bulb was the first brain region to serve as a model for the identification of noradrenalin (NA) as a central neurotransmitter (see Bloom, 1971). Iontophoresis of NA produces a depression of mitral cell activity. Interpretation of this and similar findings must take into account the local synaptic arrangements, as noted above.

DENDRITIC PROPERTIES

In olfactory bulb neurons, as in the motoneuron, an understanding of synaptic integration must be based on an understanding of the electrotonic properties of the dendrites. Because of the prevalence of dendro-dendritic synapses, the bulb is a model for the study of dendritic properties in relation to dendrodendritic interactions. We will see that these interactions include most of the types found in other brain regions where dendrodendritic synapses occur.

MITRAL CELL   In studying the mitral cell, it soon becomes apparent that its dendritic tree is not one homogeneous entity, as in the case of the motoneuron. Rather, the mitral dendritic tree is divided into several distinct anatomical entities, and each entity has its own distinct function. The glomerular dendritic tuft is primarily concerned with reception and processing of the olfactory input; it is analogous in this respect to the entire dendritic tree of a thalamic relay neuron. The primary dendritic shaft has as its main function the transfer of information from the glomerular tuft to the cell body; it is analogous in this respect to a retinal bipolar cell. The secondary dendritic branches, finally, are exclusively concerned with interactions with the granule cells.

These divisions are so distinct that it seems as if the mitral cell is not one but three cells, with transfer between them taking place through intraneuronal continuity rather than interneuronal synapses. This means that we must assess dendritic properties in relation to the different functions of each of these entities.

Let us begin with the *glomerular tuft*. We have seen that it forms a small dendritic tree within an olfactory glomerulus. The initial trunks of the tuft have relatively small diameters of 1–3 μm. Let us assume that each dendritic trunk divides in such a way as to conform to the 3/2 power constraint on the diameter, as discussed in Chapter 5. Each trunk will thus give rise to a small equivalent cylinder, which taken together will form an equivalent cylinder for the entire tuft. Then, assuming a range of values for electrical parameters that is typical of neurons, we can obtain an estimate from the graph of Fig. 5.2 of a characteristic length of 150–600 μm for the case of 1-μm diameter trunks and 300–1000 μm for 3-μm diameter trunks.

The significance of these estimates is seen when they are compared with the actual extent of the tuft, which is some 150–200 μm. The estimates are thus considerably higher than the actual extents of the tufts. The electrotonic length ($L = x/\lambda$) of an equivalent cylinder for the tuft might, therefore, be estimated at less than 1, and possibly less than 0.5. Note that this is even shorter than the electrotonic length of the equivalent cylinder for the motoneuron dendritic tree. Thus, the smaller branches of the tuft are counterbalanced by their shorter lengths, an expression of the scaling principle previously mentioned in Chapter 7. Because of the short electrotonic length of the tuft, current flow through the tuft must be relatively effective by passive means alone.

Next to be considered is the *primary dendrite*. This is a single unbranched process, and it is, therefore, easy to make a model for it. From the graph of Fig. 5.2, it can be seen that likely estimates for the characteristic length of a typical primary dendrite of 6 μm diameter fall in the range of 300–1500 μm. Since a primary dendrite has a length of some 400 μm, it appears that the electrotonic length of this example is at the most 1, and perhaps even less than 0.5. Electrotonic spread should, therefore, be relatively effective through such a process. Apparently, the relatively large diameter of the primary dendrite helps overcome the considerable distance required for the transmission of signals across the EPL. We have noted that myelin has been observed wrapped around the

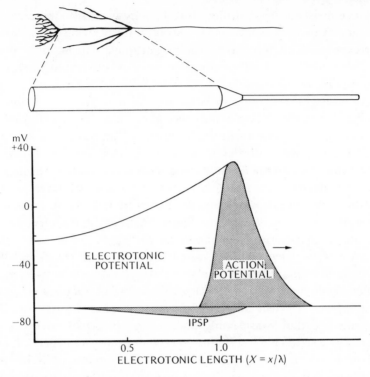

FIG. 8.10. Electrotonic model of the mitral cell, illustrating the spread of potentials in secondary dendrites.

distal primary dendrites in primates, but not in lower animals. Possibly the myelin is associated with active properties of the dendrites; alternatively, it may serve to enhance passive spread. More work is needed.

Finally to be considered are the *secondary dendrites*. The key question with regard to this compartment of the mitral dendritic tree has been the extent to which an impulse at the cell body would invade the secondary dendrites and activate the mitral-to-granule synapses. In the course of investigating the extracellular potential fields in the olfactory bulb, a biophysical model was developed for the secondary dendrites that is relevant to just this problem. This investigation provided the basis for the postulation of the existence of dendrodendritic synaptic interactions in the bulb (Rall et al., 1966; Rall and Shepherd, 1968).

The steps for modeling the secondary dendrites follow those already outlined. By these steps, an equivalent cylinder for the tree of dendrites is obtained; it is illustrated in Fig. 8.10. Individual secondary dendrites are 2–6 μm in diameter and 400–600 μm in length. Their electrotonic lengths, as well as the values for the equivalent cylinder for the entire tree, have been estimated to lie in the range of 0.5 to 1.

In the investigation of the properties of secondary dendrites, a model for the action potential was also developed, so that it was possible to simulate an experiment in which an impulse propagates into the cell body and spreads into the dendrites (Rall and Shepherd, 1968). Computational experiments were carried out in which different assumptions were made about the electrotonic lengths of the dendrites and their active and passive properties. The use of biophysical models to perform such experiments that simulate situations often inaccessible in the biological preparation itself is a powerful approach that was early stressed by Rall (1964) and has recently been explored in the cerebellar Purkinje cell and hippocampal pyramidal cell, as we shall see.

The main result obtained from the model was that impulse spread into the secondary dendrites is very effective by passive means alone. This is illustrated schematically in the diagram of Fig. 8.10. Passive spread is, in fact, so effective that it was difficult in the computations to distinguish a passively spreading impulse from an actively propagating one, in some cases; this was also true for the primary dendrites. Although this does not answer the question of whether the secondary dendrites have active properties, it does establish the point that an impulse spreading by passive electrotonus retains much of its amplitude and wave form and, therefore, can activate the mitral-to-granule synapses in much the same way a propagating impulse would. Thus, the IPSP produced by feedback from the granule cells would be expected to be distributed throughout the dendritic tree, as indicated in Fig. 8.10.

In most principal neurons, the dendritic tree receives and integrates both excitation and inhibitory synaptic actions. The mitral secondary dendrites stand out in contrast; they are specialized to receive only inhibition, that inhibition coming from only one type of intrinsic neuron, the granule cell.

GRANULE CELL   Since the granule cell lacks an axon, study of its dendritic properties is obviously crucial to an understanding of its input-output functions.

In the investigation of the recurrent dendrodendritic pathway by Rall

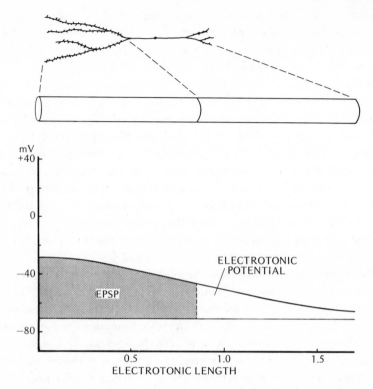

FIG. 8.11. Electrotonic model of the granule cell, illustrating the spread of potentials for case of EPSP due to a dendrodendritic input to spines in the external plexiform layer.

and Shepherd (1968), a model for the granule cell was developed and explored. The steps in its construction are summarized in Fig. 8.11. The branching tree within the EPL is represented by an equivalent cylinder; branch diameters of 0.2–0.8 μm were assumed, an electrotonic length of about 0.4 was estimated. The shaft diameter of the granule cell is of the order of 1 μm; for an average shaft length of 600 μm, an electrotonic length of 1.7 was estimated for the model of the combined tree and shaft. This is significantly longer than the estimates for the different parts of the mitral dendritic tree, but it is similar to the estimates for the motoneuron and the apical dendrites of cortical pyramidal cells.

We consider the case of synaptic depolarization of the granule spines in the EPL, as shown in Fig. 8.11. The distribution of intracellular potential in the model during the rising phase of the EPSP is shown diagrammatically. The importance of this model in the study of Rall and Shepherd was its demonstration that this synaptic depolarization gives rise to the period III extracellular potentials that are recorded in physiological experiments (Phillips, Powell, and Shepherd, 1963; see Fig. 8.5). When the mitral cell model and the granule cell model were joined in sequence, it could be postulated that the EPSP in the spines is due to a dendrodendritic input from the mitral secondary dendrites. As described in the previous section, the localization and timing indicated that the spine EPSP activates inhibitory synapses onto the same secondary dendrites, to produce the long-lasting IPSP recorded in the physiological experiments (Phillips et al., 1963).

What can be said about the properties of the granule *dendritic spines* within the EPL, spines that have both synaptic input and output? This has already been discussed in relation to Fig. 8.11 and to the computational model in Fig. 5.5. Although the stems, or necks, of the spines may be narrow (i.e. 0.2 μm) and the intervening branches thin (i.e., 0.2–0.5 μm), any reasonable assumptions about the electrical properties of the membranes lead to the conclusion that electrotonic spread from spine to spine is considerable over the short distances involved. It appears therefore that lateral inhibition can be mediated by passive spread alone through the dendritic tree in the EPL. The inhibition is spatially graded according to the electrotonic decrement of the potentials in the tree.

As in the case of the mitral cell dendrites, these considerations do not rule out the possibility of active properties of the granule dendritic membrane, in addition to electrotonic properties. Might the spines themselves have active properties, so that spread into the branches is more effective? And might the branches have active properties, for which there is evidence in cerebellar Purkinje cells and hippocampal pyramidal cells? The biophysical model for the granule cell does not rule out active spine properties, but it indicates that active properties must be limited and not lead to propagation from the branches in the EPL into the main dendritic shaft. These questions have been discussed at greater length by Rall and Shepherd (1968) and Shepherd (1972a).

Finally, what may be said with regard to other inputs to the granule cell, particularly the centrifugal inputs from the AON and AC? These inputs make synapses on the shaft and deep processes, and the question arises of how the EPSPs from these inputs spread to activate the output synapses in the EPL. For inputs to the deep processes, perhaps 1 to 2 characteristic lengths (λ) away from the EPL, it would appear that the effect on the synapses in the EPL would be limited if spread through the shaft were by passive means alone. Certainly the amount of activation must be much less than with direct activation of the spines by the reciprocal synapses. The centrifugal inputs, however, have been shown to be capable of giving rise to substantial extracellular field potentials, indicating that spread through the granule shafts is, in fact, effective. Whether this is by virtue of very large EPSPs, or whether spread is assisted by active properties, is not known. Similar questions will arise when the properties of the apical dendrites of pyramidal cells in the hippocampus and neocortex are discussed.

PERIGLOMERULAR CELL   The PG cell has already been discussed as an example of the short-axon cell, a type we will encounter in many parts of the brain. Being small, the PG cell has been relatively inaccessible to experimental studies, and there is yet no biophysical model as in the cases of the mitral and granule cells. For a first approximation to its over-all electrotonic properties, the dendritic tuft may be regarded as a smaller version of the mitral dendritic tuft described above. Taking into account both the smaller diameters and the shorter lengths of the branches, it seems reasonable to conclude that an equivalent cylinder for the PG cell tuft would be similar to that for the mitral tuft, i.e., $L = 0.5$–1.0. This is, again, an expression of the scaling principle for dendritic trees of different size.

   PG cell functions appear to be exquisitely dependent on levels of input activity. At threshold there is mainly straight-through excitation of mitral cells by receptor axons; long-lasting facilitation is sometimes detectable (Getchell and Shepherd, 1975a,b). As input activity increases, the activation of PG cells, both by direct olfactory axon input and indirect dendrodendritic synapses, begins to bring about inhibitory feedback from the PG cell dendrites. Small EPSPs probably mediate only local input-output paths through the dendrites; moderate EPSPs will lead to more extensive inhibitory actions within a glomerulus, large EPSPs, by spreading to the axon hillock, set up impulses which mediate inhibition of dendrites arising from neighboring glomeruli. Thus, several levels of interaction can be identified within the glomerular layer, governed by the amplitudes of EPSPs and their electrotonic spread within the PG cell dendrites. Functionally, these interactions enhance transmission at detection thresholds, and provide the lateral inhibition necessary for discrimination between odors at higher odor concentrations. The PG cell dendritic tree thus provides for *multiple-state-dependent input-output functions.* Similar properties have been postulated for thalamic short-axon cells, and may apply to other types of cells.

9

RETINA

The retina is a thin sheet of nervous tissue at the back of the eye, wherein takes place the reception of visual stimuli and the initial stages of processing of information in the visual pathway. The retina differs from the olfactory bulb and from other sensory centers in that the receptors are a part of the neuronal region itself. There is also the obvious difference in geometry between the sheet-like retina and the bulb-like bulb. The flattened conformation of the retina is dictated by the distribution of visual receptors, which in turn is determined by the optics of the eye. These overt features of the retina are striking, but their functional significance can only be assessed in light of an understanding of the internal synaptic organization.

In terms of its main cell types and layers, the retina retains a remarkably similar structure throughout the vertebrate series. It varies considerably, however, in the amount of processing of the visual input carried out within it. On this basis, one distinguishes between simple retinas, in which there is relatively little processing, and complex retinas, in which there is a great deal of processing. This division is notable in not following an evolutionary progression; frogs and rabbits, for example, have complex retinas, whereas primates, including man, have simple retinas (Dowling, 1968; Michael, 1969). The difference reflects the extent to which various types of processing are postponed to higher levels in the central visual pathways.

NEURONAL ELEMENTS

The over-all similarity in the construction of vertebrate retinas belies the fact that the neuronal elements are differentiated into subtypes, some of which are absent, or show wide variation, in different parts of the same

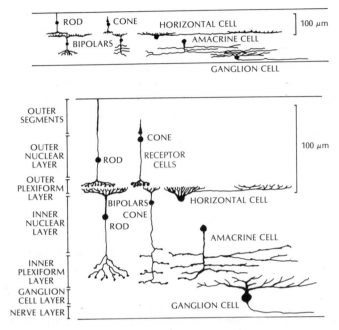

FIG. 9.1. Neuronal elements of the mammalian retina (same scale as diagrams for other regions).

FIG. 9.2. Neuronal elements, scale enlarged ×5 in the vertical axis, to show more clearly the cell morphology and layers.

Inputs: rod and cone receptors

Principal neuron: ganglion cells

Intrinsic neurons: bipolar, horizontal, and amacrine cells.

Retinal layers indicated at the left.

retina, as well as in different species. It is thus impossible to summarize the neuronal elements of the vertebrate retina in one diagram. Our recourse will be to illustrate the main elements of one part of a simple retina, that of the primate, and briefly note comparisons with the elements of complex retinas. The treatment is much oversimplified, and the interested reader should consult Cajal (1911), Polyak (1941), Boycott and Dowling (1969), and Stell (1972) for details.

The neuronal elements of the primate retina are shown in Figs. 9.1 and 9.2. Figure 9.1 is drawn to the same scale as the other diagrams in this book. It emphasizes an important feature of the retina, its extraordinary thinness. The over-all depth is less than 300 μm; apart from the receptor layer, the span of the neuronal elements themselves is less than

200 μm. This is less than the thickness of a single layer in most other regions of the brain. The nerve cells are small and their processes are very limited in the vertical dimension, although in the lateral dimension they may reach extents comparable to those in other brain regions. In the study of synaptic organization, the thinness of the retina cannot be overemphasized. It is the key to understanding the morphology of the neurons and the properties of their dendrites.

INPUTS The sensory input to the retina is, of course, light. As is well known, the *visual receptors* are of two types: *cones* and *rods*. Cones are specialized for reception of bright light, as in daylight, whereas rods are specialized for reception of dim light, as at night. In most species, the cones also contain the specific pigments that provide for color vision, but there are exceptions to this structure-function relation (see Cohen, 1972).

The receptor cell bodies form a sheet, the outer nuclear layer (ONL) (Fig. 9.2). Although the receptors are not strictly a part of the neuronal systems of the retina, their properties are crucial to an understanding of retinal organization, as will be pointed out in due course.

The receptors provide the input to the neuronal systems of the retina, analogous to the afferent inputs to the ventral horn and the olfactory bulb. The retina shares with the olfactory bulb the property of having an input of only one sensory modality, although the inputs from cones responding to different wavelengths of light (e.g., color) may be considered submodalities. The input is sent through the process that connects the receptor site in the outer segment through the cell body to the synaptic terminals. In the peripheral part of the retina, this process is vertically oriented and very short (25–50 μm); near the center of vision (fovea), the neuronal elements to which the receptors connect are laterally displaced, so that the processes may run for considerable lengths (up to 0.5 mm). The process is thin (0.5–1.0 μm in rods, 1–2 μm in cones). It is usually referred to as an axon, but, in fact, its fine structure does not permit it to be positively classified as axon or dendrite. This problem of identification will recur with the other elements of the retina.

The receptor terminals are localized within a layer called the outer plexiform layer (OPL) (Fig. 9.2). In the primate, the cone terminals are large and flattened (5–6 μm across in the central region, up to 15 μm across in the periphery) and are called *pedicles*. Rod terminals on the other hand are small and round (2–4 μm across) and are called *spherules*. This distinction applies generally to other vertebrates, although, in lower forms, the terminals may be more extensive and arborized, and pedicles may arise from rods. The OPL is extremely thin, scarcely more than 10 μm in the primate, as well as in most other species; the terminals of the receptors are thus extremely restricted in vertical extent, more so than for the input to any other region of the brain in our study.

In addition to this afferent input there is in some species a *central* (centrifugal) input from the brain. These fibers run in the optic nerve and terminate in the deeper layers of the retina (Cowan, 1970). These fibers are present in birds, although they are not numerous; in most vertebrate species they are absent or rare. The retina is thus almost exclusively concerned with the processing of its single afferent input; it is unusual among neuronal centers in this respect.

PRINCIPAL NEURON   The output of the retina to the brain is carried in the axons of *ganglion cells*. Their cell bodies lie in a sheet at the inner margin of the retina (see Fig. 9.2). They vary widely in size and in dendritic arborization. The smallest is the so-called *midget ganglion cell*, found near the fovea in the primate. The cell body is 12–15 μm in diameter; each gives off a single dendritic trunk, several microns thick, that extends vertically only some 20–30 μm, ending in several club-shaped terminals scarcely 5 μm across within the inner plexiform layer (IPL). These tiny cells are unique to primates; their cell bodies are among the smallest of principal neurons in the nervous system, and their dendritic "trees" are among the smallest of any neuron. By virtue of their position near the fovea and their restricted extents and synaptic connections (see below), they provide for the greatest visual acuity.

The largest ganglion cells, by contrast, have cell bodies 20–30 μm in diameter and a trunk (4–8 μm thick) that arborizes over a field of 200–300 μm diameter. Such a cell is termed a giant ganglion cell with *diffuse* dendritic tree. Ganglion cells of intermediate size (cell bodies 15–30 μm across) may have diffuse trees of varying extents (as in the example in Fig. 9.2), or they may have dendrites that branch sparingly at one distinct level; in the latter case, they are called *unistratified* ganglion cells. In nonprimate species, ganglion cells may have several distinct levels of branching in their dendritic trees and are referred to as *multistratified* ganglion cells. These cells are characteristic of complex retinas (Maturana, Lettvin, McCulloch, and Pitts, 1960). In some lower forms, the dendritic trees may extend more than 2 mm (Stell and Witkovsky, 1973).

In the cat, there are three main types of ganglion cell, termed α, β, and ω, with cell body diameters of about 30, 20, and 15 μm, respectively (Boycott and Wässle, 1974). These correspond to the physiological classes Y, X, and W, as discussed later in the chapter.

The axons of the ganglion cells pass along the inner surface of the retina and emerge to form the optic nerve. It is especially notable that within the retina the axons give off no recurrent collaterals. The ganglion cell is one of the few types of output neuron in the nervous system that lacks such collaterals. The optic nerve projects to the lateral geniculate nucleus of the thalamus, which is described in Chapter 11; there are also projections to the tectum (superior colliculus).

INTRINSIC NEURONS   There are three main types of intrinsic neuron in the retina, each clearly differentiated.

Horizontal cells are the most superficial in location (see Fig. 9.2). In the primate, their cell bodies are 10–15 μm in diameter; each gives rise to 10 to 15 trunks of varying thickness (1–5 μm). In the central region, the dendritic fields extend only 25 μm in diameter; in the periphery they extend over 100 μm (Boycott and Dowling, 1969; Kolb, 1970; Boycott and Kolb, 1973). The dendrites terminate within the outer plexiform layer. Several of the processes may be especially long and thin. One such process is commonly longer (several hundred microns) and thinner (1 μm diameter) than the rest, and unbranched; by these criteria, it is referred to as an axon. Although these processes are rarely impregnated in Golgi stains throughout their extent, arborizations of terminals, as is illustrated in Fig. 9.2 are presumed to arise from them. Boycott and his co-workers have provided evidence that the "dendritic" terminals connect only to cone pedicles, whereas the "axonal" terminals connect to rod spherules (see also Fig. 9.7 below).

In other vertebrate species, there may be more than one type of horizontal cell; the processes may extend for considerable distances (500 μm or more), and it is often impossible to identify an axon, whether by Golgi impregnation, dye injection, or electron microscopy. In addition to this problem, the horizontal cells have appeared to many observers to be more like glial cells than neurons. In internal fine structure, they have been reported to lack the Nissl substance and the Golgi apparatus typical of neurons and to possess, on the other hand, some of the morphological features of glial cells (e.g., glycogen granules). Some workers have considered them specialized glial "controller" cells. Most modern workers regard them as neurons, on the basis that they have synaptic connections, generate synaptic responses, and are part of a system for processing sensory information. The horizontal cell thus provides a good example of the problem of defining not only the different parts of the neuron but also the neuron itself.

Bipolar cells are oriented vertically and obviously provide the necessary link between the receptor cells and the ganglion cells. They are differentiated into two main types, one of which connects to cone pedicles, the other to rod spherules. A cone bipolar cell is illustrated in Fig. 9.2. It has a small cell body (8–10 μm in diameter), which has earned it the inevitable eponym *midget*. A single peripheral trunk (several microns in diameter) ascends vertically to terminate in enlargements some 5–6 μm across; these are much the same dimensions as those of the cone pedicles to which it connects. Depending on the connection to the pedicle, the midget bipolar cells are classified as *invaginating* and *flat;* some of the latter have branches to several cones. We will see the significance of these classifications when we consider the synaptic connections. A single deep process (1–2 μm thick) descends some 50 μm or so from the cell body and ends in several knoblike terminals in the IPL.

A rod bipolar cell is also illustrated in Fig. 9.2. This also has a small cell body, a somewhat stouter peripheral trunk, and a number of terminals within the OPL, connecting to many rod spherules. The single deep process arborizes sparingly and terminates in knoblike appendages in the IPL.

In different vertebrate species the bipolar cells show many variations, in terms of size, extent of branching, and overlap in connections from the rods and cones (see Witkovsky, 1971; Witkovsky and Stell, 1973). In complex retinas, there may be elaborate arborizations in the IPL, with the branches stratified into several layers and with laterally extending fields of several hundred microns.

It is usual to regard the outer bipolar cell process as a dendrite and the inner process as an axon. Both, however, are similar in fine structure, and there is apparently no axon hillock. One therefore has a problem of identification not unlike that for the receptors and horizontal cells. There seems to be agreement at least that the fine structure of the bipolar cell is characteristic of a neuron.

Amacrine cells are found in the deeper levels of the retina. Their cell bodies are located in the inner nuclear layer (INL), which also contains the bipolar and horizontal cell bodies. There are several subtypes. One has a cell body of 8–10 μm in diameter, and a stout descending trunk, several microns thick, which immediately arborizes into a number of terminals. These are termed *narrow-field diffuse* amacrine cells; the field of arborization is typically only 25 μm in diameter. Another type gives off several thin (1–2 μm diameter) dendritic trunks, which branch sparingly and spread over a field of 100 μm or so, although some branches may reach greater lengths. These are termed *wide-field diffuse* cells. A third type has branches confined to one layer in the IPL; these are called, appropriately, *unistratified* cells. There is a resemblance between these branching patterns of amacrine cells and those of ganglion cells. In complex retinas, the amacrine cells show a rich diversity of types, particularly of the *multistratified* variety; an example is shown in Fig. 9.2.

We have noted the difficulty of identifying an axon in the horizontal and bipolar cells. The amacrine cell has, in fact, been the traditional example in the retina of a cell without an axon. The earliest studies by Cajal and others, using the Golgi method, established this fact, and it has been confirmed repeatedly in modern studies. The analogy with the granule cell of the olfactory bulb in this respect has long been recognized. There is little doubt that the amacrine cell is a neuron, and the fine structure of its processes is consistent with the designation dendrite.

A new type of cell, termed an *interplexiform cell*, has recently been identified (Ehinger, Falck, and Laties, 1969). The cell body lies among the amacrine cells, and its processes connect to both the outer and inner plexiform layers. It will be described further in the section on neurotransmitters.

If we take an overview of this community of neurons, it is noteworthy that not only are the neurons differentiated into types, but the types are further differentiated into subtypes, on the basis of distinctive patterns of branching and connection. The retina is unusual in this respect. In the ventral horn, for example, the motoneurons vary widely in size but not in their basic branching patterns; even the gamma motoneurons, which are functionally distinct, appear for the most part as smaller editions of the alpha motoneurons. Much the same can be said of mitral and tufted cells in the olfactory bulb. The Purkinje cells in the cerebellum have a particularly monotonous appearance. In general it appears that in most local regions of the brain the neurons of a given type differ mainly in terms of size. In the retina, some of the subtypes are related to the rod and cone systems; this is clearly seen in the horizontal and bipolar cell populations, as well as in certain ganglion cells. Some of the subtypes of amacrine and ganglion cells, however, are not obviously related to these systems; they appear to be related, instead, or in addition, to the processing of other aspects of the visual input.

The retinal neurons bear little similarity to the neurons we have encountered in the ventral horn and olfactory bulb, and will meet in other parts of the brain, with respect to either their small size or their peculiar shape. Does this mean that the retina is *sui generis?* That comparisons with the organization of other regions cannot be made? The peculiarities of the retinal neurons are deceiving in this respect, for they become understandable once one has a grasp of synaptic connections and dendritic properties, and of the functions they serve within the spatial confines of the retina.

CELL POPULATIONS In man, the following estimates have been made: 100,000,000 rod receptors; 5,000,000 cone receptors, 1,000,000 ganglion cells. These give input-output ratios for the retina of 100:1 for rods and 5:1 for cones. The latter, presumably, reflects the high acuity associated with the cone systems. In the human fovea, in fact, where visual acuity is highest, it is believed that the ratio of cones to ganglion cells is less than 1:1. The convergence ratios vary widely for different input-output subsystems within the retina, as has been discussed by Stell (1972).

The numbers of neuronal elements vary considerably in different species. Estimates of the number of optic nerve fibers in some representative species are given in Table 9.1. The figures are a direct measure of the numbers of ganglion cells giving rise to the fibers. It may be seen that there is a general tendency toward larger populations and myelination of the fibers, but there are wide differences between closely related species within that overall framework.

The significance of such numbers depends on many factors, and it is not so obvious as it may appear. For example, Bruesch and Arey (1942) set the 1,000,000 optic nerve fibers against the total of all other craniospinal nerves, and concluded "that 38% of all the fibers entering or leaving the central nervous system do so by way of the optic nerve." This was considered to be a quantitative evaluation of the "predominant

Table 9.1

Quantitative estimates of numbers of optic nerve fibers (from retinal ganglion cells) in different vertebrates.

Lamprey	5,000 (100%)*	Pigeon	1,000,000
Goldfish	53,000	Rat	75,000 (22%)*
Mudpuppy			
(*Necturus*)	360 (100%)*	Cat	100,000
Frog	29,000 (47%)*	Macaque	1,200,000
Chick	400,000	Man	1,000,000

From Bruesch and Arey (1942).
*Percent unmyelinated fibers.

role of vision in human activities"; Granit (1955) cited this figure to the effect that "we are exceptionally visual animals." But the calculation, for some reason, neglected the 50,000,000 olfactory nerve fibers; if they are included, is it evident that we are "exceptionally olfactory" as well? And consider further that there are only some 30,000 auditory fibers to carry the input from the ear to the brain. Is this evidence that the auditory input is insignificant by comparison? Although these numbers are important in reconstructing the mechanisms of information processing in the different sensory systems, they must be viewed with great perspicacity in assessing the relative roles of the systems in the lives of the species.

We may mention, finally, that numbers for intrinsic neuronal elements are hard to come by. It may be estimated that the ratio of bipolar to ganglion cells is of the order of 2:1; of horizontal cells to ganglion cells is 5:1; and of amacrine cells is 10–100:1. These are only very crude estimates, and they vary with the species and complexity of the retina. It is at least clear from these ratios that the populations of intrinsic neurons are relatively large and that a great deal of processing goes on through the connections that they make, particularly at the amacrine cell level. In this respect the retina is similar to the olfactory bulb and different from other regions with relatively low ratios of intrinsic to input and output elements.

SYNAPTIC CONNECTIONS

The study of synaptic connections in the retina has been an extremely active area of research. The identification of terminals has been aided by the sharp differentiation of cell types and the localization of synapses in the outer and inner plexiform layers. The development of techniques for serial reconstructions of electron micrographs (Sjöstrand, 1958; Missotten, 1965; Allen, 1969; Kolb, 1970) and for fine structural analyses of Golgi-stained neurons (Stell, 1964, 1967) has put identification on a sound basis, and has permitted quantitative analyses of some connections to be made. We will again focus our attention on the salient features of the primate retina (for reviews, see Dowling and Boycott, 1966; Stell, 1972).

OUTER PLEXIFORM LAYER The OPL contains the terminals from the receptor cells, bipolar cells, and horizontal cells. A cone pedicle is shown in (A) of Fig. 9.3 and a rod spherule in (B). Note the size of the cone pedicle; it is among the largest terminal structures in the nervous system (compare the terminals of mossy fibers in the cerebellum). That these large structures should arise from the small receptors illustrates the fact that terminal size is not necessarily related to cell body size.

The receptor terminals have invaginations that envelop the terminal processes of both bipolar and horizontal cells. The patterns of connections between the terminals are characteristic for rods and cones. In primates, the invaginations in the *rod spherule* contain a central process of the dendrite of a rod bipolar cell, flanked by two processes from the "axonal" arborizations of horizontal cells. This is shown in Fig. 9.3 (A). The three processes within an invagination have been termed a *triad* (Missotten, 1965; Stell, 1967), not to be confused with our use of that term to apply to general principles of organization (see below). *Cone pedicles* have invaginations in which a dendrite from an invaginating midget bipolar cell is flanked by two processes from the "dendritic" arborizations of horizontal cells [Fig. 9.3 (B)]. Clustered around the bipolar cell dendrite are terminals from several other bipolar cells of the flat midget and flat variety. This may be said to form a *synaptic complex*, in the sense in which that term is used elsewhere in the brain (see Chapter 10). The careful reconstructions of Kolb (1970) have shown that, in the central retina, a single invaginating midget bipolar cell connects to a single cone pedicle by means of 10 to 25 triads. The multiple and exclusive nature of this synaptic relationship is remarkable, although not unique; we have previously noted the multiple contacts of Ia terminals onto motoneuron dendrites. Flat midget bipolar cells connect to approximately 6 cones, whereas rod bipolar cells connect to 10 to 50 rod spherules.

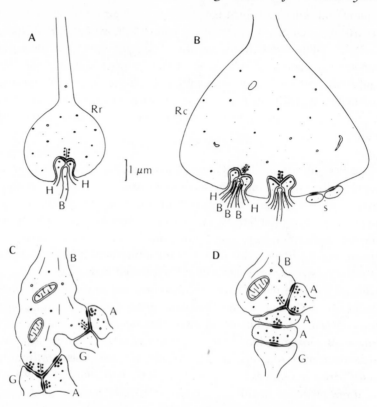

FIG. 9.3. Synaptic connections in the primate retina. (A) Connections in the outer plexiform layer, of a rod receptor (Rr) onto bipolar (B) and horizontal (H) terminals. (B) Connections of a cone receptor (Rc); note also superficial (s) contacts. (After Kolb, 1970; Cohen, 1972.) (C) Connections in the inner plexiform layer, between bipolar terminals and amacrine (A) and ganglion (G) cell dendritic terminals. (After Dowling and Boycott, 1966; Allen, 1969.) (D) For comparison with (C), connections in the inner plexiform layer of a complex retina (frog). (After Dowling, 1968.)

Let us now consider the synaptic junctions more closely. Within the receptor terminal, and opposite the point at which a bipolar and horizontal cell triad of processes meet, is a so-called *synaptic lamella* (Ladman, 1958) or *ribbon*, surrounded by a cluster of vesicles. This is indicated in Fig. 9.3 (A,B). There is a moderate amount of densification of the pre- and postsynaptic membranes in the vicinity of the ribbon. The horizontal cell processes of the triad are in direct apposition to the terminal membrane, but the central bipolar cell process is some 800–1000 Å distant, e.g., roughly 0.1 μm (Dowling and Boycott, 1966). It is not known, in fact, whether synaptic transmission occurs directly from the terminal to the bipolar cell process, or indirectly through the horizontal cell processes. These junctions are, therefore, quite distinctive; they are specialized synapses, in the sense we have previously discussed (Chapter 2). It is clearly at this site that information transfer takes place, and the synaptic ribbon with its vesicles is taken as presumptive evidence that the transfer takes place at least in part by chemical means.

Many other types of synapses are found in the OPL. There are contacts by the flat bipolar cells on the outer faces of the terminals; these are termed *superficial* contacts. In lower vertebrates, simple ("conventional") synapses are observed from horizontal cells to bipolar cells, and between horizontal cells. Gap junctions are present between horizontal cells in some retinas, particularly in fish (Yamada and Ishikawa, 1966), and in the A-type of horizontal cell in the cat (Kolb, 1977); that is significant relative to physiological evidence for electrotonic coupling between horizontal cells in those retinas (see below). Finally, there is evidence in some retinas for contacts between receptors and from horizontal cells back onto receptors (see Stell, 1972, for review). The retina is special in this respect; synapses back onto the input elements are not found in the other regions of the brain in our study.

INNER PLEXIFORM LAYER The second level for synaptic connections is the IPL, which contains the terminals of bipolar, amacrine, and ganglion cells. Ribbon synapses are again encountered, here located within the bipolar cell terminal (Dowling and Boycott, 1966; Dowling, 1968). It is noteworthy that ribbon synapses are found within two cell types that are disparate in morphology and have distinct yet very closely linked functions. Note also a large terminal arising from a small neuron; a bipolar cell terminal may be up to 8 μm in diameter. The presynaptic ribbon in a bipolar terminal is situated opposite the point where two postsynaptic processes meet; hence, the junction is called a *dyad*.

The identity of the postsynaptic processes varies according to the complexity of organization. In simple retinas (e.g., primate), one of these terminals is from an amacrine cell, the other is from a ganglion cell. Typically, the amacrine cell has, in addition, a synapse back onto the bipolar terminal. The term *reciprocal synapse* was first used to describe this arrangement (Dowling and Boycott, 1966), and it has been generally accepted in describing the similar arrangements of side-by-side synapses in other parts of the brain. Amacrine cells also have synapses onto ganglion cell dendrites. These patterns of connections are illustrated in Fig. 9.3 (C). By serial reconstructions, Allen (1969) has shown that a single elongated terminal of a bipolar cell has as many as 23 synaptic ribbons, at which sites connections are frequently made to more than two other processes. Stell (1972) has noted that these complex clusters of processes resemble, in certain respects, the synaptic glomeruli of other parts of the nervous system.

In complex retinas (e.g., frog), all the processes opposite a ribbon may belong to amacrine cells, and there are numerous amacrine-amacrine synapses of the simple ("conventional") type. It has been inferred that, in these retinas, the bipolar cells connect to the ganglion cells not directly but through several amacrine cells, as illustrated in Fig. 9.3 (D). The term *serial synapse* was first used by Kidd (1962) to describe these sequences. The finding of amacrine-amacrine synapses is very important evidence that an intrinsic neuron can have synapses onto other intrinsic neurons of the same type. The complexity of the amacrine-amacrine sequences appears to be directly related to the complexity of information processing (Dowling, 1968).

We may conclude that the synaptic connections in the retina show a great diversity of types. Some can be characterized as specialized terminals and synapses, others as simple terminals and synapses. Since many of the intrinsic neurons lack a clearly defined axon, the terminology for the types of synapses, in terms of the processes that take part in the synapses, is not settled. One extreme position would be that all the synapses can be regarded as dendrodendritic, or at least equivalent to that type of connection. At the other extreme, some of the synapses would be regarded as axodendritic, as, for example, from the bipolar terminal onto the ganglion cell and amacrine cell dendrites [Fig. 9.3 (C)]. But this immediately requires that one label as dendroaxonic the reciprocal synapses from the amacrine cell to the bipolar terminal. It also requires that one label as axon a process that does not generate an action potential (see later). Thus, under any set of definitions, one obtains types of synaptic orientation that violate the functional canons of the traditional neuron doctrine, as outlined previously in Chapter 1.

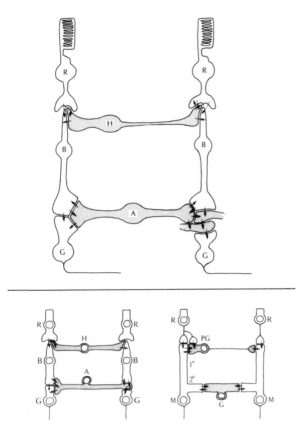

FIG. 9.4. Basic circuit diagram for the vertebrate retina. Abbreviations as in Fig. 9.3. (Modified from Dowling, 1968.) *Below,* comparison between the synaptic organization of the retina and olfactory bulb.

BASIC CIRCUIT

The knowledge of synaptic connections between the clearly defined neuronal types of the retina leads directly to a summary of organization in a basic circuit diagram, as in Fig. 9.4 (A).

To summarize briefly: in the OPL, the receptors connect to both bipolar and horizontal cells through the ribbon synapses. A horizontal cell may, in turn, have synapses with bipolar cells, with other horizontal cells, and also back onto receptor terminals. In the IPL, the bipolar terminals connect to both ganglion cells and amacrine cells through their ribbon synapses. The amacrine cells have reciprocal synapses back onto the bipolar terminals and other synapses onto ganglion cells. This pattern is characteristic for simple retinas, as shown in Fig. 9.4 (A). To the right in the figure are shown the serial synapses through the amacrine cell processes that are characteristic of complex retinas.

It can be seen that the main framework of the retina is one of vertical and horizontal pathways. There are vertical pathways from receptors through bipolar cells to ganglion cells, and horizontal pathways between the vertical paths. The horizontal connections are separated rigidly into two levels, or tiers. At the first level, the OPL, the horizontal cells are related to processing of the receptor input to the bipolar cells. At the second level, the IPL, the amacrine cells are appropriately situated to control the output from the ganglion cells.

In terms of this framework, the retina appears to be organized on principles similar to those of the olfactory bulb. A diagram for the bulb is included for comparison [Fig. 9.4 (B)]. The framework of vertical and horizontal connections and the two-tier separation of the horizontal connections are obviously similar. The horizontal cells are analogous to the PG cells in being at the level of input processing, whereas the amacrine cells are analogous to the granule cells in being at the level of output control. Note that the amacrine cells and granule cells both lack axons and both take part in reciprocal synaptic connections with the vertical pathway at the output level.

These similarities indicate that the over-all outline of synaptic organization in the retina is not unique. It is useful to view the retina in this light, for it is one of the steps that is necessary in the development of common principles that apply throughout the brain.

Let us now consider the organization of the retina more closely, using the diagram of Fig. 9.4 as our guide. In discussing the olfactory bulb, we introduced the principle that the input elements to a region are related in some way to both the vertically and the horizontally conducting elements in that region; the three types of elements form, it was suggested, a synaptic triad. In the retina, the ribbon synapses of the receptor terminals provide a simultaneous input to both the horizontal cells and the vertically conducting bipolar cells. This type of synaptic arrangement is similar to that in the cerebellum and thalamus, and appears to provide for a more synchronous and possibly more stereotyped transfer to the vertical and horizontal pathways than is the case in the olfactory bulb. This might be essential for the transfer of spatio-temporal patterns and sequences in the retina.

The position of the bipolar cell as the vertical conducting element from input to output levels is clearly shown in the diagram of Fig. 9.4. In this function, the bipolar cell is analogous to the primary dendrite of the mitral cell in the olfactory bulb. Note that we have compared, in this way, the function of an entire neuron (the bipolar cell) with the function of only part of another (the mitral cell). Consider, as an alternative, that the anatomically bounded cell is the actual unit of function. Then the entire mitral cell must be comparable to the entire bipolar cell, since both are the first-order neurons in their respective pathways. This comparison is obviously of limited value. In the analysis of the functional significance of synaptic organization, therefore, functional entities must be identified regardless of anatomical boundaries, a principle that has already been introduced in discussing the neurons of the olfactory bulb.

If we next consider the connections of the bipolar cells in the IPL, it can be seen that the relation of the ribbon synapses to the terminals of ganglion cells and amacrine cells is similar to the triadic pattern in the OPL. In complex retinas, this input is largely to the amacrine cells alone, i.e., the intrinsic elements (see Fig. 9.4). The break, as it were, in the vertical pathway at this level, provides for more degrees of freedom than is possible in the case of direct continuity from primary dendrite to mitral cell body in the olfactory bulb [see Fig. 9.4 (B)]. These greater degrees of freedom are effected by increased synaptic interconnections involving the intrinsic elements, as is shown by the high degree of correlation between the functional complexity of the retina and the number of amacrine-amacrine synapses (Dowling, 1968).

The amacrine cells exert their control over the ganglion cells in three ways: through synapses onto the bipolar cell terminals, by synapses directly onto the ganglion cells, and by amacrine-amacrine connections. The control mediated by the amacrine-bipolar synapse (which is, in fact, part of the reciprocal pair) is of particular interest, since it is presynaptic in position relative to the ganglion cell. It is, thus, part of the functional repertoire of the IPL that the amacrine cells can control the ganglion cell output through both presynaptic and postsynaptic connections. The fact that the ganglion cell is entirely postsynaptic in position (i.e., its dendrites have no presynaptic functions) means that, by itself, it is a relatively simple integrative unit, like the motoneuron, as compared with a neuron like the mitral cell of the olfactory bulb. Its true complexity, however, is seen when it is considered as part of the larger multineuronal functional units it forms with the bipolar and amacrine cells.

The synaptic connections at the two levels in the retina provide many pathways for feedback and feedforward interactions. Compared to other local regions, the retina is notable in being devoid of internal feedback loops through axon collaterals from the output neurons and external feedback loops from other parts of the brain. It is as if the retina has quite enough to do, thank you, handling the visual input alone. In the OPL, the connections are specific in many retinas for rod and cone systems, although this is not shown in the basic diagram of Fig. 9.4 (A). In the IPL, a given synaptic connection may be part of either, or both, systems, as well as part of other systems that process more complex aspects of the visual stimulus. It seems highly likely that many of these pathways overlap, and that a synapse is multifunctional in the sense previously discussed in Chapter 8.

SYNAPTIC ACTIONS

It is a great advantage in the investigation of the retina that one can not only activate it with a specific stimulus (light) but activate it discretely, with stimuli closely controlled in spatial extent and temporal course. No other region of the brain provides these advantages for the experimenter to the extent that the retina does. One can, therefore, analyze the retina using light stimuli rather than electrical shocks, and the results are correspondingly more closely relevant to the processing of natural stimuli. The basic types of stimuli used are a spot and a surrounding rim (annulus) of light.

The disadvantage in the study of the retina is the small size of the neuronal elements; analysis had to await the development of refined techniques for intracellular recording and staining (see Svaetichin, 1953; Tomita, 1965, 1972; Werblin and Dowling, 1969; Kaneko, 1970). The results that are considered typical for synaptic actions in the different types of neuron in the retina are illustrated in Fig. 9.5. In describing them, we will begin with the receptors and work inward to the ganglion cells.

Intracellular recordings from a *receptor cell* (R) are shown in Fig. 9.5. The salient features are, first, that the resting membrane potential is very low (10–30 mV); second, the response to a spot of light is a slow potential transient (not an impulse); and third, the potential is in the

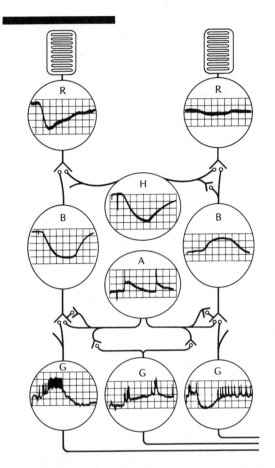

FIG. 9.5. Synaptic actions in the vertebrate retina, as recorded intracellularly from neurons in *Necturus* (mudpuppy). *Left*, responses recorded at the center of a spot of light (bar above). *Right*, responses in the surround. Voltage calibrations, one scale division equals 1 mV (R); 2 mV (H, B, and G); 5 mV (A). Time calibration, one division equals 200 msec. (From Dowling, 1970, after Werblin and Dowling, 1969).

hyperpolarizing direction. Rod receptors respond in graded fashion proportional to light intensity. Cone receptors are of three types depending on their peak sensitivities to blue, green, and red light.

It is a characteristic of many sensory receptors that they respond to their specific stimulus by a depolarization; the mechanism for this depolarization involves a conductance increase similar to that for an EPSP.

The hyperpolarizing responses of receptor cells in the vertebrate retina were therefore astonishing when revealed in the early electrophysiological investigations (see Tomita, 1965, 1972). The explanation appears to lie in the fact that, in the resting state, there is a constant leak of electrical current from the light-sensitive region of the receptor (the outer segment), which keeps the resting membrane potential at its relatively low level. The effect of a sudden light stimulus is to reduce this current and hyperpolarize the cell. There is evidence that the dark current is carried principally by Na ions, and that light acts by reducing the permeability to Na at some membrane site in the outer segment (Penn and Hagins, 1969; Toyoda, Nosaki, and Tomita, 1969).

Horizontal cells (H in Fig. 9.5) also give slow responses to light stimuli. As in receptor cells, the responses arise from low resting potentials. These were the first intracellular recordings from the retina (Svaetichin, 1953); the responses are termed S (slow) potentials. The responses are of two types: the luminosity type (L), a hyperpolarization of the cell to all wavelengths of light, and the chromaticity type (C) (not indicated in Fig. 9.5), in which the response may be hyperpolarizing or depolarizing, depending on the wavelength of light.

What is the mechanism for synaptic transmission from the receptors to the horizontal cells? Figure 9.5 shows that the potential change in the presynaptic terminal of the receptors is a hyperpolarization and that the postsynaptic potential change in the horizontal cells is also a hyperpolarization. This poses a difficult problem, because, as Hodgkin (1971) has pointed out, there are no known exceptions to the rule that transmitters are released by depolarization of the cell membrane (see Chapter 3). This requires the postulate that the receptors release transmitter continuously in the dark and that light suppresses this release. There is evidence that this is, in fact, the case. In response to light, the horizontal cells undergo a decrease in conductance similar to that of the receptor cells (Toyoda et al., 1969), so that it appears possible that the mechanism of the response of horizontal cells may be similar in principle to that of the receptors, as described above.

It should be clear to the reader at this point that the hyperpolarizing responses in receptors and horizontal cells are due to a mechanism that is different from that of the hyperpolarizing IPSPs found in many neurons in other parts of the brain. They are produced by a turning off of a depolarizing conductance channel (i.e., Na), whereas the IPSP is produced by a turning on of a hyperpolarizing conductance channel (i.e., Cl). That, at least, is the mechanism that has been postulated for the horizontal cells (see Trifonov, 1968), although recently other possibilities have been considered (Nelson, 1973). See Chapter 3 for a discussion of these and other synaptic mechanisms. The postsynaptic hyperpolarizing potential in the horizontal cell is, thus, presumed to be produced by a sudden interruption of synaptic depolarization from the receptors, rather than by an active inhibitory process.

Bipolar cells, like receptors and horizontal cells, also generate only slow potentials in response to a light stimulus (see B, Fig. 9.5). The latency of onset of the response is similar to that of the horizontal cell, which is consistent with the idea that the receptor terminal, through its ribbon synapse, provides for simultaneous transmission to both cell types. The responses also arise from resting potentials that are relatively low, in the range of 30–40 mV. The responses may be hyperpolarizing (example, left, Fig. 9.5) or depolarizing (right, Fig. 9.5). Different bipolar cells show different polarities in their responses to a central spot and a surrounding annulus of light flashed on the retina. The bipolar cell is the first in the sequence of neurons within the retina to show marked center-surround antagonism by opposite polarities of response in relation to spatial aspects of a stimulus.

Amacrine cells respond to light stimuli with graded depolarizing potentials upon which may be superimposed one or two spikes (A, Fig. 9.5). Amacrine cells are therefore the first in the sequence of neurons within the retina to respond with depolarizations resembling the EPSPs of other neurons in the brain, and the first to generate impulse activity. The case of an amacrine cell that responds to both the ON and the OFF of a spot of light with slow potentials and single impulses is shown in the example in Fig. 9.5. Amacrine cells vary in whether they respond at ON or OFF and in the grading of the amplitudes of the responses. The responses are relatively transient compared with the more sustained responses of the other cell types described earlier.

Ganglion cells respond to light stimuli with various combinations of EPSPs, IPSPs, and impulse discharges, all of which resemble their counterparts in other output neurons of the brain. Resting membrane potentials are relatively low (40–50 mV). Ganglion cells are the first (and only) neurons in the sequence within the retina to show spontaneous impulse activity. Some ganglion cells respond with a steady discharge to a central spot of light, and are inhibited by a surrounding annulus (left and right G, Fig. 9.5); it has been suggested that these ganglion cells may receive their input primarily by way of direct connections from the bipolar cells, which have similar receptive field organization (see Dowling, 1970). Other ganglion cells show transient responses at both the onset and cessation of a light stimulus (center G, Fig. 9.5); this is similar to the pattern of responses in amacrine cells, and suggests that such ganglion cells are driven predominantly through amacrine cells.

Figure 9.5 gives only a slight hint of the range of responses that has been recorded in ganglion cells. In simple retinas, the ganglion cells respond primarily to stationary spots and annuli of light, as was shown in the classical experiments of Kuffler (1953). In complex retinas, the ganglion cells are less responsive to simple and stationary stimuli and more responsive to complicated aspects of the stimuli (Barlow, 1953; Maturana et al., 1960). For example, a ganglion cell may respond only to a moving spot of light, or to movement in one particular direction. Or it may respond, not to a spot of light, but to an edge of light and dark; to evoke a maximal response, the edge may have to be convex or concave.

The nature of these responses suggests that the retina abstracts specific aspects of the stimuli and that ganglion cells are tuned, as it were, to these aspects. Since such responses are not seen in the more peripheral retinal elements (receptors and horizontal and bipolar cells), it means that the tuning must come about through synaptic interactions mediated by the amacrine cells in the IPL (but see next section). This is consistent with the fact, noted above, that complex retinas are characterized by a well-developed IPL, containing dendritic trees of ganglion and amacrine cells with complicated branching patterns, and a multiplicity of connections between the amacrine cells. Within this neuropil are established the excitatory and inhibitory feedforward and feedback pathways that are the basis for the functional properties of the ganglion cells.

In the cat, a distinction has been made between Y cells, which summate light stimuli nonlinearly and respond best to transient stimuli, and X cells which summate light stimuli linearly and respond with tonic discharges (Enroth-Cugell and Robson, 1966). Careful study has shown that Y cells are large ganglion cells with large fast-conducting axons, and that X cells are medium-size ganglion cells with small, slowly conducting axons (Boycott and Wässle, 1974; Cleland and Levick, 1974). The two categories are superimposed on the classical on-center, off-center classes as originally defined by Kuffler (1953). We will see that the Y and X distinction has a functional significance that carries through the relay in the lateral geniculate nucleus (Chapter 11) and into the visual cortex (Chapter 15).

NEUROTRANSMITTERS

One would expect that a region as well studied as the retina would have quickly yielded up the identities of its transmitters, but the record thus far is somewhat puzzling. Part of the difficulty seems to be the multiple interconnections, both chemical and electrical, between the cells, and part seems to be the inability to activate the synaptic circuits synchronously and selectively by input volleys evoked electrically in the manner used in other systems.

In the outer plexiform layer, there is evidence that the receptors synthesize acetylcholine from labeled choline (Lam, 1972), suggesting that the receptors may be cholinergic onto bipolar and horizontal cells. Various studies have supported this idea (Gerschenfeld and Piccolino, 1977; Negishi, et al., 1978), but other studies suggest a role for amino acids (Dowling and Ripps, 1973), and still others suggest a combination of both, including the possibility of cholinergic interactions between horizontal cells (Marshall and Werblin, 1978). Species differences may be an important factor in these studies.

Traditionally, a cholinergic transmitter has been long suspected at synapses in the inner plexiform layer. Specific cholinesterase staining is associated with amacrine cells (Nicholls and Koelle, 1968), and choline acetyltransferase activity is concentrated in the inner plexiform layer, where it has been ascribed to some, but not all, of the amacrine cell population (Ross and McDougal, 1976). Some amacrine cells take up ^{3}H-GABA (Neal and Iversen, 1972; Marshall and Voaden, 1975). A role for GABA has also been suggested by experiments in which the GABA antagonists, picrotoxin and bicuculline, caused a reduction of the surround effect of the receptive fields of Y, but not X, cells (Kirby and Enroth-Cugell, 1976). Thus, it appears that the amacrine cell population is subdivided into biochemical subtypes, similar to the PG cells in the olfactory bulb. Perhaps, as Kirby and Enroth-Cugell note, "part of the reason that X and Y cells are so different pharmacologically is because X cell surround signals are mediated by horizontal cells . . . while those of Y cell surrounds are mediated by amacrines."

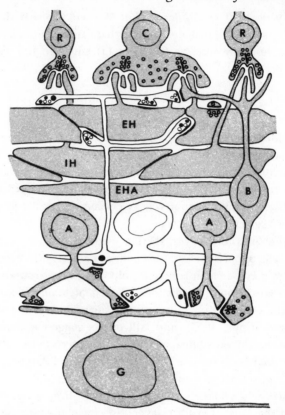

FIG. 9.6. Schematic diagram showing synaptic connections of interplexiform cell (shaded) in the goldfish retina. (Redrawn from Dowling et al., 1976.)

A sixth cell type in the retina, the interplexiform cell, was first detected using histofluorescence methods (Ehinger et al., 1969). Dowling, Ehinger, and Hedden (1976) showed that, in the goldfish, these cells receive synapses from amacrine cells in the IPL, and make synapses onto other amacrine cells in that layer, as well as onto horizontal and bipolar cell processes in the OPL (see Fig. 9.6). Their physiological studies suggested that this cell is dopaminergic, and has a direct depolarizing action on horizontal cells that reduces their antagonistic surrounds. The reader may compare this with the actions of dopamine reported in sympathetic ganglia and in the neostriatum. Subsequent studies have suggested that there is considerable species variation in this cell, with respect to synaptic connections and types of transmitter (see Kolb and West, 1977). It appears that this is yet another type of amacrine cell, which can perform different types of feedback operations in different species, using different transmitters. Thus, it is an example of the flexible relation that exists between structure and function in synaptic circuits, as discussed in the introductory chapters.

DENDRITIC PROPERTIES

It has been shown that the intrinsic neurons of the retina are remarkable not only for their small size but also for the paucity or lack of morphological axons. Therefore, the study of these neurons can be said to involve largely a study of their dendritic properties. It has also been shown that there is a dramatic absence of impulse traffic within the retina. This means that the spread of activity through the retinal neurons is determined by electrotonic properties. Knowledge of these properties is, therefore, especially important in the study of the retina, as the necessary basis for reconstructing functional organization.

It would be hoped in the light of these remarks that electrotonic models were available for retinal neurons, but this is unfortunately not the case. We will only be able to note some preliminary steps toward the construction of models and to discuss some implications of dendritic structure and function.

BIPOLAR CELLS There are two main aspects of bipolar function, one local and integrative, the other transmissive. The local role is carried out at both input (OPL) and output (IPL) levels in the retina. At both levels, the bipolar cell branches have synaptic inputs as well as outputs, so that a single branch or terminal functions to some extent as an input-output unit. The degree of autonomy of such units depends on the amount of electrotonic current spread between them. In view of the rather limited branching fields, it would appear that there is fairly effective spread of local synaptic inputs to neighboring branches; a local synaptic input would, therefore, lead to output that was graded in both intensity and in local spatial extent.

The other aspect of function is the role of the bipolar cell in transferring signals vertically from input to output level. We have noted the analogy to the mitral primary dendrite in this regard. The transfer in the bipolar cell is apparently exclusively by passive electrotonic spread.

There is no electrotonic model available for the bipolar cell, but insofar as it can be considered as a single process extending from OPL to IPL, one can indicate how such a model might be developed. Experimental measurements (Nelson, 1973) suggest that electrical properties of the bipolar cell place it between the middle and lower lines of the graph of Fig. 5.2. Assuming a diameter of 1 μm, the process would have a characteristic length of 150–300 μm. Since the bipolar cell is approximately 100 μm in vertical extent, its electrotonic length (L) would be considerably less than 1, and it could be concluded that spread would be very effective through it.

At higher levels of input intensity, the transfer from OPL to IPL is quite effective, as evidenced by the large potentials recorded from the cell body. Transfer in the opposite direction, from IPL to OPL, however, is presumably also effective, and this is relevant because of the inputs from the amacrine cells onto the bipolar terminals in the IPL. To what extent can the responses to these inputs spread back through the bipolar cells, to influence synaptic outputs from the bipolar terminals in the OPL? If it is assumed that this kind of "backtalk" must be held to a minimum, then one has the interesting proposition that the dendritic properties of the bipolar cell represent a compromise between minimizing transfer in this direction while maximizing it in the other. There are possibly similar principles underlying the properties of other dendrites within the overlapping multifunctional local circuits in the brain.

HORIZONTAL CELLS   In the early work on S potentials, it was clear that the recording electrode was within a confined space, but whether it was a cell body or an extracellular compartment was difficult to determine. Various explanations were tendered for an extracellular compartment whose resting potentials could be the negative sum of the neighboring cells. The image conjured up by Naka and Rushton (1967) was that of a river, "flowing through that crowded community into which all cells can empty their electrical effluence. The latter is a rather versatile concept, but degrading. One likes to have one's electrode in the council chamber not in the sewer." Fortunately, the electrode has been found to be in dignified company (Werblin and Dowling, 1969; Kaneko, 1970; Baylor et al., 1971).

We have noted the strategic position of the horizontal cell terminals, which are interposed, to a certain extent, between the receptor terminal and the bipolar cell dendrite [Fig. 9.3 (A,B)]. It is possible that the horizontal cell processes have both presynaptic and postsynaptic positions and function, therefore, as local input-output units. Spread of synaptic potentials within the processes is presumably by passive means alone, graded in intensity and spatial extent, as in the bipolar cell terminals.

The horizontal cells also provide for the transfer of local inputs to other parts of their branching trees by passive electrotonic spread. In the primate horizontal cell, the single long slender "axon" is particularly enigmatic. If one is indeed justified in labeling it an axon, then it stands as a rare example of an axon that does not conduct action potentials. The length (several hundred microns) and diameter (1 μm or so) are not inconsistent with effective spread by passive means alone. If both "dendritic" and "axonal" arborizations have local input-output relations, however, as discussed above, then the arborizations will function independently of each other to a certain extent. It is possible, therefore, that the primate horizontal cell provides separate branching systems whose functions are not necessarily sequential, as is implied by "dendritic" and "axonal" labels, construed in their classical sense.

The preceding remarks anticipated the study of Nelson et al. (1975) in an interesting way. They recorded intracellularly from the type B horizontal cells in the cat and showed that the cell body receives input primarily from cones, whereas the axonal ramification receives input primarily from rods (see Fig. 9.7). Nelson et al. calculated the attenuation of signals due to electrotonic decrement in the long thin axon ($L = 2-3 \lambda$) and to the large conductance load offered by each ramification to any signal reaching it. They concluded that the axon serves more to isolate the two parts of the cell than to connect them functionally. "It is intriguing," they note, "that in the teleost retinas entirely separate horizontal cells have evolved for rods and cones, whereas in mammals one cell of the axon-bearing variety appears to perform both functions. A possible advantage in having single neurons with electrically isolated regions is that the number of integrating units within the brain can be increased without adding more cells. It would therefore not be surprising if similar arrangements were present elsewhere in the central nervous system."

In lower vertebrates, the input resistance (R_N) of horizontal cells has been reported to range from 1–30 MΩ (see Witkovsky, 1971). In the fish it is clear that spread of electrical current through the horizontal cells is effective, for it has been possible, in recent experiments, to inject small

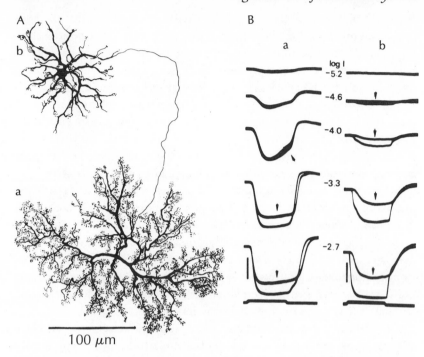

100 μm

FIG. 9.7. Horizontal cell of the cat. (A) Type B horizontal cell with cell body and dendritic arborization (a), and a long, thin axon giving rise to a large axonal arborization (b). Calibration bar: 100 μm. (B) Intracellular responses of axonal arborization (b) and cell body (a) to large spots of light and two different wavelengths at increasing intensities (log I). When traces superimpose, only rod receptors contribute to the responses; where they differ, some cone input is implied. Arrowhead indicates response to 400 nm light; other response is to 658 nm light. Note different relations of responses to wavelength and intensity (see text). (From Nelson et al., 1975.)

amounts of current into a horizontal cell and thereby influence the activity of distant ganglion cells. This influence is mediated through electrical synapses between the horizontal cells, and synaptic pathways through bipolar cells and, possibly, amacrine cells as well. Electrotonic considerations relevant to this case have been discussed by Marmarelis and Naka (1972). Such considerations also apply to the electrically coupled A-type horizontal cells in the cat.

AMACRINE CELLS   Amacrine cells have a predominantly lateral orientation, resembling that of horizontal cells. They differ, however, in that they are clearly neuronal in morphology; they generate depolarizing synaptic potentials, and they appear to have limited impulse-generating properties.

The amacrine cell processes occupy both presynaptic and postsynaptic positions within the IPL [see Fig. 9.3 (C, D)], and those processes, therefore, function as local input-output units. As in the horizontal cells, spread of synaptic potentials between branches is presumably effective and graded in intensity and in spatial extent.

The nature of the local feedback onto the bipolar cell terminal, through the reciprocal synapse (see Fig. 9.3), is one of the puzzling aspects of amacrine cell function. An analogy with the reciprocal synapses in the olfactory bulb has been suggested (Rall et al., 1966; Dowling and Boycott, 1966; Stell, 1972). In the olfactory bulb, the reciprocal synapses of granule cells provide for inhibitory feedback onto the mitral cells; this feedback is triggered by the initial impulse in the mitral cell, and the feedback occurs in the aftermath of the impulse. In the retina, the input from the BP terminal is a slow potential; since the amacrine cell responses tend to be transient, it has been suggested (Werblin and Dowling, 1969) that the reciprocal synapse could mediate inhibitory feedback onto the bipolar cell terminal to shut off the bipolar input after the initial excitation.

Since the amacrine cell is placed at the interface between hyperpolarizing and depolarizing elements in the retina, it raises the possibility that the amacrine cell could, through postsynaptic depolarization at all its terminals, oppose the excitatory input from the bipolar cells, on the one hand, while exciting amacrine and ganglion cells, on the other. The interface thus extends the range of possible mechanisms for amacrine cell modulation of synaptic transfer at this level. Even given these differential effects, it seems necessary to postulate different actions at some amacrine cell synapses to account for the IPSPs in ganglion cells (Fig. 9.5).

The amacrine cell is also faced with the problem of providing for transmission to distant parts of its branching tree. The lateral field may extend up to 1 mm in diameter in some retinas. Few estimates of electrical parameters of the amacrine cells have been made, and it is clearly premature to suggest any kind of electrotonic model (see Nelson, 1973). It would appear that attenuation might be severe through the entire extent of an amacrine cell, but the amacrine cell, nonetheless, may be assumed to provide for such spread, since the experimental evidence implicates it in the lateral processing that underlies the extensive center-surround fields of ganglion cells, as well as other properties in more complex retinas (see Dowling, 1970). It may be that a limited amount of impulse activity assists in promoting lateral spread. This is analogous to the role of dendritic spikes in cerebellar Purkinje cells and hippocampal pyramidal neurons.

GANGLION CELLS   The ganglion cell dendrites are, as far as is known, exclusively postsynaptic in position. This means that, like motoneuron dendrites, their local role is concerned with integration of synaptic inputs preparatory to transmission to the cell body and axon hillock. It is assumed that this integration takes place by passive spread; no evidence of active properties of the dendrites has been reported. The dendritic trees of the smallest ganglion cells, in the foveal region, are quite limited in extent, so it may be presumed that spread of synaptic potentials within them is very effective. This, of course, is consistent with their role of providing for the highest acuity in the visual periphery.

In complex retinas, the dendritic trees of ganglion cells have complicated patterns; as indicated in Fig. 9.2. The possibility that different functional classes may be correlated with different patterns of dendritic arborization was investigated by Maturana et al. (1960) in their classical study of visual processing in the frog. They obtained evidence that the number of distinct levels of stratification of dendritic branches did, in fact, provide a basis for explaining the functional classes of ganglion cell responses. The idea seems reasonable. However, West and Dowling (1972) found in an electron microscopical study of Golgi impregnated ganglion cells that cells with the same branching pattern may differ widely in their synaptic connections with amacrine and bipolar cells. This implies that ganglion cells of the same anatomical type have different functional properties.

These results should not be taken to mean that dendritic geometry is not important in assessing structure-function relations within the brain; it means that these relations must be assessed with caution. Particularly to be resisted is the notion that a specific function is correlated with a specific structure. To illustrate this point, consider (as is obvious) that the amacrine and ganglion cells have become differentiated in complex retinas to subserve complex functions. Does this imply a unique relation between the geometrical patterns of these retinal cells and those specific functions? It is easy to show that this cannot be the case, for, in animals (e.g., primates) with simple retinas, abstraction of visual stimuli is postponed to the cerebral cortex, an expression of the encephalization of nervous control. This means that, within the cortex, neurons that are radically different from the retinal neurons in size, shape, and branching pattern nonetheless perform steps of sensory processing similar to those performed by the retinal neurons. We will review that evidence in discussing the neocortex. It must be concluded, therefore, that a flexible relation exists between structure and function in the neurons of the brain and that *similar functions may be subserved by different structures*. One may also conclude that the obverse is true: *different functions may be subserved by similar structures;* the extraordinary range of properties of neuronal dendrites may be taken as evidence of this. Recognition of these facts about structure-function relations is necessary in formulating the principles underlying the synaptic organization of different regions of the brain.

10

CEREBELLUM

The cerebellum, an outgrowth from the brainstem, is an important part of the brain that is present throughout the vertebrates. Its relative size and position can be seen in the diagram of Fig. 1.2. It is a largely central region, the first that we take up in our study. From its strategic position, it makes connections with many brain regions, motor, sensory, and other. Some relations with motor systems are shown in Figs. 12.1 and 16.1. Because of this it is not nearly as easy to determine its specific functions as it is for such regions as the olfactory bulb and retina, with their single afferent inputs, or the spinal ventral horn, with its single motor output.

Studies of animals with cerebellar ablations, and of humans with traumatic injuries and disease, indicate that the cerebellum is involved in at least three broad functions: (1) maintenance of posture and balance, (2) maintenance of muscle tone, and (3) coordination of voluntary movements. Although these functions express themselves as motor acts, they nonetheless also depend heavily on specific sensory inputs. Posture, for example, requires information from spindle receptors about the state of muscle contraction. Balance requires information from the vestibular canals. Coordinated movements require many additional inputs: somatosensory, visual, etc. The cerebellum must therefore be looked upon as an organ for sensori-motor coordination, not merely as a motor appendage.

Like the olfactory bulb and retina, the cerebellum is a laminated region in which the basic internal structure is similar throughout. The structure does vary considerably in vertebrate phylogeny, as has been summarized by Llinás and Hillman (1969). There are also various anatomical subdivisions of the cerebellum, which are covered in neuroanatomy textbooks. Our concern will be restricted to the lateral hemisphere in the mammal, in order to illustrate general principles of cerebellar organization.

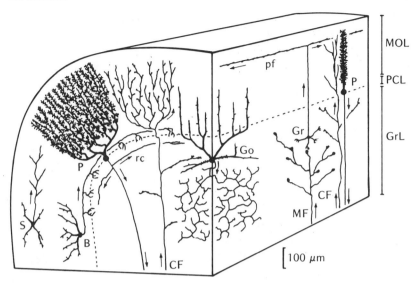

FIG.10.1. Neuronal elements of the mammalian cerebellum.
Inputs: mossy fibers (MF) and climbing fibers (CF).
Principal neuron: Purkinje cell (P), with recurrent collateral (rc).
Intrinsic neurons: granule cell (Gr); stellate cell (S); basket cell (B); Golgi cell (Go).
Histological layers are shown at the right: molecular layer (MOL), Purkinje cell body layer (PCL), granule layer (GrL).

NEURONAL ELEMENTS

The cerebellum is a highly convoluted structure, its layers being thrown into numerous folds. It resembles in this respect many nuclear regions in the brainstem, as well as the cerebral cortex of higher mammals. Convolutions in the cerebellum, as elsewhere, increase the amount and extent of the region, presumably in response to increasing demands for the functions performed therein.

Within the convolutions a rigid geometry dominates the organization to an extent unusual in other central brain regions. This is an outstanding characteristic of the cerebellum and must be incorporated, along with the convolutions, in the description of the neuronal elements. In order to do this a three-dimensional diagram is commonly constructed, as in Fig. 10.1. This diagram preserves the same scale of magnification used in the other diagrams of this book. In most of the cerebellum the convolutions are oriented transversely to the longitudinal axis of the animal.

We follow in the main the classical account of Cajal (1911), the acount of Eccles, Ito, and Szentágothai (1967), Szentágothai and co-workers (Palkovitz, Magyar, and Szentágothai, 1971), and the compendium of Palay and Chan-Palay (1974).

INPUTS The cerebellum receives its input from fibers arriving through the depths of the cortex. It resembles in this respect the neocortex and differs from other "cortical" regions—olfactory bulb, olfactory cortex, and hippocampus, as well as retina—in which the afferent component of the input arrives at the outer surface.

It is usual to divide the input into two types. One is the *climbing fiber*, so called by the manner in which it ascends through the cortical layers. It is thinly myelinated and has a diameter of 1–3 μm. Within the deeper, granule layer (GrL, Fig. 10.1), it loses its myelin and arborizes into long branches, which ascend through the cortex. Some collaterals are given off within the granule layer; most terminate within the superficial, molecular layer (MOL, Fig. 10.1). The branching field is very extensive across a convolution (folium) but very restricted along it; in this it resembles the dendritic tree of the Purkinje cell (see below).

The other type of input fiber is the so-called *mossy fiber*. These fibers also arrive through the depths, but they extend only into the granule layer. They are somewhat larger in diameter than the climbing fibers and much more numerous. On their way, they branch repeatedly, so that one fiber may supply several folia and several areas within one folium. Within the granule layer they lose their myelin, branch several times, and terminate in the characteristic, large, mossy-like terminals that give them their name. There is no particular orientation in the field of mossy fiber branches.

The sources of the two types of input fiber are different. The climbing fibers originate mainly in the *inferior olivary complex* (see Eccles et al., 1967), a region that, in turn, receives input from all three levels of the brain: spinal cord, brainstem, and cerebral cortex. The mossy fibers, on the other hand, have much more widespread origins. The vestibular nerve, which carries sensory information about balance from the *vestibular canals*, has some axons that end in mossy terminals in a part of the cerebellum known as the flocculus. An important source is the nearby *pontine nuclei* of the brainstem, which in turn receive direct connections from the cerebral cortex. Other sources are the *spinal cord* (through the spino-cerebellar tracts), the *reticular nuclei*, and the *vestibular nuclei*. Some of these inputs show a preference for terminating at different levels within the granule layer. In addition to these input sources, the locus coeruleus in the brainstem sends noradrenergic fibers to the cerebellum (Bloom, Hoffer, and Siggins, 1971; Olson and Fuxe, 1971).

It may be noted that we have not described the inputs in terms of a division between afferent and central, or central and centrifugal, as can be done in most other regions of the brain. The vestibular and spino-cerebellar inputs, arriving through mossy fibers, are analogous to the sensory afferent inputs of other regions. The other mossy fiber inputs, and the climbing fiber inputs, would by this analogy be comparable to the central inputs of other systems.

The differences between the climbing fiber and mossy fiber terminals seem remarkable, if not unique, but it should be recalled that the afferent and central inputs to the olfactory bulb are also markedly dissimilar. It is also remarkable that so many different functional "modalities" are funneled into the cerebellum through the same rigidly stereotyped structure of the mossy fiber terminal.

PRINCIPAL NEURON   The output from the cerebellum is carried through the axons of the *Purkinje cells*. Although it is sometimes said that every cell of the brain is unique, the Purkinje cell is "more unique", if that is possible, than most. The cell bodies are arranged in a single sheet about 400 μm below the surface, at the junction of the molecular and granule layer. As shown in Fig. 10.1, each Purkinje cell has a large dendritic tree that is flattened in one plane, so that it looks like a pear tree espaliered against a garden wall. In its branching field and plane of orientation, the dendritic tree is similar to the climbing fiber branches.

The Purkinje cell bodies have diameters ranging from 20 to 40 μm. Each has a stout dendritic trunk (up to 10 μm or so in diameter) that gives rise to a sequence of primary, secondary, and tertiary branches. The branching tree stretches across the molecular layer to the surface, so that in vertical and horizontal extent it is 400 μm or so, whereas across its plane of orientation it is little more than the diameter of its branches (see Fig. 10.1). The smaller dendritic branches are profusely invested with *spines* or thorns; these are basically similar in outward appearance to

the spines of olfactory granule cells and of pyramidal cells in the hippocampus and neocortex. It has been estimated that a single Purkinje cell
has upwards of 100,000 spines. This is only the first of many amazing
numerical counts we will mention that have been obtained in the analysis
of cerebellar elements and circuits.

The rigidity of cerebellar geometry is clearly expressed in the Purkinje
cell dendritic tree, the single sheet of cell bodies, and the relatively homogeneous size and shape of the Purkinje cells. No subgroups (as seen in
olfactory mitral and tufted cells or the varieties of retinal ganglion and
cortical pyramidal cells) have as yet been described. Compared to other
output neurons, Purkinje cells, therefore, appear as a very stereotyped
population.

The Purkinje cell axons give off numerous recurrent collaterals within
the folium of origin. The branches of the collaterals form a plexus at the
level of the Purkinje cell bodies. As shown in Fig. 10.1, the branches
spread predominantly across the folium, in the plane of the Purkinje cell
dendritic tree. The collaterals are myelinated up to their terminals.

The axons descend through the granule layer, wherein they gain a
myelin sheath and carry the output away from the cerebellum. The
remarkable feature of this output is that most of it goes to three nearby
nuclei that are packed into the depths of the cerebellum; they are referred to collectively as the *deep cerebellar nuclei*. In the parts of the
cerebellum with which we will be concerned, all the axons terminte in
these nuclei; hence, the cerebellar output is relayed through them to the
rest of the brain. The Purkinje cell axons are, therefore, relatively short,
no more than a few millimeters in length in small animals.

The deep nuclei act as relays from specific parts of the cerebellum to
specific parts of the brain. The newest part of the cerebellum, the neo-
cerebellum, projects through its Purkinje cell to the dentate nucleus. In
higher mammals this nucleus is deeply convoluted, in correlation with
the enlarged neocerebellar hemisphere. It projects mainly to the *ventral
lateral nucleus* of the thalamus, where integration with the projection from
the basal ganglia occurs (see Figs. 12.1 and 16.1). It also projects to the
red nucleus (a motor integration center with connections to the spinal
cord) and to a part of the *reticular nuclei*. Since the dentate and other deep
nuclei also receive inputs from branches of the climbing and mossy fibers
on their way to the cerebellum, it is obvious that we must include the
deep nuclei in studying the functional organization of the cerebellum.

INTRINSIC NEURONS   There are three main types of intrinsic neuron in the cerebellum, all distinct from the Purkinje cells and from each other.

Granule cells fill the granule layer (see Fig. 10.1). The cell bodies are very small (6–9 μm in diameter). Each gives rise to three to five dendrites, which are less than 1 μm in diameter and no more than 30 μm in length. The cell bodies and their dendrites are thus among the smallest in the brain. Each dendrite terminates in a claw-like expansion that is the site of synaptic connections.

The granule cell gives rise to a thin axon (1 μm or less in diameter) that ascends several hundred microns through the granule layer into the molecular layer. Here it divides, in a T-shaped fashion, to give rise to two branches that run horizontally through the molecular layer. These branches have their own name of *parallel fibers*, from the fact that they are all arranged in parallel in the axis of the folium. In this orientation they run perpendicularly through the Purkinje cell dendritic trees, as is shown in Fig. 10.1. The parallel fibers are unmyelinated, with diameters of only 0.2 μm near the surface of the molecular layer; these therefore resemble olfactory nerve axons. Their diameter gradual increases to about 1 μm in the depths of the molecular layer. Each parallel fiber branch is 2–3 mm in length, i.e., several times longer than the ascending axon from which it arises (Brand et al., 1976).

It should be stressed that the cerebellar granule cell differs morphologically in almost every respect from the olfactory granule cell and from the granule cells of the dentate gyrus and cerebral cortex, each of which also differs radically from the others. The term "granule" has no general significance as thus employed; it only describes the dot-like appearance of the small cell bodies in the primitive preparations of the histologists of the nineteenth century.

Golgi cells are relatively large neurons, with cell bodies about the same size as Purkinje cells. The cell bodies are scattered throughout the superficial part of the granule layer. Each gives off several large and rather straight-appearing dendrites; most of them ascend and branch in the molecular layer, although a few are directed to the granule layer (see Fig. 10.1). The field of arborization is unoriented and very wide, perhaps three times as wide as a Purkinje cell dendritic tree (i.e., up to 1 mm across). There are few dendritic branches, and the branches are only sparsely invested with spines. The axon is striking in appearance. It arises from the cell body or a dendritic trunk and immediately, within a few microns, begins dividing repeatedly, giving rise to a dense arborization of short branches that span the entire granule layer. It is surely one of the most fantastic arborizations of any axon in the brain. In breadth, the field of branching approximates the extent of the dendritic tree. The branches end in clusters of terminals, which resemble the claw-like terminals of the granule cell dendrites.

In the molecular layer are several types of *stellate cells*, so called because of the star shape of their dendritic tree. The most highly differentiated type is the *basket cell*. These cell bodies are situated in the deeper part of the molecular layer. Each is some 20 μm in diameter. The dendritic tree extends for 100–200 μm. The branches bear spines, and the tree is oriented across the folium, much as the Purkinje cell dendrites are. Each cell gives rise to an axon, 1–2 μm in diameter, that is oriented across the folium. During its course it gives off branches, which entwine the Purkinje cell bodies in a basket-like form, which gives these cells their name (see Fig. 10.1). A single basket cell may give rise to as many as ten baskets, to as many Purkinje cells, in its course over a distance of 1 mm or so. The terminals envelope the cell body and also the initial segment of the Purkinje cell axon, making contacts that are described in the next section.

Other varieties of stellate cell are found more superficially in the molecular layer. The cell bodies and dendritic trees are generally smaller than those of the basket cells. The axons tend to run in the same horizontal plane, but the branches are simple and short and oriented vertically (see Fig. 10.1). There is a gradation of transitional forms, from the basket cells to the simplest and smallest stellate cells near the surface of the molecular layer.

It may be noted that none of these intrinsic neurons strictly satisfies the classical definition of a short-axon cell, that is, a cell whose axon ramifies in the vicinity of the cell body. On the other hand, they do satisfy our working definition of a cell whose axon distributes within the same histological region (i.e., the cerebellum). But within this very general classification, the cerebellar short-axon cells are markedly different in form and function from other short-axon cells and from each other. We will see that the granule cell is actually a type of relay neuron in the input pathway from mossy fibers to Purkinje cells. The Golgi cell, with its distinctive dendrites and fantastically arborized axon, is a unique type of intrinsic neuron. Only the stellate cells of the molecular layer are recognizable as short-axon cells that resemble their counterparts elsewhere in the brain.

CELL POPULATIONS The cerebellum has been a favorite subject for the geometricians and arithmeticians of the brain. If the geometry is striking, the arithmetic is no less than astounding. Rolled out into a flat sheet, the cortex of a cerebellar hemisphere of man would cover a surface approximately 2 × 100 cm (see Braitenberg and Atwood, 1958). This is some two-hundred times the area of the retina, and almost one-third of the area of a hemisphere of the entire cerebral cortex. Within the cortex of a cerebellar hemisphere are approximately seven-million output neurons (the Purkinje cells); this is seven times the estimate of retinal ganglion cells in man, and more than one-hundred times the estimate of olfactory mitral cells. From these numbers alone one would anticipate that the cerebellum must provide a dominant input to the brain. Recalling our discussion of neuronal populations in Chapter 9, would one say that we are "exceptionally cerebellar animals"?

The populations of input fibers are no less remarkable. There is a roughly one-to-one ratio of climbing fibers to Purkinje cells. Because of this, there is little or no convergence or divergence in this input pathway. The mossy fibers, on the other hand, are far more numerous. No figures are available, but they must outnumber the climbing fibers by several orders of magnitude, which puts their numbers in the billion range. Compared with the figures mentioned in Chapter 9, this is far more input than any sensory system provides. It thus appears that the two types of cerebellar inputs stand at extremes, one at the limiting minimum of convergence and divergence, the other at the maximum.

It is in the population of granule cells that the arithmeticians come into their own. Consider the estimate of 2.4 million cells/ mm^3 in man (Fox and Barnard, 1957); this works out to be approximately 20 billion granule cells in one cerebellar hemisphere, or 40 billion in both hemispheres. It is commonly stated that the human brain contains 10 billion nerve cells, as evidence of its fantastic complexity; clearly those statements do not take into account the granule cells of the cerebellum!

The other two types of intrinsic neuron are much less numerous; in fact, they tend to be scarce or absent in lower vertebrate species. In mammals, the ratio of Golgi to Purkinje cells is only about 1:10, whereas the numbers of stellate and basket cells are probably of the same order, or somewhat greater, as the Purkinje cells. If we consider the granule cell to be a relay neuron, then the populations of intrinsic neurons, i.e., Golgi, stellate, and basket cells, can be seen to be quite modest in number. The dendritic trees and extensive axonal arborizations of these cells mean that their convergence and divergence ratios vis-à-vis the Purkinje cells are much greater than the numbers of cell bodies would indicate, however. For a detailed study of neuronal populations, and convergence and divergence ratios, in the cat, the reader is referred to a study of Palkovits et al. (1971) (summarized in Eccles, 1973).

This brief account will serve to indicate that the cerebellum is characterized by extraordinarily large populations of some of its neuronal elements, which are, in addition, packed in together at a very high density. The significance of these population figures depends on an accurate knowledge of the internal circuits of the cerebellum. Further quantitative data will, therefore, be mentioned in conjunction with the basic circuit diagram.

SYNAPTIC CONNECTIONS

In the cerebellum, as in the olfactory bulb and retina, the distinct cell types and lamination greatly expedite the identification of synaptic connections. Indeed, as in the olfactory bulb and the retina, the main types of connection were inferred from Golgi stained preparations by the classical histologists of the late nineteenth century (see Cajal, 1911). Studies with the electron microscope have confirmed most of these inferences and revealed important details of synaptic structure (see Eccles et al., 1967; Llinás and Hillman, 1969; Mugnaini, 1970; Rakić and Sidman, 1973; Palay and Chan-Palay, 1973).

We begin with the afferent input, and consider the connections made by the mossy fibers. As shown in Fig. 10.2, the mossy terminals, as viewed under the electron microscope, appear as enlarged swellings, termed *rosettes*. The rosette is one of the largest terminal structures in the brain; the medium-sized example shown in Fig. 10.2 is some 10 μm in width and 20 μm in length. This terminal structure is, therefore, larger than the cell bodies of most small neurons in the brain.

Tightly grouped around a rosette are numerous terminals, the whole cluster being surrounded by a single layer of glial membranes. The glial membranes thus demarcate a specific group of terminals, which is termed a *glomerulus*. Within a glomerulus, the mossy rosette makes synaptic connections onto dendritic terminals of granule cells, as shown in

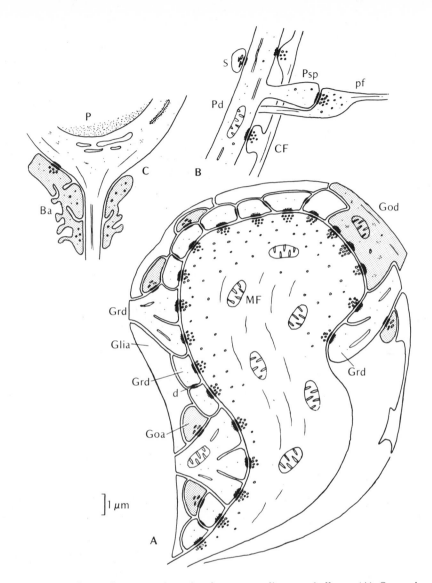

FIG. 10.2. Synaptic connections in the mammalian cerebellum. (A) Synaptic glomerulus in the granule layer, showing axodendritic connections between a mossy terminal (MF), granule dendrites (GrD), and Golgi dendrites (God); also from Golgi axons (Goa) onto granule dendrites. Note the desmosomes between the granule dendritic terminals; note also the surrounding glia. (B) Molecular layer, showing axodendritic connections from parallel fibers (pf), climbing fibers (CF), and stellate cells (S) onto a Purkinje cell dendrite (Pd) and dendritic spines (Psp). (C) Specialized terminal of a basket cell axon (Ba) onto the cell body, axon hillock, and initial axonal segment of a Purkinje cell (P). (After Eccles et al., 1967; Palay and Chan-Palay, 1974.)

Fig. 10.2. These are type I chemical synapses. The rosette also has synapses of a distinctive type onto Golgi cells; because the surface of the Golgi cell is wrinkled like a Spanish chestnut, these synapses have been termed *en marron* (Chan-Palay and Palay, 1971b). A third type of connection within the glomerulus is from axon terminals of Golgi cells onto granule cell dendrites; these are more characteristic of type II chemical synapses. In many cases, a granule cell dendritic terminal receives a connection from both a mossy rosette and a Golgi axon. The granule dendritic terminals are interconnected by desmosome-like membrane specializations. It has been estimated that a single glomerulus contains 100 to 300 dendritic terminals from some 20 granule cells.

The term *glomerulus* has already been used to describe the large areas of neuropil in the olfactory bulb, and we will encounter it again in our description of the organization of the thalamus and the cerebral cortex. It is, therefore, one of those terms likely to give rise to confusion, and it is appropriate to consider it more carefully. What we are basically dealing with is a *synaptic complex*, which may be defined (see Shepherd, 1972a), in the most general sense, as *a set of specific synaptic connections between axonal and dendritic terminals, which terminals may themselves be interconnected*. This generalizes previous definitions (see Szentágothai, 1970; Pinching and Powell, 1971) to cases of dendrodendritic, axoaxonic, and dendroaxonic, as well as axodendritic connections. *Glomerulus* may then be defined, again in the most general sense, as *a synaptic complex enclosed in glial membranes or otherwise set apart*. The olfactory glomerulus, involving many axonal and dendritic terminals, might appropriately be termed a *macroglomerulus;* this term might also apply to the barrels in the neocortex. The cerebellar and thalamic type, on the other hand, involving only a small number of terminals, could be termed a *microglomerulus*. The synaptic complex formed in relation to single olfactory axon terminals is analogous to the synaptic complex of the cerebellar and thalamic microglomeruli, although it lacks the well-defined glial enclosures of the latter. The synaptic patterns within the cerebellar glomerulus will be compared with these other cases when we describe the basic circuit, below; a detailed comparison with the thalamic glomeruli is provided in Chapter 11.

Within the molecular layer of the cerebellum are three major types of connection onto the Purkinje cell dendrites. First, the parallel fibers, arising from the granule cell axons, have synapses onto the spines of the Purkinje cell dendrites, as is shown in Fig. 10.2. These connections are type I chemical synapses. The presynaptic process is simply an enlargement of the parallel fiber as it passes by the spine; this is an *en passage* or a *crossing-over* synapse. This is the only type of synapse made by the parallel fibers; such synapses are also made onto the dendritic spines of the basket, stellate, and Golgi cells in the molecular layer.

The second major type of connection onto the Purkinje cell dendrites is made by the climbing fibers. This type also may be regarded as a variety of *en passage* synapse, but at right angles to the parallel fibers, as the climbing fiber ascends along the Purkinje cell dendrites. These are also type I chemical synapses and are made on small somatic spines (Larramendi and Victor, 1967) and on the trunks rather than the branchlets of Purkinje cell dendrites; thus, the two types of input are highly specific for different sites on the Purkinje cell and its dendritic tree.

A third type of connection is made by the axon terminals of stellate cells onto the surfaces of the Purkinje cell dendrites. These are type II chemical synapses (see Fig. 10.2).

A distinctive type of synaptic connection is found near the Purkinje cell axon hillock. As we know, the basket cell axon entwines the Purkinje cell body. Electron microscopy shows that the terminals are of unusual design, as illustrated in Fig. 10.2 (C) (see Eccles et al., 1967). On the cell body near the axon hillock, the basket cell terminals establish contacts which generally fall into the category of type II chemical synapses. In addition, further terminals which surround the axon hillock and initial segment are given off. These contain synaptic vesicles, but there is little specialization of the apposed membranes. The terminals have numerous villi-like protuberances, which interdigitate with glial cells (the Bergman glia). Thus is formed a cap around the axon hillock region of the Purkinje cell, reminiscent of the cap around the corresponding region of the giant motor cells (Mauthner cells) of the fish spinal cord.

Despite their differences, climbing fibers and mossy fibers have some synapses onto Golgi cells and granule cells that are similar in structure. Chan-Palay and Palay (1971b) have pointed out the interesting implication that the form of a terminal is determined by the postsynaptic site.

Two characteristics of the synaptic connections in the cerebellum are especially significant in comparison with other brain regions. One is that there are synapses from recurrent collaterals of the Purkinje cell axons onto the cell bodies and dendritic trunks of neighboring Purkinje cells. The presynaptic terminals contain flat and round synaptic vesicles, but the synapses have been reported not to conform to either of Gray's types (Chan-Palay, 1971). Such recurrent connections of an output neuron onto itself, as well as onto intrinsic neurons, have also been reported in certain parts of the cerebral cortex. We will discuss further the general significance of this type of connection in those chapters. In other regions of the brain, the recurrent collaterals of the output neuron connect mainly to the intrinsic neurons; examples are the olfactory bulb, the thalamus, and, probably, the ventral horn of the spinal cord.

The other characteristic is that all the synapses thus far described are of the axosomatic or axodendritic type. No dendrodendritic synapses of the chemical type have been described, although there are densities of the opposed membranes of granule cell dendrites within the glomerulus (see Fig. 10.2). Nor have axoaxonic connections been observed, with the exception of the special type formed by the basket cell terminals onto the initial segment of the Purkinje cell. This limited stock of synaptic types is in contrast to the greater variety of connections in many other parts of the brain.

BASIC CIRCUIT

The synaptic organization of the cerebellum is summarized in the basic circuit diagram of Fig. 10.3. The first diagram (A) preserves the topographical orientation of the cerebellum and includes as much of the internal circuits as is feasible. Diagrams (B) and (C) are rearrangements of the neuronal elements which are oversimplified in order to emphasize aspects that are of interest compared to the organization of other regions in the brain.

In general, it may be said that the main plan of the cerebellum is laid down by the two input pathways and their relations to the output neuron. This plan is emphasized in the simplified diagram of Fig. 10.3 (B, C), in which the inputs are shown arriving from above, in order to facilitate comparison with the input-output connections in other basic circuit diagrams. If we take first the climbing fibers [cf. Fig. 10.3 (A)], they make synapses directly onto the Purkinje cells; as we shall see, this is an excitatory pathway. This is therefore analogous to the monosynaptic input to motoneurons, and the olfactory input to mitral cells, in having direct access to the output neuron. The climbing fibers also make connections onto the stellate (S) and basket cells (B) [Fig. 10.3 (A, C)], the intrinsic neurons of the molecular layer that control the Purkinje cell

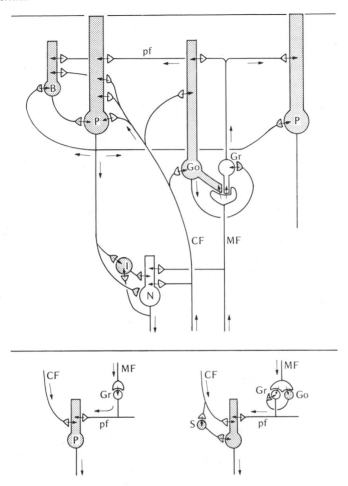

FIG. 10.3. Basic circuit diagram for the mammalian cerebellum. Abbreviations as in Fig. 10.2. Note deep cerebellar nuclear cells, including the principal nuclear cell (N) and intrinsic neuron (I). *Below*, simplified diagrams to emphasize the two main input pathways in the cerebellum, for comparison with other brain regions. *Right*, these pathways shown with their associated intrinsic neurons.

output. We thus recognize the basic elements of a synaptic triad in this pattern of connections. The intrinsic neurons are differentiated into two distinct subtypes; one of these types—the basket cell—receives axon collaterals from the output neuron it controls; this recurrent pathway is similar to pathways in the ventral horn and olfactory bulb.

The mossy fiber input to the Purkinje cells is an indirect one, being relayed through the granule cells (Gr); this is analogous to the disynaptic input to motoneurons in the ventral horn. The granule cell functions, therefore, as a relay neuron in the vertical path onto the Purkinje cells. As will be shown later, the mossy fiber is excitatory to the granule cell, and the granule cell (through its parallel fiber) is excitatory to the Purkinje cells. Thus, the granule cell is not interjected into the vertical pathway to convert an excitatory to an inhibitory input, as in the case of many interneurons in the spinal cord, for example. In this sense, the granule cell is a true relay neuron (cf. Cajal, 1911; Llinás and Hillman, 1969) rather than a type of interneuron or short-axon cell for local processing. It may characterized as a local, in contrast to a long-distance, output neuron.

This view is supported by the fact that in certain animals (e.g., electric fish) the granule cells do not lie in a layer within the cerebellar cortex but instead are clustered as a nucleus of cells at the base of a folium (ridge) (Nieuwenhuys and Nicholson, 1969). This arrangement suggests an essentially nuclear function for the population of granule cells and further shows that an ostensibly cortical structure, such as the cerebellum, may contain neurons that have a nuclear type of organization. The implication here is that the molecular layer is the true cortical part of the cerebellum and that the functional demands on the parallel fiber relay in higher vertebrates require the granule cells to be as close as possible to the molecular layer. The structure of the molecular layer is nonrepeating in relation to the output neuron (Purkinje cell) that spreads across it, in line with our previous discussion of one of the principles of cortical organization.

Seen in this light, the granule cells form what may be termed a *staging* or *pre-processing station* for input to the cerebellar cortex. This position can be appreciated more fully in the simplified diagrams of Fig. 10.3 (B, C), in which the mossy-granule cell relay has been reoriented to feed into the cerebellum as a separate entity from above. In this position, it can be compared with the interneuronal relays in the spinal cord and with the dentate relay to the hippocampus; it can also be compared with the thalamic relay to the neocortex.

Let us now consider more closely the synaptic arrangements in the mossy fiber input pathway. The excitatory connections, as already described, are found in all vertebrates. The additional connections made by intrinsic neurons provide the basis for the more complex cerebellums of higher vertebrates.

In the granule layer, the mossy fiber rosette makes synapses onto both the granule cells and the Golgi cells (GO) as shown in Figs. 10.2 and 10.3. We recognize here the elements of a synaptic triad; the input fiber (rosette), the output neuron (granule cell), and the intrinsic neuron (Golgi cell). The pattern is one of simultaneous input to the dendrites of both output and intrinsic neurons, but with no connections between the dendrites of those neurons. The cerebellar glomerulus is thus a synaptic complex which provides for a very simple stereotyped pattern of connections within the synaptic triad. In Chapter 11, we will compare this pattern of organization with the synaptic triads in the olfactory bulb, retina, and thalamus.

As can be seen in Fig. 10.3 (A, C), Golgi cells function as intrinsic neurons in controlling input-output relations between the mossy terminals and the granule layer branches; thus, there are both local circuits (within the granule layer) and longer circuits (through the molecular layer) for feedforward and feedback inhibition. Through these circuits, the Golgi cell regulates the granule cell relay to the Purkinje cells. With regard to the Purkinje cells, then, the Golgi cells are at the level of input processing.

In the molecular layer, the parallel fibers of the granule cells make connections onto the dendrites of Purkinje cells and also onto the dendrites of basket and stellate cells. The basic pattern of this synaptic triad is a rigid, near-simultaneous sequencing of input to both output and intrinsic neurons, with no dendrodendritic interactions between the latter. It is especially significant that the output and intrinsic elements in this synaptic triad are the same as those for the climbing fiber input, although the pattern of input connections to them are distinctly different.

Let us now consider some quantitative data. If we put together the estimates that a single mossy fiber has 40 rosettes, that each rosette connects to the dendritic terminals of 20 granule cells, and that a single granule cell (through its two parallel fiber branches) connects to 100–300 Purkinje cells, we obtain a combined divergence ratio of roughly 1:100,000–300,000 in going from one mossy input fiber to the Purkinje cell. The Purkinje cells, for their part, have upwards of 100,000 dendritic spines, each spine with its parallel fiber synapse onto it, and this is, therefore, roughly the number of parallel fibers, and, hence, individual granule cells, that converge onto it.

These factors for convergence and divergence between input and output are greater than those known for any other region of the brain. It is as if the extreme limits of these factors had been explored, and the mossy fiber-granule cell-parallel fiber-Purkinje cell system devised as an answer. The implications of this system are that the input arriving over an individual mossy fiber is disseminated to a population of granule cells, that the activity relayed by this granule cell population passes in a "beam" of parallel fibers to the Purkinje cells, and that this beam (spreading in opposite directions from the origin of the two parallel fiber branches) activates the Purkinje cells in a rigid temporal sequence. The input from one mossy fiber must be tiny relative to the total convergence onto a given Purkinje cell. An important consequence of this last point is that summation of granule cell inputs must be a requirement for eliciting responses over this route.

If the Purkinje cells are thus buffered, as it were, from the mossy fiber input, they are, by contrast, exposed as directly as possible to the climbing fiber input. As already noted, the convergence and divergence factors for this input are close to one. In addition, a single climbing fiber has perhaps several hundred synapses onto the single Purkinje cell over which it climbs. It is as if, in the face of the massive mossy fiber system, the climbing fibers had been devised to provide a means by which a single afferent fiber could have the most secure and effective means of eliciting a response in a Purkinje cell. We will see that this inference from anatomical considerations is supported by the extraordinary potency of this synaptic connection.

It should again be emphasized that the connections summarized in Fig. 10.3 occur within a rigidly geometrical framework. The horizontal and vertical aspects of organization that we have pointed out in the basic circuits for the olfactory bulb and retina are carried to a high degree of perfection in the lattice-like arrangement of the cerebellum. From this organization emerges the interesting fact that, when we trace activity through any of the pathways within the cerebellum, there is the clear implication that the temporal sequences are closely determined by the spatial geometry. Let us quote from Braitenburg and Atwood (1958), two of the pioneers of quantitative cerebellar studies:

> The morphological evidence is strongly suggestive that one of the main properties of the cerebellar cortex might be the transformation of spatial into

temporal patterns and vice versa. . . . Activity arising at one moment in a vertical cross-section of the molecular layer will reach different Purkinje-cell trees after different time intervals, depending on their distance. Conversely, the arrival of such a front of activity at any one Purkinje cell implies events in different loci at different times in the past, depending on the distance. Basically, therefore, equations relating certain input patterns to certain output patterns would be expected to contain time and distance interchangeably.

This should not be taken to imply that space and time are not also interrelated in other neuronal systems; it implies only that they are interrelated to a particularly rigid and stereotyped degree in the populations of the neurons within the cerebellum. We will discuss similar examples of this type of organization in the olfactory cortex and hippocampus.

DEEP CEREBELLAR NUCLEI It has already been mentioned that the Purkinje cell output from the cerebellum is directed to the nearby deep cerebellar nuclei. This is indicated in Fig. 10.3 (A). This input to the deep nuclei is inhibitory; it will be discussed further in the next section. Both the mossy and climbing fibers give off collaterals to the deep nuclei. The deep nuclei contain populations of output and intrinsic neurons that form synaptic triads with the inputs from the cerebellum and from the other parts of the brain (Angaut and Sotelo, 1973; Chan-Palay, 1973). Recently, serial synapses have been described (Hamori and Mezey, 1977). Most of these details have had to be omitted from Fig. 10.3 (A) for the sake of simplicity.

SYNAPTIC ACTIONS

Physiological analysis of synaptic actions in the cerebellum has been carried out using several methods: single volleys set up by an electrical shock (Granit and Phillips, 1956; Eccles et al., 1967); natural stimulation of sensory afferent pathways (Murphy, MacKay, and Johnson, 1973; Eccles, 1973); and single neuron activity monitored during movements performed by awake animals (Thach, 1970). We will describe the results obtained by the use of single volleys and indicate briefly their relevance to the natural control of movement.

Let us first consider the synaptic actions of a *parallel fiber volley*, set up by an electrical shock delivered to the surface of the cerebellum. At this surface location, the electrode stimulates a narrow "beam" of parallel

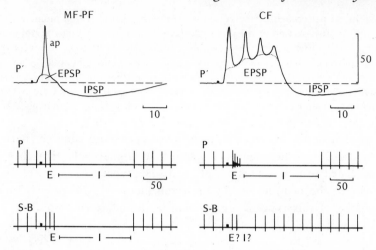

FIG. 10.4. Main types of synaptic actions in the mammalian cerebellum.

Left, MF-PF, synaptic actions elicited by a volley in the mossy fiber-parallel fiber pathway. P′, intracellular recording of a simple response in a Purkinje cell. P, extracellular recording, slower time base. Excitatory and inhibitory periods indicated by E and I, respectively. S-B, extracellular recording from stellate or basket cell.

Right, CF, synaptic actions elicited by a volley in the climbing fiber pathway. P′ and P, a complex response in a Purkinje cell. S-B, ? response in stellate or basket cell. (After Granit and Phillips, 1956; Eccles et al., 1967; Thach, 1967.)

fibers that passes through the folium. The response of a Purkinje cell, recorded intracellularly, is shown in Fig. 10.4 (P′, column MF-PF). The response consists of a brief EPSP, lasting some 5–10 msec, ascribed to the beam of active parallel fibers making excitatory synapses onto the dendritic spines of the Purkinje cell. This brief EPSP, in turn, generates a single impulse, or sometimes two or three. The response to input from the parallel fibers has been termed a simple spike (Thach, 1967).

The EPSP evoked by the parallel fibers is usually followed by a long-lasting hyperpolarization, as shown in Fig. 10.4. This has been described as a "prolonged, graded and chloride-sensitive hyperpolarization—the necessary and sufficient criterion for synaptic inhibition" (Llinás and Nicholson, 1971). In these respects, it resembles the IPSPs recorded from other output neurons in the brain. The entire depolarizing-hyperpolarizing sequence is, in fact, a characteristic response of principal neurons in different brain regions to a single input volley, as is pointed out in other chapters.

In other regions of the brain, IPSP's are due to feedforward and feedback connections of the intrinsic neurons (see Fig. 7.6). In the cerebellum it is believed, largely on inference from anatomy, that the Purkinje cell IPSP is mainly caused by a feedforward pathway through the stellate and basket cells. These cells are, indeed, activated by the parallel fiber volley; they respond with a discharge of spikes as is shown in Fig. 10.4 (SA, left column). The prolonged spike discharge to a single volley implies a prolonged excitatory action on these cells, suggesting that special factors (slow buildup, sequestration of transmitter, temporal dispersion) control the time course of transmitter action at these synapses from the parallel fibers (Eccles et al., 1967).

With regard to feedback connections, we have seen examples of this in the Renshaw circuit of the spinal cord and the dendrodendritic recurrent pathway in the olfactory bulb. The situation is different in the cerebellum, by virtue of the fact that the synaptic actions of the Purkinje cells are inhibitory. This has been shown for the output of the Purkinje cells to the deep cerebellar nuclei (see below), and, largely by inference from Dale's Law (but see Chapter 4), it has been assumed that the Purkinje cell axon collaterals are also inhibitory to the stellate and basket cells within the cerebellar cortex. Thus, rather than exciting the intrinsic neurons through recurrent collaterals, the Purkinje cells are presumed to inhibit them; since the intrinsic neurons are inhibitory to the Purkinje cells, the action of the recurrent pathway is to disinhibit the Purkinje cells, rather than to inhibit them. An inhibitory feedback pathway also exists through the recurrent collaterals back onto the Purkinje cells themselves, so it is obvious that the control of Purkinje cell excitability is the outcome of a very complex process of inhibitory interactions.

The synaptic actions elicited by a *mossy fiber volley* are similar in basic outline to those described above. The actions are neither as strong nor as limited in space, as would be expected from their dispersion by the relay through the large population of granule cells. The physiological evidence is consistent with the scheme in which the mossy rosette is excitatory to the granule and Golgi cells, and the latter are inhibitory to the granule cells. The Golgi cells thus function as inhibitory interneurons at the granule level, providing feedforward and feedback pathways as described for the basic circuit in the previous section. From the widely ramifying axonal plexi of the Golgi cells, it would appear that each Golgi cell creates a compartment of inhibited granule cells; these compartments apparently do not overlap (see Eccles et al., 1967). It is possible that the compartments are analogous to the glomeruli of the olfactory bulb and the barrels in the neocortex, in the sense of constituting subdivisions of neuropil with a structural and functional unity. The term macroglomeruli has been discussed above as applicable to such compartments.

Let us turn now to the action of a *climbing fiber volley* set up by an electrical shock to the inferior olivary nucleus. The Purkinje cell response consists of an intense and prolonged depolarization, which generates a large initial spike followed by several small ones (see Fig. 10.4, P′, column CF). This was originally termed an *inactivation response* by its discoverers (Granit and Phillips, 1956); it has also been termed a complex spike (Thach, 1967), in contrast to the simple spike response to mossy fiber input. This response is similar to the inactivation bursts of hippocampal pyramidal cells.

The mechanism for the complex burst in the Purkinje cell was first explained in the following way (see Eccles et al., 1967). The volley of impulses not only propagates through the climbing fibers but also invades their axon collaterals within the inferior olive. Through these collaterals, a sequence of activation of inferior olive cells takes place, which provides a rapid series of impulses in the climbing fiber and, consequently, a rapid sequence of EPSPs in the Purkinje cells. More recently, intracellular recordings from the inferior olive cells have shown that these cells respond with a prolonged depolarization and burst of impulses, rather similar to the complex spike of the Purkinje cell. In these studies, there is evidence that the prolonged depolarization occurs in the dendrites of these cells and that it is this depolarization that underlies the brief burst of impulses in the climbing fibers and, hence, in the Purkinje cells (Crill, 1970). Gap junctions exist between inferior olive cells (Llinás et al., 1973), so that electrical interactions may also play some role in the discharges of these cells (see Chapter 3 for discussion of these electrical synapses). There is also evidence that the prolonged depolarization of the Purkinje cell may be intrinsic to the membrane of the Purkinje cell itself (Fujita, 1969), and due to dendritic spikes generated by calcium currents (Llinás and Hess, 1976; see Fig. 10.5 below).

Whatever the outcome of these analyses, two interesting points emerge. One is that the climbing fiber synapse is extremely "potent", a physiological property that correlates with the dense innervation of the Purkinje cell by the climbing fiber. The other is that the inferior olivary cell is, to some extent, matched in its physiological properties to the Purkinje cell.

Like the simple spike response, the complex spike is also followed by a prolonged inhibition, which takes the form of a long-lasting hyperpolarizing IPSP, as shown in the intracellular recording of Fig. 10.4 (P', column CF). In P, below, is an extracellular recording, on a slow time base, that shows the excitatory-inhibitory sequence as it is interposed in the resting background discharge.

The IPSP following the complex spike has been attributed to the action of local circuits. In addition to its connections to the Purkinje cells, the climbing fiber also activates stellate and basket cells, which provide feedforward inhibition to the Purkinje cells. The climbing fibers also activate to some extent the Golgi cells, which may inhibit, in turn, the granule cell excitatory input. Some of the suppression following the complex spike may be an expression of the intrinsic properties of the Purkinje cell membrane. After their initial excitation, the stellate and basket cells are themselves inhibited, presumably through Purkinje cell axon collaterals (see Fig. 10.3). These collaterals probably provide for similar inhibitory effects on the granule and Golgi cells (see Fig. 10.3).

If we take an overview of these synaptic actions, an especially striking aspect is that, whereas the actions of the input fibers (including the granule cell-parallel fibers) are all excitatory, the actions of the cells within the cerebellum are all inhibitory. This has the important consequence, as pointed out by Eccles et al. (1967), that sustained activity in response to an input is not possible within the cerebellar circuits. There are no pathways that provide for re-excitatory or reverberating activity, as have been described for the spinal cord or the cerebral cortex. Some complex sequences involving disinhibition (e.g., through Purkinje cell axon collaterals onto the inhibitory neurons) can take place, but these are apparently not sustained for long.

This aspect takes on further significance with respect to an outstanding characteristic of the cerebellar neurons, that they all have high rates of resting impulse discharge. In awake monkeys, for example, it has been found that Purkinje cells in the anterior lobe discharge at rates of 3 to 125 impulses/sec, with a mean discharge rate of 70 impulses/sec (Thach, 1972). This is in sharp contrast to the low rates, in the range of a few impulses per second, that are characteristic of output neurons in many other regions of the brain; motoneurons, as already noted, are, in fact, often silent in the absence of external input. The activity of Purkinje cells is closely correlated with the mossy fibers, which have similar high rates of resting discharge (see Jansen, Rudjord, and Walløe, 1970; Eccles, 1973). The high excitability of Purkinje cells thus derives from the synaptic drive to them, rather than from the "size principle" deduced from motoneurons. Similar considerations apply to the activity of intrinsic cerebellar neurons.

It is important to realize that the synaptic actions of cerebellar inputs take place against the high-frequency background. As a consequence, both the excitatory and inhibitory aspects of the responses are significant. For example, a slight increase in resting discharge of a Purkinje cell engendered by a mossy fiber input might be difficult to detect, but an inhibitory pause following that input might be quite obvious. The extreme, high-frequency burst elicited by the climbing fiber, followed by suppression, reflects the specialization of this input for eliciting a clearly detectable Purkinje cell response no matter what the resting background discharge; at higher discharge levels, the inhibitory phase may well be the more detectable and significant part of the response.

DEEP CEREBELLAR NUCLEI It has already been noted in discussing the basic circuit of Fig. 10.3 that the cerebellar cortical output carried by the Purkinje cells is entirely directed to the deep nuclei. The work of Ito and his colleagues (Eccles et al., 1967) established that this input is inhibitory; the Purkinje cells have inhibitory synapses on the deep nuclear cells, which respond with IPSPs. The Purkinje cells are the only output neurons we will study that have an inhibitory output, and it means that the cerebellar cortical output has to be viewed through inverted spectacles, so to speak, in assessing its significance. By virtue of this output it is possible to regard the Purkinje cell as a species of interneuron, which has become displaced and has acquired elaborate internal circuits to control its own input-output relations.

The significance of the Purkinje cell input to the deep nuclei must also be assessed relative to the other inputs to the deep nuclei. A review of the synaptic organization of the deep nuclei is beyond our present scope, but anatomical and physiological studies are consistent with the following picture: both mossy and climbing fibers have connections onto both the principal and intrinsic neurons, and these connections are excitatory. Opposed to these are the inhibitory inputs from the Purkinje cells and from intrinsic nucelar neurons. Figure 10.3 (A) gives an outline of these connections, from which some impression of the dynamic control of the nuclear output may be obtained.

The deep nuclear cells are matched with the Purkinje cells in having high rates of resting impulse discharge, ranging from 1–87/sec, with a mean of 37/sec in awake monkeys (Thach, 1972). Thus, as in the Purkinje cells, suppression of the resting discharge (by Purkinje cell input) is especially significant.

As more has been learned about the cerebellum and the deep nuclear cells, it has become clear that the relations between them are quite complex. One view that has emerged, consistent with the inhibiting function of the Purkinje cells as discussed above, is that of the cerebellar cortex as a massive accessory processing apparatus superimposed on the input-output relations of the nuclear cells with the rest of the brain. Thach (1972) has pointed out the possibility that "a step increase in the mossy fiber input might cause first a high frequency burst in the nuclear cell, and second a lowering of nuclear cell frequency as the inhibitory restraint built up in the slower Purkinje cell loop." By this means, a differentiated, rate-sensitive output from the nuclear cells could be achieved that would be similar to the kind of dynamic differentiation that is characteristic of rate-sensitive receptor cells (cf. Ottoson and Shepherd, 1971). Such rate-dependent transients might be important in the initiation of muscle movements or the control of rapid movements. This is clearly not the only possible function of the cerebellar control of the deep nuclei, and the elucidation of these functions is a most exciting challenge for future work (cf. Eccles, 1973).

NEUROTRANSMITTERS

Studies of GABA uptake (Hökfelt and Llungdahl, 1972) and GAD localization (McLaughlin et al., 1974) indicate that the Purkinje cells are GABAergic at their synapses in the deep nuclei and also at their axon collaterals within the cortex. The inhibitory neurons within the cortex— stellate, basket, and Golgi cells—also appear to be GABAergic. Basket cell inhibition of Purkinje cells, as well as the inhibition caused by iontophoretically applied GABA, is blocked by bicuculline, a GABA antagonist (Curtis and Felix, 1971). The evidence for GABA is backed up by a variety of biochemical studies of GABA content and GAD activity (see Roberts, 1975). This uniformity among different cells using the same neurotransmitter within a region is unusual, as can be ascertained by reviewing the diversity of transmitters among different neuronal types in other regions described in this book.

There is little direct evidence concerning the excitatory transmitters for the mossy and climbing fibers. Glutamate is a possible transmitter for the fibers of the granule cells; it excites Purkinje cells when applied to the molecular layer (Chujo, Yamada, and Yamamoto, 1975). High-affinity uptake of glutamate and aspartate is sharply reduced in the cerebellums of hamsters infected with a virus that selectively destroys granule cells (Young et al., 1974). In synaptosomal preparations, the release of glutamate is stimulated by K^+ depolarization, dependent on Ca^{2+} and antagonized by Mg^{2+}, thus fulfilling the usual criteria for a neurotransmitter (Sandoval and Cotman, 1978). The fibers from the locus coeruleus are noradrenergic. There is evidence that they inhibit Purkinje cells by a conductance-decrease synaptic mechanism mediated by cyclic AMP (Yamamoto, 1967; Bloom et al., 1971; Bloom, 1975; but see Lake and Jordan, 1974). This type of mechanism was discussed in the introductory chapters, and has also been postulated for the NA input to the spinal cord and the hippocampus.

DENDRITIC PROPERTIES

We confine our attention to the Purkinje cell, and by noting that all the evidence to date indicates that the Purkinje cell dendrites are exclusively postsynaptic in position. This means that the properties of the dendrites will be relevant to local integration of synaptic inputs and transfer of the potentials to the axon hillock.

ACTIVE PROPERTIES   The Purkinje cell has been a focus of interest with respect to the question of active impulse properties of dendrites. The first studies were made in tissue cultures, in which growing Purkinje cells send out long and relatively undifferentiated "dendritic" processes. With a stimulating microelectrode at one end of a process, and a recording microelectrode at the other end, evidence was obtained for a spike-like response that spread like an impulse through the dendrite (Hild and Tasaki, 1962). Such studies have great potential for the analysis of neuronal properties; but the fact that the neurons are embryonic, poorly differentiated, and essentially deafferented suggests the need for caution in extrapolating the results to the adult *in vivo* situation.

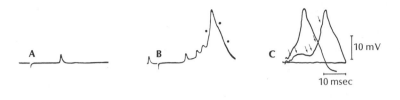

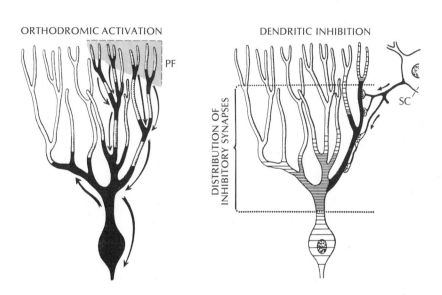

FIG. 10.5. Properties of Purkinje cell dendrites. (A, B) Microelectrode recording from within a dendritic trunk, showing responses to a parallel fiber volley of increasing strength. Note "dendritic" potentials as small spikes and bumps (dots). (C) After treatment with tetrodotoxin and 3-aminopyridine, to block Na currents. Note persistence of long-duration depolarization and notches, suggesting Ca spikes in dendritic branches. (C from Llinás and Hess, 1976; others from Llinás and Nicholson, 1971.) *Below*, schematic diagrams to illustrate *orthodromic activation* of dendritic spikes at dendritic branch points and *dendritic inhibition* by stellate cells.

Direct study of dendritic properties has been attempted by a combination of intracellular recordings and intracellular staining; such a study has been carried out in the alligator cerebellum, in which the stain has shown an intradendritic location for some of the recordings (Llinás and Nicholson, 1971). A representative result is shown in Fig. 10.5, in which responses are shown to parallel fiber volleys of increasing strength (A)-(B).

The small spikes and bumps in these recordings were interpreted as all-or-nothing spike-like activity within one dendritic tree. The Purkinje cell dendrites are considered to have patches, or "hot spots", of excitable membrane; with a weak synaptic input, the patches fire singly (A) or asynchronously; with strong input they fire synchronously and summate thereby to give a large intradendritic action potential (B). It is presumed that the patches occur at branch points in the dendritic tree (Lorente de Nó and Condouris, 1949). As shown diagrammatically in Fig. 10.5 (orthodromic activation), the action potentials at branch points are presumed to spread electrotonically in a "pseudosaltatory" fashion, from branch point to branch point, toward the cell body, where they summate to produce an impulse that propagates down the axon. This explanation for intradendritic impulse activity in Purkinje cells is similar to that for spike-like activity in chromatolytic motoneurons, for fast prepotentials in hippocampal pyramidal neurons, and for small spikes in immature neocortical neurons. As shown in (C), there is evidence that the dendritic spikes are generated by calcium currents (Llinás and Hess, 1976).

The spread of activity in the Purkinje cell dendritic tree has been further analyzed by Pellionisz and Llinás (1976) in a computational model. In the example shown in Fig. 10.6, a parallel fiber volley elicits a large EPSP in one-half of the dendritic tree; the traces show the spread of the EPSP into the rest of the cell, and the superposition of impulses triggered at the axon hillock and spreading back through the cell body into the dendrites.

What is the functional significance of active properties in the dendrites of Purkinje cells and other neurons? In addition to making distant synapses more effective vis-à-vis the impulse output from the axon hillock, impulse conduction in dendritic trees probably depends upon the proper amounts and timing of excitation and inhibition at successive branch points within the tree. As Rall (1970b) has pointed out, "such multiple possibilities of success or failure, at many different points of bifurcation, could lead to elaborate sets of contingent probabilities which would provide a single neuron (if it has suitable input patterns over the dendritic branches) with a very large logical capacity." The Purkinje cell provides a particularly vivid illustration of these possibilities.

DENDRITIC INHIBITION   The inhibitory neurons onto the Purkinje cells are differentited into two types, stellate and basket cells. The stellate cell

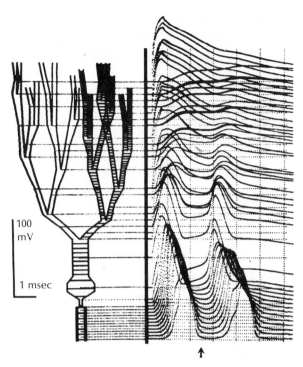

FIG. 10.6. Electrotonic compartmental model of Purkinje cell, illustrating response elicited by parallel fiber volley to one-half of dendritic tree. Traces on the
right are recordings from compartments; arrow indicates 2.5 msec after onset of
response (vertical line). (From Pellionisz and Llinás, 1977.)

inhibition is directed to the Purkinje cell dendritic tree and, thus, provides yet another example of inhibition that has a dendritic, rather than a
somatic, location. In line with the comments on electrotonic properties
in Chapter 5, and the discussion of similar situations in the motoneuron,
mitral cell, thalamic relay neuron, and prepyriform pyramidal neuron,
we may presume that this siting is dictated by the dynamic relationship
between the inhibitory and excitatory inputs to the dendritic tree. Figure
10.5 also shows a model of this concept. The diagram shows that the
stellate cells may be able to effect "a selective inhibition of particular
dendritic segments of a Purkinje cell" (Llinás and Nicholson, 1971). In
the view of these workers, the large changes in local conductance that
accompany dendritic inhibition should produce a "functional amputa-
tion" of particular dendritic branches.

In contrast to the stellate cells, the basket cells deliver their inhibition to the axon hillock region of the Purkinje cells. In this position, it is optimally placed to strangle, as it were, the Purkinje cell output. For the Purkinje cell to be amputated by one neuron and strangled by another makes it appear to keep rather rough company. Perhaps a more felicitous image is "inhibitory sculpturing" (Eccles, 1964), that by the stellate cells being primarily a spatial shaping of activity within the dendritic tree, that by the basket cell being more in the temporal domain of impulse firing. This is with respect to the individual Purkinje cell; with respect to the population of Purkinje cells, both types of inhibition contribute to the spatiotemporal patterning of a multineuronal functional ensemble.

DENDRITIC SPINES A prominent feature of Purkinje cells is the profuse investiture of the dendritic branchlets with spines. We have seen that the parallel fiber synapses are exclusively to these spines, whereas the climbing fiber synapses are exclusively to the trunks and branches. This difference in synaptic input sites has a profound implication; it shows that the spine is not simply a devise for increasing the surface area of dendritic membrane but, rather, is differentiated as a specific anatomical site for a specific synaptic connection and function. A similar conclusion has been reached for the spines of neocortical pyramidal neurons.

The Purkinje cell dendritic spines are notable in being entirely postsynaptic in position; there are no synapses from them onto neighboring neurons. In this respect, they resemble the spines of cortical neurons and differ from the spines of olfactory granule cells and thalamic intrinsic neurons.

The fact that the Purkinje cell spines are only postsynaptic in position means that their input-output functions are simpler than those of the presynaptic spines of olfactory granule cells and thalamic intrinsic neurons. The only output from such a spine is by current flow through the spine stem. Llinás and Hillman (1969) pointed out that there must be a very high longitudinal resistance through the stem, with the consequence that even a small amount of postsynaptic current flow would give rise to a large postsynaptic potential (cf. Fig. 5.5). Furthermore, this high resistance lessens the shunting effect of a synapse on activity spreading past into the dendritic trunk. It can thus be seen that in the cerebellum, as elsewhere, a spine functions as a semi-independent input-output unit, and the elaboration of spines, therefore, serves to increase the complexity of the contingent probabilities that were mentioned above.

CONCLUDING REMARKS   The cerebellum and the retina provide an interesting comparison. Retinal processing is carried out almost exclusively within the domain of graded potentials, whereas cerebellar processing is carried out largely in the frequency domain. The fractionation of cerebellar circuits into an immense number of pathways, combined with the fractionation of temporal sequences into very brief intervals, appear to be the means by which the cerebellum, operating in the digital mode, achieves finely graded input-output relations like those of the retina, operating in the analog mode. Perhaps the fact that the cerebellum operates in the frequency domain reflects its close association with motoneuronal output, which, perforce, must be carried in a frequency code by impulses in the motoneuron axons to the muscles. Another close similarity is that both regions process information against a background of steady activity; the transient responses, therefore, are in the form of perturbations of ongoing activity. This apparently is a more precise mode of information transfer than is transmission by excitatory responses against little or no background. Since background activity may be adjusted under different behavioral conditions, information may be transmitted about steady states, and transient inputs are interpreted relative to those states.

Despite all the interest that has been focused on the cerebellum, and all the data obtained, one is still left with the question, as Thach (1972) has put it: What does the cerebellum do? The best answer, at present, seems to be that it helps initiate and maintain some types of movement and posture and that some of the Purkinje cells may have specific relations to specific movements and postures. The activity of Purkinje cells has been clearly correlated with the initiation of voluntary movements (Thach, 1970); as shown in Fig. 10.7, the impulse discharge changes in advance of the onset of a flexion movement of the wrist in an awake, behaving monkey. The discharge persists during the movement, suggesting that it is also related to the maintenance of the voluntary muscle contractions. Related findings will be discussed in the chapters on basal ganglia and motor cortex.

A theory of cerebellar function has been proposed by Marr (1969), and its interest for present concerns lies in the fact that it is formulated at the level of synaptic organization and hinges very much on the properties of the dendritic spines. The central hypothesis in this theory is that the synapses of the parallel fiber onto the Purkinje cell dendritic spines are

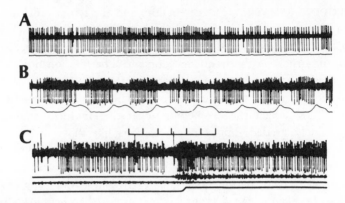

FIG. 10.7. Relation of Purkinje cell activity to movement in awake monkey. (A) At rest. (B) During alternating movement at the wrist. (C) In relation to triggered flexions of the wrist. Bottom trace, movement; middle traces, electromyographs. Note pause followed by increased simple spike discharge in relation to onset of movement, and a complex spike during the pause. Time bar; 100 msec divisions. (From Thach, 1970.)

modifiable; it is proposed that such modification, in the form of increased efficacy, comes about if a climbing fiber input to the Purkinje cell occurs at the same time as the parallel fiber input to the spine. The context of a movement is conveyed to a Purkinje cell by the pattern of mossy fiber-parallel fiber inputs to the spines; the Purkinje cell "learns' the appropriateness of its output for a movement by being triggered by the climbing fiber input; that learned behavior is stored ("memorized") by means of the increased efficacy of the parallel fiber synapses. As a result of the increased efficacy, the parallel fiber inputs themselves can activate the Purkinje cell and provide for its participation in the appropriate movement contexts.

It is beyond our present concerns to pursue the theory in greater depth. What is relevant to note here is that it basically involves a conditioning pardigm, in which one kind of input is not effective unless it is "learned" in conjunction with another input. We will mention a similar hypothesis in relation to the inputs to the hippocampus and motor cortex. The conditioning paradigm has, of course, a long history in concepts of brain function, and, as formulated at the level of synaptic organization, it has invariably required the postulate that there is some change in synaptic efficacy through use (see Hebb, 1949). We have already pointed out (Chapter 4) that this is an active field of neurophysiological investigation and that there are some suggestive leads, but few conclusive results. The fact that the Purkinje cell response to a parallel fiber volley includes a long-lasting inhibition, perhaps due to persistent transmitter effects, might indicate the possibility of long-lasting changes at the synapses onto the spines, but, beyond that, the appetite of the theory outruns the nutriment of the data. The much more labile synaptic actions in the hippocampus and neocortex seem more likely on the face of it to provide for learned behavior.

11

THALAMUS

The thalamus is one of the key relay and integrative centers of the brain. It is most conspicuously the gateway to the neocortex, and as such it has evolved in close relation to the cortex. It is, therefore, like the cortex, most highly developed in mammals and, especially, primates. Pathways from all the major sensory systems (from the muscles, deep tissue, and skin; from the eye, the ear, and the taste buds, as well as from the olfactory cortex) send their fibers here, to terminate on cells that in turn relay these inputs to the neocortex. Each part of the thalamus, in turn, receives fibers from the area of cortex to which it projects. Because of these relationships, the thalamic nuclei are integral parts of *thalamocortical systems* as well as *ascending systems*.

Each sensory pathway has its specific thalamic nucleus; Fig. 11.1 shows in schematic fashion the position of each. The lateral geniculate nucleus (LGN) provides the relay for the visual input coming from the retina. The medial geniculate nucleus (MGN) provides the relay for the auditory input that arrives through multisynaptic pathways originating in the cochlea of the inner ear. The ventrobasal complex (VBC) is the center for somatosensory input arising in the skin, deep tissues, and muscles of the body, and relayed thither through the lower brain stem (see Fig. 1.1).

Each thalamic nucleus provides for the transmission of its specific modality, as well as for convergence and integration of one or more other modality or input. The diagram of Fig. 11.1 illustrates a point that is important with regard to synaptic organization, and that is the very different positions of the thalamic relays in these pathways; there appears to be little similarity in the stages of processing prior to the thalamic level in these three systems. The thalamus is, thus, a processing

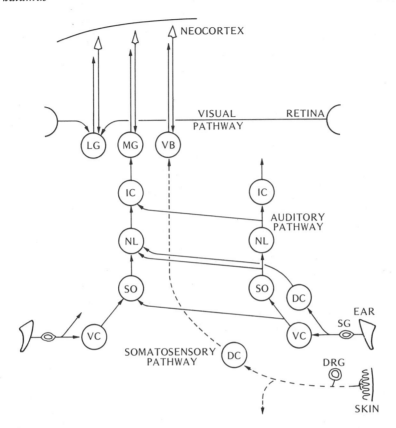

FIG. 11.1. Schematic diagram of different positions of the thalamic relay nuclei in their respective sensory pathways to the neocortex.

Visual pathway: lateral geniculate nucleus (LG).

Auditory pathway: spiral ganglion (SG); dorsal cochlear nucleus (DC); ventral cochlear nucleus (VC); superior olive (SO); nucleus of the lateral lemniscus (NL); inferior colliculus (IC); medial geniculate nucleus (MG).

Somatosensory pathway: dorsal root ganglion cell (DRG); dorsal column nucleus (DC); ventrobasal complex (VB).

station for inputs from widely differing sources within the brain, a key fact for understanding its integrative position and for comparing it with other regions.

In addition to these *specific central relay nuclei,* there are *specific central nuclei* that provide relays to the cortex from the cerebellum and the hypothalamus. Still others receive inputs from various parts of the reticular formation and, in turn, project widely to the neocortex; they are often referred to as *nonspecific thalamic nuclei*. The term "nonspecific", used in this and other contexts, is largely a reflection of our ignorance of their connections and functions. As more is learned about them, the terms "diffuse", "multimodal", or "specific" may become applicable in many of these cases.

It should be evident from even these brief remarks that the thalamus is, in fact, a most complex group of relay centers. When we single out the specific sensory relay nuclei for study, as we shall now do, we must keep in mind that they constitute scarcely one-eighth of the total thalamic volume. It might appear that even the three sensory relay nuclei are too disparate to be discussed together in one chapter. In the face of this it is, therefore, all the more remarkable that in the studies of recent years, many workers have reported similarities in the synaptic connections and functional properties of the neurons in these three nuclei. It is, thus, precisely at the level of synaptic organization that evidence for common principles in the construction of these centers has been gained. In reviewing that evidence, we will focus on the LGN, and compare the findings there with those in the MGN and VBC. The specific central nuclei related to the basal ganglia are discussed in the following chapter.

NEURONAL ELEMENTS

In depicting the neuronal elements of the sensory relay nuclei of the thalamus, we first encounter the problem that the input (through the afferent fibers) arrives from "below" (caudally), while the output is directed to the cortex "above" (rostrally). This is the reverse of the diagrammatic convention we have sought to develop as a basis for comparisons between different regions. It is perhaps just as well to be reminded by this that the brain is too complicated to permit simple generalizations about the geometrical relations of its constituents. It will hopefully be least confusing to depict the thalamic neuronal elements in their true relations, as just described, and then follow our customary procedure when we come to the basic circuit, in order to facilitate comparisons there with the circuits of other regions. Our description of the neuronal elements in the LGN is based on the accounts of Guillery (1971), Famiglietti and Peters (1972), Rafols and Valverde (1973), and Grossman, Lieberman, and Webster (1973).

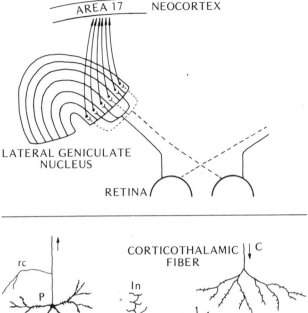

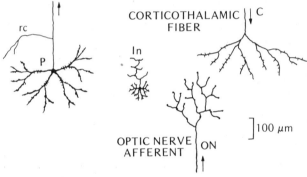

FIG. 11.2. (A) Relation of layers in the geniculate nucleus to inputs from ipsilateral and contralateral retinas. (B) Neuronal elements of the lateral geniculate nucleus.

Inputs: optic nerve afferent (ON); central fiber from cortex (C).

Principal neuron: thalamocortical relay neuron (P), with a recurrent axon collateral (rc).

Intrinsic neuron: (In) (shown with a short axon).

INPUTS   The *afferent input* is through the specific sensory fibers. For the LGN, these are the axons of the optic nerve that arise from the ganglion cells of the retina. In most mammals, the axons that arise from the cells in the lateral parts of the retina pass to the LGN of the same side, while those from the medial part of the retina cross in the optic chiasm to the LGN of the other (contralateral) side; this arrangement is indicated very schematically in Fig. 11.2.

In the optic nerve the axons vary in diameter (1–10 μm); in higher vertebrates most or all of the axons are myelinated (see Chapter 9). The larger axons come from Y ganglion cells in the retina, and project to both the LGN and the superior colliculus (cf. Hoffmann, 1973). The smaller axons arise from X ganglion cells and project only to the LGN.

Within the LGN, the axons from the two eyes terminate in separate layers; this is shown, again very schematically, in Fig. 11.2 (see also Fig. 15.8). Within its layer, the axon arborizes repeatedly to form many short branches, each of which ends in a knob-like terminals, as is shown in Fig. 11.2. The axonal branches are described as thick and myelinated up to very close to the terminal. The field of arborization is relatively restricted, of the order of 100–200 μm in diameter. This restricted field is assumed to be a necessary basis for preserving the high degree of spatial acuity in the visual system.

The other type of input to the thalamus is the *central input* from the neocortex. This comes through axons from cortical pyramidal cells. The axons are termed *corticothalamic fibers.* As already noted, these fibers arise largely in the same areas of the cortex to which the sensory nuclei project. They may thus be regarded as centrifugal fibers feeding back to their input source. These axons are described as fine and thinly myelinated. Within the LGN, they branch more sparingly but more widely than the specific afferents. The branches have a distinctive appearance, in that they give off many short side branches during their course; see Fig. 11.2. These corticothalamic fibers are the main type of central input we will consider; other central inputs include fibers from *other thalamic nuclei* and, to varying extents, from such *brainstem* regions as the reticular system.

PRINCIPAL NEURON   The output from the thalamic relay nuclei is carried in the axons of cells that, rare among principal neurons, have remained noneponymous; they are usually referred to as *relay,* or *thalamocortical, cells.* They take on a variety of forms in the different nuclei, but, in general, they appear, as in Fig. 11.2, as multipolar neurons, with four to eight dendrites that radiate outward in several directions. As principal neurons go, they are of small-to-medium size: the cell body varies in diameter from 15–30 μm, whereas the dendritic trunks vary from 1–8 μm in diameter. The dendrites are generally sparsely branched near the cell body, but they often have more branches peripherally. This gives them a tufted appearance (Ramón-Moliner, 1962), although this is not so marked as for glomerular tufts of olfactory bulb neurons. Clusters of small appendages—knobs, thorns, spines—arise from the proximal and intermediate dendritic branches, as is shown in Fig. 11.2. The tree attains extents of 100–300 μm from the cell body. In the LGN the principal neurons divide into Y and X classes on the basis of size, corresponding to their inputs from the retinal ganglion cells.

The axon of the principal neuron may, or may not, give off collateral branches; this is still a matter of controversy (see Grossman et al., 1973). As we will see, such collaterals have figured prominently in concepts of functional organization of the thalamus, but it appears from the anatomical evidence that collaterals are not in general highly developed (cf. Schiebel and Schiebel, 1970), and in the monkey LGN they have been reported to be absent (Le Vay, 1971). In view of this fact, it seems particularly significant that the retinal ganglion cells, which provide the input to the LGN, are also conspicuous for their lack of axon collaterals (Chapter 9). This sequence of principal neurons in the visual pathway therefore provides a contrast to the well-developed systems of such collaterals in the output neurons of many other brain regions (e.g., mitral cells, motoneurons, Purkinje cells, cortical pyramidal cells).

The thalamocortical cell axons immediately enter the white matter of the cerebrum and travel to their projection sites in the neocortex. Within the white matter, they mingle with fibers of many other systems and, therefore, have not been accurately characterized as to numbers and diameters. Most if not all of them are presumed to be myelinated.

INTRINSIC NEURONS A variety of small neurons has been described within the LGN of different mammals (Tömböl, 1967; Guillery, 1971; Famiglietti and Peters, 1972; Rafols and Valverde, 1973; Grossman et al., 1973). In general they are all subsumed under the term *short-axon cell*, or *Golgi type II neuron*. Some of these are very small (cell body 6–8 μm in diameter); an example is shown in Fig. 11.2. The dendritic trunks are relatively thin (1–3 μm in diameter), and the dendritic fields are limited to diameters of 50–150 μm. The dendrites are notable for giving rise to clumpy, claw-like appendages along their course and at their terminals. Other intrinsic neurons are larger, with cell bodies 10–20 μm in diameter, and dendrites that are correspondingly thicker and longer. In some species, the intrinsic neurons are described as bipolar in form, with their dendritic trees spanning the layer in which they lie (Rafols and Valverde, 1973).

The axons of the intrinsic neurons are thin and unmyelinated. They branch and terminate after a relatively short trajectory, which is rarely more than 200 μm. These axons are among the shortest in any region we will study; taken together with the cell body size, these neurons are among the smallest of any region. In some cases, the axonal field is in the vicinity of the cell body and closely overlaps the field of its own dendritic tree. Such a cell meets the classical definition of a short-axon cell, as one whose axon terminates in the vicinity of its cell body. In other cases, the axonal and dendritic fields do not overlap [see Fig. 11.2 (B)]; these fall under the category of short-axon cell as redefined in Chapter 8.

It has been reported that in monkey LGN the intrinsic neuron lacks an axon altogether (Le Vay, 1971), which would put it in the category of an *anaxonal* cell together with the retinal amacrine cell and the olfactory granule cell. This is a significant finding, particularly in relation to the evidence regarding the synaptic connections of thalamic intrinsic neurons, as we shall presently see. As negative evidence, it awaits further study and confirmation.

The neuronal elements in the other thalamic nuclei are equivalent to those in the LGN, although there are many different patterns of dendritic and axonal arborizations. The reader may consult Morest (1971) for description of the MGN nucleus and Ralston and Herman (1969) and Scheibel and Scheibel (1970) for the VBC. Of particular interest is the fact that, just as in the LGN, axon collaterals of principal neurons, and axons of intrinsic neurons, are difficult to visualize. Even taking account of the difficulties of Golgi impregnation of thin unmyelinted axons, it appears that these constituents may be absent in some nuclei of some species (see Scheibel, Davies, and Scheibel, 1972).

CELL POPULATIONS   The number of optic nerve fibers to the LGN in man is approximately 1,000,000 (see Chapter 9). The total number of neurons in the LGN has been estimted to be approximately 1,000,000. The majority of these are principal neurons (see below), so it is permissible to conclude that the convergence ratio of afferents onto principal neurons is not much more than one. This approaches the strict 1:1 ratio of climbing fibers to Purkinje cells in the cerebellum, but stands in contrast to the much larger convergence ratios in most other regions of the brain (for example, retina, olfactory bulb, granule layer of cerebellum). Since the afferent fiber arborizations are relatively restricted, the input-output relations in the LGN are relatively point-to-point in the spatial domain. As already noted, this is assumed to be essential for the transmission of precise spatiotemporal patterns relayed thereto from the retina.

Some figures for relative numbers of principal and intrinsic neurons are available from recent Golgi studies. It has ben reported that the ratio of principal:intrinsic neurons is approximately 10:1 in LGN (Le Vay, 1971), 2:1 in MGN (Morest, 1971), and 4:1 in VBC (Ralston and Herman, 1969). The remarkable feature of these ratios is, of course, that they reflect relatively small populations of intrinsic neurons in all the sensory relay nuclei. In fact, HRP studies indicate that in some species nearly all the cells in the LGN are labeled following a cortical injection. The relatively small sizes and extents of the intrinsic thalamic neurons further restrict the possibilities for convergent and divergent arrangements vis-à-vis the principal neurons. These considerations, by themselves, indicate that the degree of processing carried out within the relay nuclei is likely to be rather modest.

SYNAPTIC CONNECTIONS

Electron-microscopic study of the synaptic connections in the thalamus has developed in three stages. First was the discovery that the main sites of synaptic connection are in tight clusters of terminals, called variously *synaptic nests, islands,* or *glomeruli.* Their general similarity to the synaptic glomeruli of the cerebellum was early noted (Szentágothai, 1963). The second stage involved the identification of the terminals within the glomerulus according to the classical criteria for axon and dendrite (see Chapter 1). This work established the basic similarity of the organization of the glomeruli in the three relay nuclei (Peters and Palay, 1966; Jones and Powell, 1969; Szentágothai, 1970). In the final, and very recent, stage, the relevance of the findings in olfactory bulb and retina has been realized, and certain of the presynaptic terminals have been re-identified as dendritic rather than axonal (Ralston and Herman, 1969; Morest, 1971; Famiglietti and Peters, 1972; Pasik et al., 1973; see also Reese and Shepherd, 1972; Ralston, 1979). For our description, we will continue to focus on the example of the LGN.

A synaptic glomerulus in the LGN is illustrated in Fig. 11.3. At or near the center is the large terminal of an optic nerve axon. Around this

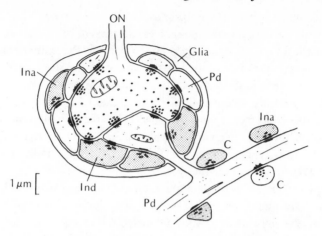

FIG. 11.3. Synaptic connections in thalamic sensory nuclei (lateral geniculate). Diagram shows a synaptic glomerulus, which contains axodendritic connections from an optic nerve terminal (ON) onto principal cell dendrites (Pd) and intrinsic cell dendrites (Ind), and dendrodendritic connections from intrinsic cell dendrites onto principal cell dendrites. Note also the axodendritic connections from intrinsic cell axons (Ina) onto principal cell dendrites. The glomerulus is surrounded by glial membranes. Outside the glomerulus are axodendritic connections from corticothalamic (C) and intrinsic cell axons onto a principal cell dendrite. (After Szentágothai, 1970; Jones and Powell, 1969; Morest, 1971; Famiglietti and Peters, 1972.)

terminal are numbers of other terminals; small glomeruli have only a few terminals; the largest have 15 to 20. The whole group or cluster is surrounded by one or more layers of glial membrane. Note that the size of a thalamic glomerulus is much smaller than a cerebellar glomerulus (Chapter 10, Fig. 10.2), and that both are microglomeruli in contrast to the macroglomeruli of the olfactory bulb and cerebral cortex.

Within the glomerulus, the optic nerve terminal makes synaptic connections onto two types of dendritic terminal. One of these is a thorn or other appendage from the dendrite of a principal neuron; this is a type I chemical synapse (see Fig. 11.3). The other, and more numerous, type is constituted by terminal "knobs" or other appendages from the dendrites of intrinsic neurons; these connections are also type I chemical synapses. In addition, these terminals have dendrodendritic synapses, of type II, onto the dendritic thorns of the principal neurons. These connections are all indicated in Fig. 11.3.

When these arrangements were first observed, the terminals that make type II synapses were assumed to be axon terminals of the intrinsic neurons, on the basis that they were presynaptic in position. With the demonstration in the olfactory bulb and retina that dendrites could occupy presynaptic positions, the identification of type II terminals in the thalamus as arising from intrinsic dendrites has become accepted. The intrinsic neurons thus receive axodendritic synapses from the optic nerve terminals, and, themselves, make dendrodendritic synapses onto the principal neuron dendrites that also receive axodendritic synapses from the same optic nerve terminal.

In addition to these main patterns of connection, reciprocal dendrodendritic synapses have also been reported (Famiglietti, 1970; Harding, 1971; Lieberman & Webster, 1973). A few terminals from the axons of the intrinsic neurons are situated toward the periphery of the glomerulus and make type II synapses onto either type of dendritic terminal (principal or intrinsic). The possibility of axoaxonal synapses within the glomerulus has not been ruled out, but in the recent studies it is assumed that they are relatively infrequent.

Outside the glomeruli, two main types of connection have been identified. The more numerous are the connections from the terminals of extrinsic axons from the cerebral cortex (corticothalamic fibers) onto the dendrites of both principal and intrinsic neurons. They are type I synapses. These terminals can be identified unequivocally because they can be seen to degenerate after ablations of the cortex. There are also type II synapses onto the principal cell dendrites from the axons of intrinsic neurons. These connections are indicated in Fig. 11.3.

The patterns of connections in the other relay nuclei bear a general similarity to those illustrated in Fig. 11.3. In the MGN, the central element is usually the dendritic terminal from the principal neuron, rather than the axonal terminal from the afferent fiber; but, otherwise, the synaptic glomeruli are reported to have the same basic construction (Jones and Powell, 1969; Morest, 1971). The same can be said of the VBC, where the glomeruli have been reported to be somewhat less clearly demarcated by enveloping glial processes than in the other nuclei (Ralston and Herman, 1969).

BASIC CIRCUIT

The organization of the sensory relay nuclei of the thalamus is summarized in the basic circuit diagram of Fig. 11.4. In brief, the large termi-

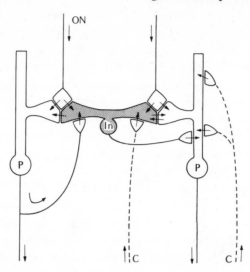

FIG. 11.4. Basic circuit diagram for thalamic sensory relay nuclei. Abbreviations as in Fig. 11.3.

nals of the afferent axons make synapses onto the dendrites of both principal and intrinsic neurons within the synaptic glomeruli. The dendrites are interconnected by dendrodendritic synapses, predominantly oriented from intrinsic to principal neurons. The intrinsic neuron also has synaptic connections through its axon (when present) onto the dendrites of neighboring principal neurons. Depending on the presence of axon collaterals, there may be additional connections from the principal neuron onto the intrinsic neurons (Fig. 11.4, dotted line). These various connections provide for feedforward and feedback pathways within the thalamus. In addition, corticothalamic fibers have synapses onto the dendrites of both principal and intrinsic neurons, providing for long feedback loops through the cortex.

Much of the basic function of the thalamus in relaying information can be seen to revolve about the synaptic glomeruli, and it is appropriate, therefore, at this point, to assess their significance in the light of what we have learned about similar arrangements in other regions of the brain. The thalamic glomeruli resemble their counterparts in the cerebellum not only in being surrounded by glial membranes, but, more importantly, in providing for specific interconnections between input, principal, and intrinsic elements. This relation was recognized by Famiglietti

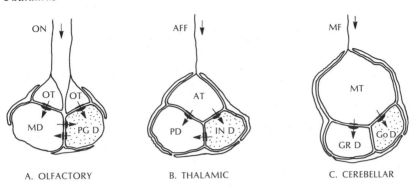

FIG. 11.5. Schematic diagrams comparing synaptic triads of olfactory bulb, thalamus and cerebellum. (A) ON, olfactory nerve; OT, olfactory terminals; MD, mitral cell dendrite; PG D, periglomerular cell dendrite. (B) AFF, afferent nerves; AT, afferent terminals; PD, principal cell dendrite; IN D, intrinsic cell dendrite. (C) MF, mossy fibers; MT, mossy terminal; GR D, granule cell dendrite; Go D, Golgi cell dendrite. (From Shepherd, 1977.)

and Peters (1972) and designated the "triadic relation," and this is precisely the sense in which we have used the term in our discussion of the synaptic organization of the cerebellum and of other brain regions.

In view of this general similarity, it is of interest to compare the synaptic triad in the thalamus with that in the olfactory glomeruli, on the one hand, and the cerebellum, on the other. Figure 11.5 summarizes the essential arrangements in the three regions. In the thalamic triad, the input synapses onto the principal and intrinsic cells arise from a single large afferent terminal. There are connections between the dendrites, oriented from intrinsic to principal cell. Thus, in both these respects, the synaptic complexity is less than in the olfactory triad, where there are separate terminals onto principal and intrinsic cells, and there are connections in both directions between their dendrites. In addition, there is a complete glial wrapping around the thalamic glomerulus. It seems reasonable to postulate that the thalamic triad provides for a simpler type of synaptic processing than in the olfactory triad.

In the cerebellar triad, a very large afferent terminal makes a great many synapses onto the relay neuron (granule cell) and intrinsic neuron (Golgi cell). No synapses are present between their dendrites. The very considerable divergence from the same input terminal, and the lack of any dendrodendritic interactions, suggests an even simpler and more stereotyped transmission of information than in the case of the thalamus.

In comparison with other regions of the brain, the organization of the thalamus shares certain features with both the OPL and IPL of the retina, principally in that the input is made simultaneously from an input terminal to both principal and intrinsic elements. At both these levels in the retina, there are interconnections between the principal and intrinsic elements as well as back onto the input terminal; these interconnections make the arrangement of the synaptic triad more complex than in the thalamic nuclei. A thoughtful comparison between the synaptic organization of intrinsic neurons in the retina and thalamus has been provided by Morest (1971).

Apart from the synaptic glomeruli, the other prominent aspect of thalamic organization is the input from the cortex. The difference between afferent input, on the one hand, and central "centrifugal" input, on the other, is very clear and unambiguous. Not only are these fiber constituents separate (as they were not in the cerebellum), but their synaptic terminations are also distinct. It appears that the corticothalamic connections are primarily concerned with modulating the thalamic principal neurons through their dendritic branches, rather than controlling the initial events in the relay through the synaptic glomeruli. Like all other regions of our present study, except the retina, the thalamus has a feeback from the sites of projection that is integrated within its local circuits.

It is, of course, possible that, under some conditions, the cortex becomes the dominant input to the thalamic relay neurons, and the afferent fibers function as long and complex delayed feedback loops from the periphery. We must, therefore, be cautious about adopting an inflexible view of which inputs provide the primary drive to a region and which inputs provide feedback modulation; the same input pathway may function in either mode under different conditions.

SYNAPTIC ACTIONS

Since the thalamic relay nuclei receive specific sensory afferents, synaptic actions can be investigated by using brief sensory stimuli, as, for example, a spot of light, a click or tone, or a brief mechanical deformation. Alternatively, an electrical shock can be delivered to the afferent pathways. By either method, a synchronous volley is set up, similar to the method of procedure in other regions of the brain. We cannot review the many studies that are relevant to the evidence for synaptic actions in

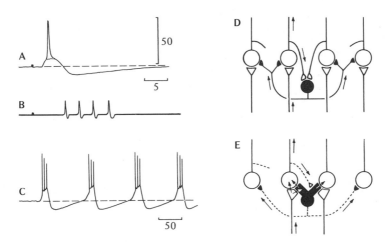

FIG. 11.6. Synaptic actions in thalamic sensory relay nuclei. (A) Intracellular recording of the response of a principal neuron to an afferent volley. (After Nelson and Erulkar, 1964; Andersen et al., 1964.) (B) Extracellular recording of the response of a presumed intrinsic neuron to an afferent volley. (After Andersen et al., 1964.) (C) Rhythmic "burst" responses of a principal neuron. (After Purpura and Cohen, 1962; Andersen and Eccles, 1962.) Intracellular voltage calibration, as in (A). (D) Schematic diagram of pathways for the generation of rhythmic activity through axon collaterals and short-axons. (Modified from Andersen and Eccles, 1962; Andersen and Andersson, 1968.) (E) Schematic diagram of possible pathways for rhythmic activity, in the light of recent evidence (see text).

all the nuclei or even in one of them. Our concern must be limited to only the basic types of synaptic actions.

The key finding is illustrated in Fig. 11.6 (A). An afferent volley produces an initial depolarization of the principal neuron. This depolarization has a brief latency, is graded in intensity, and, at threshold, gives rise to a single (or sometimes several) impulse(s) (see below); these are the characteristics of a monosynaptic EPSP. It is followed by a long-lasting hyperpolarization, during which impulse activity is completely suppressed; this suppression has the characteristics of an IPSP.

This type of excitatory-inhibitory sequence has been reported in all relay nuclei. For references for the LGN, the reader may consult Burke and Sefton (1966), McIlwain and Creutzfeldt (1967), and Kalil and Chase (1970); for the MGN; Nelson and Erulkar (1964) and Aitken and Dunlop (1969); for the VBC, Andersen, Eccles, and Sears (1964). It is particularly notable that later authors have stressed the similarity of the responses in the three nuclei (see also Purpura, 1967, 1972; Eccles, 1969).

INHIBITORY PATHWAYS   The pathway that mediates the inhibition of the principal neuron has been investigated by recording from units believed to be the intrinsic neurons. These units respond to an efferent volley at a latency that is slightly later than the spike, but earlier than the IPSP, in the principal neuron; see Fig. 11.6 (B). It has therefore been inferred that an impulse invades the axon collaterals of the principal neurons and synaptically excites the intrinsic cells, which then synaptically inhibit the principal neurons through their short axons (see Eccles, 1969). Such a pathway is analogous to the Renshaw pathway of the ventral horn, and similar pathways have been inferred in other regions, for example, the cerebellum and the hippocampus.

These physiological studies have not taken into account the recent findings regarding synaptic connections. As reviewed in the previous section, it is obvious that the dendrodendritic synapses also provide pathways for inhibition of the principal neurons. When we take into account the paucity of axon collaterals in most principal neurons and the equivocal evidence in some cases for short axons, the dendrodendritic connections within the synaptic glomeruli would appear likely to play a major role in the inhibitory control of principal neurons, particularly in their responses to afferent inputs (Morest, 1971; Shepherd, 1972b; Pasik et al., 1973). The role of afferent (lateral) inhibition as the basis for contrast enhancement in the specific sensory pathways has long been recognized (see Mountcastle, 1974). Physiologists now need to incorporate the dendrodendritic pathway into concepts of these processing mechanisms.

A similar re-evaluation is needed of the evidence for presynaptic inhibition. It was postulated that this was mediated through axoaxonal contacts from the intrinsic neurons onto the afferent terminals (Andersen et al., 1964), but the anatomical evidence suggests, instead, that the most likely pathway is through dendrodendritic inhibitory synapses from the inhibitory interneurons onto the principal neurons within the synaptic glomeruli (see Fig. 11.3).

Inhibitory potentials are also elicited in principal neurons by a volley from the area of cortex to which the neuron projects. Such potentials can still be recorded after cortical ablations, which cause the fibers from the cortex to degenerate. This was taken as evidence that this inhibition is also due to the Renshaw circuit within the thalamus (see Andersen et al., 1964). There is now the additional possibility that the antidromic impulse invades the dendrites of the principal neuron to activate excitatory dendrodendritic synapses onto the dendrites of the intrinsic neurons, which then feed back inhibition onto the principal neuron dendrites, in analogy with the sequence of mitral-granule-mitral inhibition in the olfactory bulb. But reciprocal synapses, and synapses from principal to intrinsic cell dendrites, are much less numerous in the thalamus than in the olfactory bulb.

From the experiments just cited, it has been further concluded that the inhibition caused by stimulation of the intact cortex is due to intrathalamic circuits and mechanisms (see Eccles, 1969). Recent work on the influence of the visual cortex on the LGN, however, has provided evidence for both excitatory and inhibitory effects (Kalil and Chase, 1970). The synaptic connections proposed for these effects consist of direct excitatory input to the principal neurons, and direct excitatory input to the intrinsic neurons, which are then inhibitory to the principal neurons. These connections are consistent with the basic circuit diagram of Fig. 11.4, with the exception that the latter connection is to presynaptic dendrites, rather than axons as was formerly believed.

RHYTHMIC ACTIVITY   A prominent characteristic of thalamic neurons is the tendency to rhythmic activity. This is particularly evident under conditions in which neuronal excitability is high. As shown in Fig. 11.6 (C), an afferent volley elicits, under these conditions, a burst of impulses in a principal neuron, followed by the long-lasting IPSP already described. The IPSP subsides over a period of 100 msec or so; when the membrane potential again reaches resting level, there is a rebound excitation, a burst of impulses is again generated, and the cycle repeats itself.

It was proposed that the rhythmically generated IPSPs are responsible for the phasing of the burst discharges (Purpura and Cohen, 1962) and that the IPSPs are due to feedback through a Renshaw type circuit (Andersen and Eccles, 1962). As illustrated in Fig. 11.6 (D), the essential feature of the feedback circuit is that inhibitory interneurons have connections with many principal neurons, so that a discharge in a principal neuron leads not only to feedback inhibition of that neuron but also to feedforward inhibition of neighboring neurons. By this means, a large population of neurons becomes involved in synchronous excitation and inhibition within a few rhythmic cycles.

The mechanism as just described has been termed an *inhibitory phasing of neuronal discharge* by Andersen and Eccles (1962). It has served as a model for the generation of the alpha rhythm of the electroencephalogram (EEG) (see Purpura, 1967; Andersen and Andersson, 1968) and for the generation of rhythmic potentials by inhibition in other regions, for example the hippocampus. That it depends on pathways within the thalamus has been inferred from the fact that the rhythms persist after cortical ablation, which has been taken as evidence against the possibility of reverberatory thalamocortical circuits. That it depends on an intrathalamic pathway through axon collaterals and intrinsic cell axons has been postulated on the basis of an analogy with Renshaw inhibition in the spinal cord. But we have described in the olfactory bulb a possible mechanism for inhibitory phasing of neuronal discharge through exclusively dendrodendritic interactions between mitral and granule cell dendrites. The demonstration of dendrodendritic connections in the thalamus, as reviewed above, thereby provides alternative, or additional, pathways for rhythmical activity in the thalamus that now require physiological investigation. A tentative scheme to indicate how the dendrodendritic connections may be incorporated into the postulated circuits of the thalamus is shown in Fig. 11.6 (E).

DENDRITIC PROPERTIES

PRINCIPAL NEURON The evidence thus far indicates that the principal neurons of the thalamic relay nuclei are primarily postsynaptic in position. This means that in these neurons, as in other such neurons we have considered elsewhere, the dendrites provide for local integration of synaptic inputs, and transmission of the integrated potentials to the axon hillock. An electotonic model for assessing the properties of the dendritic tree in relation to these functions is unfortunately not available. The thalamic relay neurons are rather small, so that the acquisition of information about electrical parameters, upon which a model could be used, will not be an easy task.

There are a few clues to dendritic properties meanwhile. One clue is that, apart from details of gemoetry, the dendritic tree of the thalamic principal neuron is not unlike that of a smaller version of a motoneuron or of the glomerular tuft of an olfactory mitral cell. By again making use of the concept of a scaling principle, it may be postulated that an equivalent cylinder for the dendritic trees of thalamic principal neurons would have an electrotonic length (L) in the same range of 1 to 2. We have seen that this is consistent with the transfer of signals through a dendritic tree by passive means alone, and it could be suggested, therefore, that this is also the case in the thalamic neurons. There is, in any event, little evidence for active properties of the dendrites, in terms of fast prepotentials or the like, as in cerebellar Purkinje cells or hippocampal pyramidal neurons. It is relevant to note, however, that following a period of inhibition the principal neurons become hyperexcitable, a phenomenon that is termed *post-inhibitory exaltation;* this is a possible additional component in the mechanism for the generation of rhythmic activity (cf. Purpura, 1967; Andersen and Andersson, 1968).

There is an interesting difference when the dendritic tree of the principal neuron is compared with the glomerular tuft of the olfactory mitral cell. In the thalamus, the afferent inputs are to the appendages on the more proximal dendrites, whereas the central (cortical) inputs are to the more distal branches. In the olfactory glomerulus, on the other hand, the afferent inputs are to the more distal branches and the interglomerular and centrifugal inputs are to the proximal branches. The relative placements of afferent and central inputs are thus different in the two cases, yet both have as primary functions the relay of specific sensory information and modulation by central pathways. This may serve as a useful caution against correlating particular functions with particular positions of synaptic inputs in a dendritic tree.

An interesting point bearing on dendritic properties is raised by the fact that the thalamic principal neurons respond to an afferent volley with an excitatory-inhibitory sequence [see Fig. 11.6 (A)] similar to the response of the principal neurons of many other regions to an afferent volley. This similarity has seemed all the more remarkable in the face of the quite different sizes and shapes of the dendritic trees in the different neurons. To account for this most peculiar paradox, Purpura (1967) has suggested the principle that the major determinants of response patterns are the nature and distribution of postsynaptic potentials, rather than the size, configuration, and orientation of the dendrites. A somewhat similar conclusion was inferred from the study of ganglion cell dendritic patterns in the retina.

This may seem inconsistent with our emphasis on the importance of dendritic properties and dendritic branching patterns in assessing the input-output dynamics of a neuron or neuronal part. Is it also at variance with such a statement as that of Peters et al. (1976): "the form of the dendritic tree provides a topographic map of the world as seen by a particular cell"? Probably not. One of the important results of our inquiry into dendritic properties is that the dendritic trees of most neurons are within 1 to 2 space constants of the cell body where recordings are usually made. Thus, regardless of the size or configuration of a neuron and its dendrites, postsynaptic potentials spread rather effectively through the tree, a fact that is implicit in the notion of a scaling principle. The summated response to a synchronous volley of many afferent fibers does not reflect the different sites of input in the tree. Under natural conditions, however, the contributions of individual inputs, weighted and shaped by the electrotonic properties of the dendritic tree, may be assumed to stand out more clearly within the integrative fabric of the neuron. Yet even under these conditions, the point raised by Purpura has some relevance. The particular geometry of a dendritic tree is the starting point for assessing dendritic function, but the final goal is the dynamic properties of the interactions within the dendrites.

INTRINSIC NEURONS   We have seen that the dendrites of the intrinsic neuron are presynaptic as well as postsynaptic in position. The dendro-dendritic synapses from the presynaptic dendrites are not an occasional finding; they are a major type of connection, and we have reviewed the suggestion that, in some species, they may be the only output from the intrinsic neuron, if an axon is not present. This means that, as in the olfactory bulb and retinal neurons with presynaptic dendrites, the dendrites have a local input-output role to play as well as providing for longer-range transmission of signals within the dendritic tree.

These roles have been discussed in explicit and lucid form by Ralston (1971). Figure 11.7 is an illustration of the model he has suggested for dendritic functions in the intrinsic neurons. The starting point is the fact, which we have noted, that the dendritic terminals are at a distance from the cell body and axon hillock. This makes it possible for a dendritic terminal to receive synaptic input without the postsynaptic potential being of sufficient amplitude to spread to the axon hillock to generate an impulse. Ralston noted the possibility that the local postsynaptic

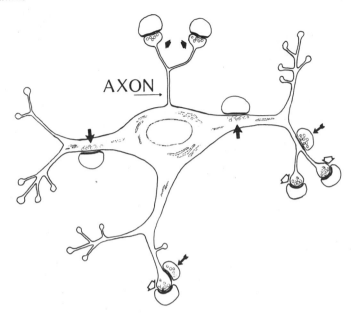

AXON

FIG. 11.7. Schematic diagram of an intrinsic neuron in the thalamus, to illustrate input-output relations in dendritic branches (large solid arrows) and dendritic terminals. Terminals can act as semi-independent functional units, receiving axonal input (solid, tailed arrows) and giving rise to local dendrodendritic synaptic output (open arrows). (From Ralston, 1971.)

potential would be adequate to activate local dendrodendritic synapses onto neighboring dendrites. Each of the terminals or branches might be capable of releasing its transmitter, graded by the amount of local synaptic deplarization, regardless of the activity of other dendritic branches; thus, each would function as an "independent synaptic unit". In contrast, when an action potential was initiated in the axon hillock, it might invade the proximal dendritic branches, causing synchronous release of transmitter from those synapses, but it probably would not reach the finer branches. In this way, several levels of output activity are possible in the synaptic output from the dendritic tree of the intrinsic neuron.

This model must now be tested in physiological experiments. As it stands, it is entirely consistent with the evidence for dendritic spread of an impulse in the olfactory mitral cell, with the evidence for graded transmitter release from retinal neurons and olfactory granule cells, and with the evidence for dendrodendritic synaptic interactions in the distal terminals of the periglomerular cell dendrites, as described in Chapter 8. The model of Fig. 11.7 may thus be taken, by and large, as a working model for the periglomerular cells in the olfactory bulb and for short-axon cells, with presynaptic dendrites, in other parts of the brain. The concept of independent synaptic units is further consistent with the suggestion that dendritic terminals form identifiable *functional units*.

12

BASAL GANGLIA

The telencephalon consists of an outer mantle of cortex and an inner system of nuclear structures, referred to collectively as the basal ganglia. Their remoteness, complicated anatomy, and elusive functions have made the basal ganglia seem to be the nervous counterpart of a puzzle wrapped in a mystery inside an enigma. Responding to the challenge, neuroscientists have been picking at the puzzle, and it is possible to discern, however dimly, some outlines of the synaptic organization of these regions.

The anatomical locations and main connections of the basal ganglia are illustrated schematically in Fig. 12.1. Embryologically the *caudate* and *putamen* arise together; though separated along most of their extent by the fibers of the internal capsule, they have essentially the same structure. Together they are referred to as the *neostriatum*, or simply *striatum*. The neighboring *globus pallidus* is the major recipient of the striatal output, and is divided into lateral and medial segments. The lateral segment projects to a small region called the *subthalamic nucleus*, which in turn connects to the medial segment. The medial segment has a complicated set of output sites that include specific parts of the thalamus, substantia nigra, and pontine tegmentum. In the brainstem, the *substantia nigra*, though formally not one of the basal ganglia, is functionally closely related by virtue of its input from the striatum and globus pallidus, and its output back to the striatum and to the parts of the thalamus which project to the striatum. This is only a capsule summary of the main connections of the basal ganglia, as a prelude to the detailed account that follows.

Historically our understanding of the functions of the basal ganglia has been drawn heavily from clinical studies of the effects of certain diseases.

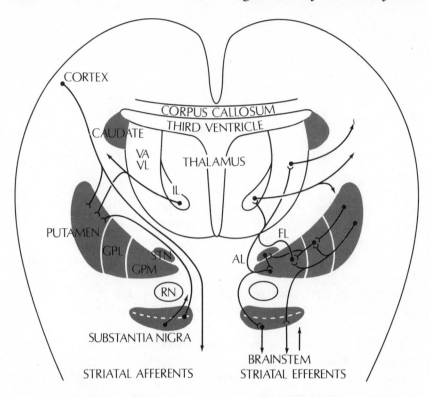

FIG. 12.1. Schematic frontal section of human brain, showing main connections and relations of the basal ganglia. Globus pallidus, lateral segment (GPL); medial segment (GPM). STN, subthalamic nucleus; AL, ansa lenticularis; FL, fasciculus lenticularis. Thalamic nuclei: VA, ventral anterior; VL, ventral lateral. RN, red nucleus. Connections of caudate are similar to those shown for putamen.

Thus, in Parkinson's disease there is a degeneration of the dopamine-containing cells in the substantia nigra, with loss of dopamine there and in the striatum to which the cells project. This disease is associated with a variety of disturbances, including muscular rigidity, restriction of movement, and tremor. Other types of movement disorder are athetosis (slow writhing movements), chorea (rapid coordinated muscle jerks), and ballismus (violent flinging movements). Each is associated with pathological changes in parts of the basal ganglia, thalamus, or cortex. In some cases surgical intervention can alleviate the symptoms. From these clinical experiences has arisen the concept that the basal ganglia are a part of the extrapyramidal motor system, concerned with coordination of motor control.

Laboratory studies have broadened this view. The early studies were unrewarding, in that neither restricted lesions nor electrical stimulation could be shown to produce clear effects on motor behavior. However, more systematic experiments have revealed a variety of effects. These involve not only distortions of posture and coordination, but also impairments of initiation and performance of movements oriented toward the tactile and visual environment. Other experiments have shown disruptions of performance in complex behavior, such as delayed responses to a visual discrimination test. Single-unit studies have provided evidence that multiple sensory inputs converge onto the basal ganglia, and that neuronal firing patterns are related to slow, voluntary movements of the extremities. Finally, neuropharmacological investigations of cholinergic neurons in the striatum and the introduction of dopamine-precursor (levodopa) therapy for the treatment of parkinsonism have given birth to new concepts of the balance between neurotransmitter systems in the control of basal ganglia functions. The reader is referred to the symposium on the basal ganglia edited by Yahr (1976) for reviews of these subjects.

Of the several components of the basal ganglia, the striatum is a key structure. We shall therefore focus our study on the organization of the striatum, with briefer allusion to the globus pallidus and substantia nigra.

NEURONAL ELEMENTS

The importance of lamination, as an aid in identifying cell types and connections, has often been stressed in this book. Perhaps no region better illustrates this point than the striatum, where this aid is so conspicuously lacking. The structure of both caudate and putamen appears relatively homogeneous; fibers, cell bodies, and synaptic neuropil are everywhere intermingled. As a consequence, work on the identification of neuronal elements has proceeded slowly, and many of the points are still tentative.

Modern work, combining Golgi methods of electronmicroscopy, began with the papers of Kemp and Powell (1971a–e) and Fox and his collaborators (Fox et al., 1971), with important contributions from histofluorescence techniques (Ungerstedt, 1971). Recently, HRP tracing (Grofova, 1975) and electrophysiological analysis (Kocsis and Kitai,

1977) have provided new and powerful tools to supplement the traditional anatomical methods.

INPUTS There are three main sources for inputs to the striatum, as
shown in Fig. 12.1. The largest input comes from the *cerebral cortex*.
Most of the cortex sends fibers, and there is a topographic organization
(anterior cortex to anterior striatum, etc.) though with considerable
overlap. The projections are mainly ipsilateral, with contralateral connections from some areas (supplementory motor area and area 5; cf.
Kemp and Powell, 1971e).

The second source of inputs is the *intralaminar nuclear complex* of the
thalamus. This complex is usually considered to be nonspecific in modality and diffuse in connections, but, as we have noted elsewhere, such
characterizations largely reflect our ignorance. The intralaminar complex
probably receives collateral fibers from ascending sensory and brainstem
pathways, and in turn has a topographic projection to the striatum, the
centromedian nucleus sending fibers to the putamen and the more anterior nuclei to the caudate.

The third input arises from the *substantia nigra* in the midbrain. Classical degeneration methods gave little evidence of these fibers, and they
were first clearly revealed by the histochemical fluorescence technique
(Fuxe, 1965). Subsequently it has been shown that the fibers contain
dopamine, and arise from cell bodies in the cell body layer (pars com-
pacta) of the substantia nigra. This projection also has a topographic
organization.

In addition to these main inputs, fibers to the striatum have been
reported from several brainstem sites, including the reticular formation
and the median raphe.

We have seen in many regions of the nervous system that the input
fibers have distinctive morphologies and sites of laminar termination.
Such is not the case in the striatum, and the correlation of input sources
with the types of fibers and terminals is not yet established. Kemp and
Powell (1971a) describe three main types in Golgi material, as illustrated
in Fig. 12.2. One type (a) consists of bundles of fine axons less than 1
μm in diameter; the other two of single thin (c) or thick (b) fibers which
branch and terminate. Recent studies suggest that some of the projections are not homogeneous throughout the striatum, but terminate in
clusters (Goldman and Nauta, 1977; Graybiel and Ragsdale, 1978) which

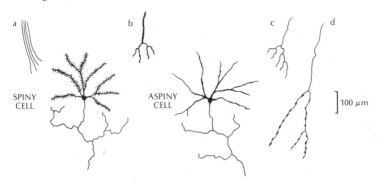

FIG. 12.2. Neuronal elements of the mammalian neostriatum.
Inputs: (a–d) as described in text.
Principal and intrinsic neurons: spiny and aspiny cells.

may define functional compartments. Also depicted in Fig. 12.2 is a dopamine-containing axon (d), though these have not been visualized in Golgi material. Each axon is believed to branch profusely; estimates of the number of terminals reach as high as several hundred thousand (Andén et al., 1966).

PRINCIPAL AND INTRINSIC NEURONS   The projection of the striatum to the neighboring globus pallidus has been known for many years, and recent work has added the projection to the substantia nigra (pars reticulata); these are shown in Fig. 12.1. A most difficult problem has been the identity of the principal neurons which give rise to these axons. Cytoarchitectonic studies in the 1920's indicated that the striatum consists of a large population of small neurons and a small population of large neurons, and it was an attractive hypothesis that the small neurons were short-axon cells acting as intrinsic interneurons, and the large neurons were long-axon cells acting as output neurons.

Modern studies have emphasized instead that most striatal cells fall into a medium-size category, with cell bodies 12–20 μm in diameter. Two types of dendritic trees have been distinguished: those that are spiny and those that are "aspiny" (smooth). These are illustrated in Fig. 12.2. The spiny cells account for 95% of the cells in the striatum, and thus include most of the previously described small neurons. The belief has been widespread that they are the interneurons, and the aspiny cells the output neurons, as previously inferred. However, this distinction

appears to be breaking down, and it is best to describe the cell types
without categorizing them as principal or intrinsic.

A *spiny cell* is illustrated in Fig. 12.2. The cell body gives rise to 5–6
dendritic trunks; these are 2–3 μm in diameter, and have a smooth
surface for their initial 10–20 μm. They then branch sparingly and reach
lengths of 150–250 μm; a few are as long as 600 μm. The branches "are
covered with the most robust spines found anywhere in the central
nervous system" (Fox et al., 1971). A density of approximately 1 spine
per μm of dendritic length has been reported (Kemp and Powell, 1971d;
Pasik, Pasik and DiFiglia, 1976). The smooth dendritic trunks and spine-
laden branches are reminiscent of the cerebellar Purkinje cell. The total
number of spines is likely several hundred to several thousand per cell—
a lot of spines compared with most other neurons, but fewer than those
on Purkinje cells by at least two orders of magnitude.

The axon of the spiny cell arises from the cell body or a dendritic
trunk. In the electron microscope one or more spines are seen arising
from the initial segment of the axon (see next section). The axon diameters are thin, probably 1 μm or less. The axon begins to give off fine
collateral branches at 50–100 μm, and has been reported to terminate
within 200 μm. On this basis the spiny cells appear to be intrinsic
short-axon cells. However, Pasik et al. (1976) have been able to follow
the axons of spiny cells as far as 500 μm, and suggest that spiny cells
may have distant connections within the striatum, or may be principal
neurons contributing to efferent pathways. Bunney and Aghajanian
(1976b) found after HRP injections into the substantia nigra that 30–50%
of the cells in the striatum are labeled, indicating that their axons project
to the injection site; these cells must be mostly spiny cells, but aspiny
cells may also be included.

The *aspiny cell* accounts for only 2–5% of the striatal cell population.
They range in size from giant (up to 30 μm in diameter) to small (as little
as 5 μm, among the smallest in the nervous system). A medium-size cell
is shown in Fig. 12.2. It typically has 4–6 dendrites which branch
sparingly and reach lengths of 150–300 μm. Some cells have dendrites
with occasional spines; others show occasional varicosities. The axon
arises from the cell body or a dendritic trunk. Some cells have a long
axon with few collaterals, others a short axon with many collaterals;
some very small cells may lack axons, suggesting a variety of amacrine
cell (Kemp and Powell, 1971a). Keeping in mind the vagaries of Golgi

impregnations, it appears that aspiny cells may be either principal or intrinsic neurons (cf. Pasik et al., 1976).

The efferent axons gather into bundles (or "pencils") and converge onto the globus pallidus "like spokes in a wheel" (not shown). The fibers in the bundles are termed "radial fibers"; they are thinly myelinated and approximately 0.7 μm in diameter. Between the globus pallidus and substantia nigra is a set of parallel bundles, called the "comb" system. The fibers in the comb teeth are nearly all unmyelinated, approximately 0.2 μm in diameter. There is evidence that the myelinated radial fibers give rise to myelinated collaterals to the globus pallidus as well as the unmyelinated axons which pass on to the substantia nigra (Yoshida, Rabin, and Anderson, 1974; Fox and Rafols, 1976). The presence of branch points and changes in diameter and myelination suggest the opportunity for some degree of information processing in the transmission of impulses through the striatal output axons.

CELL POPULATIONS In the human it has been estimated that there are 110 million small cells and 670,000 large cells in the striatum (Fox and Rafols, 1976). There are an estimated 540,000 nerve cells in the lateral segment of the globus pallidus and 170,000 cells in the medial segment. The small cells of the striatum, though numerous, are less so than the cells of the neocortex (by 2 orders of magnitude) and are fewer than the granule cells of the cerebellum by 2–3 orders of magnitude. In view of the uncertainties in identification of principal and intrinsic neurons (see above), it is not possible to compare the totals for these two cell types as in other regions. In the substantia nigra it has been estimated that there are only 3,500 dopamine-containing neurons (Andén et al., 1966), though each gives rise to an enormous number of terminals (see above).

SYNAPTIC CONNECTIONS

Under the electron microscope the spiny dendrites can be readily observed, surrounded by numerous synaptic terminals, as shown in Fig. 12.3 (A). The dendrites contain prominent neurotubules and small mitochondria. The spines vary in size and shape; many contain a spine apparatus (sa), consisting of several flattened membrane sacs. They share this feature with the dendritic spines of cerebral cortical cells, but differ from the spines of olfactory granule cells and cerebellar Purkinje cells (see below for discussion of axonal spines).

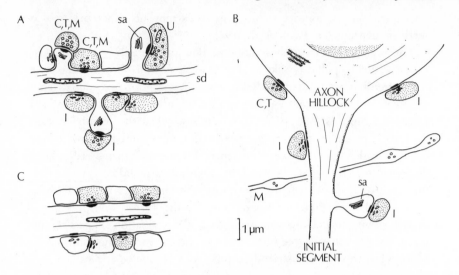

FIG. 12.3. Synaptic connections in the neostriatum. (A) Synapses onto spiny cells. Afferent terminals from C, cortex; T, thalamus; M, midbrain (substantia nigra); U, unidentified. I, intrinsic terminals; sa, spine apparatus; sd, spiny dendrite. (B) Synapses at initial segment region of striatal cell. (C) Synaptic connections in globus pallidus. (After Kemp and Powell, 1971a,b; Fox et al., 1971; Pasik et al., 1976.)

Evidence for the identification of the terminals onto spiny cells has been obtained by making lesions in the regions sending fibers to the striatum. Using this approach, Kemp and Powell (1971b,c) found that the axons from the cortex (C in Fig. 12.3) make synaptic contact primarily onto dendritic spines, and also onto dendritic shafts. These are type I synapses, with asymmetrical membrane thickenings and round vesicles. Axons from the thalamus (T) also make type I synapses onto the dendritic spines, and, to a lesser extent, onto dendritic shafts. Following midbrain (M) lesions, the identifiable terminals are very sparse, but it appears they also make type I synapses onto dendritic spines and probably also onto shafts (see also Hattori et al., 1973). All three types of input axon end in small terminals, about 1 μm in diameter. Thus, the outstanding feature of the input connections is that they are similar in synaptic type and sites of termination. Quantitatively the cortical input is the largest, followed by the thalamus and the midbrain. The cortex and thalamus also send terminals to the smooth dendritic trunks and cell bodies of the spiny cells [Fig. 12.3(B)].

Synaptic connections made by intrinsic cells (I) in the striatum have been studied following lesions in the striatum. Type I synapses are found on dendritic spines and shafts, intermingled with the extrinsic terminals. In addition, many type II synapses, with symmetrical membrane densities and flattened vesicles, are present. These are primarily onto dendritic shafts, and also, as shown in Fig. 12.3 (B), onto cell bodies, initial segments, and spines arising from initial segments. At the latter sites, the synapses are a type of axo-axonic connection. They are numerous; Kemp and Powell report nine such contacts in a 15-μm length of initial segment (cf. also Fox et al., 1971; Pasik et al., 1976). The spines arising from an initial segment often have an associated spine apparatus, and thus resemble the spines on the dendrites (see above). Thus, the spine is a particular type of branching process, and is not dependent for its form and fine structure on the type of process from which it arises. The axo-axonic synapses at these sites are similar to those in cerebral cortical cells, and clearly have an important role to play in the organization of the striatum. This is underscored all the more by the fact that the intrinsic connections in the striatum are heavy, accounting for nearly half of all synapses. Unfortunately, the sources of the intrinsic connections are not known, although collaterals of axons from spiny cells are obvious candidates.

This covers the main types of synaptic connections that have been identified with reasonable certainty. In addition, there are a few large terminals (up to 5 μm in diameter) that make type I synapses onto dendritic spines [U in Fig. 12.3 (A)]. The connections shown in Fig. 12.3 refer to the spiny neurons. The connections onto aspiny neurons have not yet been identified; they may include both type I and type II synapses, and come from both extrinsic and intrinsic sources.

As discussed in Chapter 4, there may be transmitter release and transmitter actions at sites which do not show the morphological specializations of synaptic junctions. The striatum is one of the regions where these properties may be important, particularly with regard to the dopamine-containing fibers. Transmitter released from the presynaptic terminals may act not only on the postsynaptic membrane but also on the presynaptic terminal itself. In addition, many of the dopamine fibers coursing through the neuropil have vesicle-containing varicosities that do not appear to make synaptic junctions [M in Fig. 12.3 (B)]; it is postulated that transmitter released from these sites may have a neuromodulatory action on surrounding neurons. These aspects of the organization of the striatum are discussed further in the following section.

GLOBUS PALLIDUS AND SUBSTANTIA NIGRA   It is reported that the fine structure of these two regions is similar. Dendrites cut longitudinally show tightly packed rows of synaptic terminals covering the smooth dendritic surfaces [Fig. 12.3 (C)]. Most of these terminals make type I synapses onto the dendrites; a modest proportion (10–20%) makes type II synapses (Rinvik and Grofova, 1970; Fox and Rafols, 1976). Evidence relating to dendritic synapses in the substantia nigra is discussed further in the section on neurotransmitters.

BASIC CIRCUIT

In other regions we have seen that a basic circuit usually emerges from a correlation of neuronal types of synaptic connections, confirmed or supplemented by electrophysiological analysis and studies of neurotransmitters. This tidy sequence has not taken place in the case of the striatum. The principal and intrinsic neurons have not been identified, nor have the connections between them. Even more seriously, the electrophysiological and neurochemical studies have tended to go their separate ways, and as a consequence the results in certain key respects have seemed incompatible. This of course adds a certain dash of spice, but it also frustrates the attempt to put together a basic circuit that is consistent with all the data. This is much more than an inconvenience; it means we do not yet have a grasp of the principles on which this region is organized.

A provisional scheme is indicated in Fig. 12.4, summarizing the synaptic connections in the striatum and relating them to certain key pathways involving the rest of the basal ganglia. In the striatum our focus is on the spiny cells, comprising as they do the great majority of cells in this region. We begin with the evidence that the three types of input—cortical, thalamic and nigral—all terminate primarily on the dendritic spines and, to varying extents (not indicated in the diagram), on the dendritic shafts. The diagram indicates correctly that more than one input typically converges onto a single cell. The input synapses are mainly type I (open profiles) though other types are also indicated (shaded profile). For the case of the input from the substantia nigra, we include not only the possibility of both types of synapse, but also interactions involving autoreceptors (recurrent arrows) and neuromodulatory actions at a distance (unattached terminal).

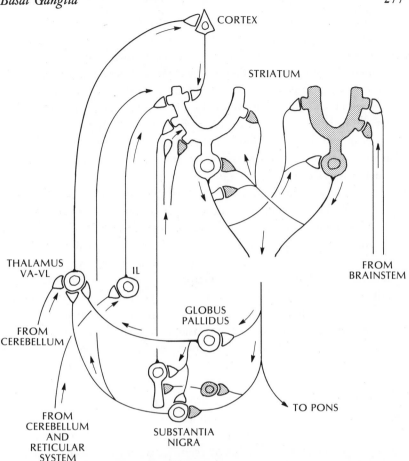

FIG. 12.4. Basic circuit diagram of the basal ganglia (see text for details).

With regard to intrinsic circuits, it appears that axon collaterals make type I and type II synapses on the spiny cells. The diagram shows one possible arrangement, with type I synapses arising from one subpopulation of spiny cells and type II synapses from another. Undoubtedly some of these intrinsic connections are also made by axon collaterals of other types of cell, including the aspiny cell. All the intrinsic connections shown in the striatum are by way of axon collaterals; possible interactions through dendrodendritic synapses are not indicated.

It should be evident that the basic circuit in Fig. 12.4 lacks certain features commonly found in other regions. Chief among these is the lack of a clear distinction between principal and intrinsic neurons. As a consequence, the usual triad of synaptic elements (input, principal, intrinsic) that is the key to the organization of most other regions cannot be identified. Without this distinction, we cannot correlate excitatory and inhibitory connections with neuronal types; nor can we specify the manner in which the inputs differentially activate these circuits, the arrangement of intrinsic circuits for controlling the output, or the cellular sources of the output. These points cover most of the basic principles that underlie the relations between structure and function in any part of the nervous system.

Despite these uncertainties, some reasonable hypotheses can at least be entertained. The diagram accurately reflects recent anatomical and physiological evidence that both extrinsic and intrinsic pathways converge onto single spiny cells. If we anticipate the physiological studies (next section), they show powerful excitatory actions by the extrinsic inputs, which correlate with the type I synapses of their axons (open terminals in Fig. 12.4). They also give evidence of excitatory-inhibitory sequences, or pure long-latency inhibition, which could be mediated by slower extrinsic inhibitory fibers or by intrinsic inhibitory circuits. Connections for both types of action are shown converging on the left spiny cell in the diagram. A simple and attractive hypothesis emerging from these considerations is that activity of the spiny cell reflects a balance between the predominantly excitatory synaptic drive by the extrinsic inputs onto the peripheral dendrites, and a predominantly inhibitory control through intrinsic synapses. The heavy concentration of inhibitory intrinsic synapses on the cell body and initial segment would be most effective in controlling impulse output, and we shall see that this is also consistent with the low frequency of impulse activity in the cells of the striatum.

Let us next consider the output connections of the striatum. The main projection is to the globus pallidus. In this position the globus pallidus serves as the main output relay station for the striatum, much as the deep nuclei serve the cerebellar cortex, a comparison to which we shall later return.

And whence projects the globus pallidus? Its output goes mainly to two nuclear complexes in the thalamus, as indicated in the diagrams of Fig. 12.1 and 12.4. In the ventral tier nuclei (anterior and lateral) the output is integrated with that from the cerebellum, and relayed to the cerebral cortex, particularly the motor area; the latter is among the cortical areas that send fibers to the striatum. In the intralaminar thalamic nuclei, the output is integrated with that from the cerebellum and from the ascending reticular system; together these become direct inputs back to the striatum. Thus, the striatal output, through the pallidum, forms closed loops that feed back onto the striatum, incorporating as they do information from cerebellar, reticular, thalamic, and cortical systems, and providing output to cortical motor systems. These are the cardinal features of the organization of the basal ganglia.

The pathways described above are only the simplest loops in which the striatum is involved. Another parallel loop passes through the substantia nigra, as shown in Figs. 12.1 and 12.4. This is by way of the striatal output to the reticular zone of the substantia nigra, thence on to the thalamus. The globus pallidus also contributes to this loop by its connections to the substantia nigra. Within the substantia nigra, intrinsic circuits and dendrodendritic interactions provide for control of the output neurons which send their axons to the striatum. Not shown in the diagrams are further types of loop circuits, such as reciprocal connections between thalamus and cortex, and connections of the globus pallidus with the subthalamic nucleus (cf. Fig. 12.1).

What is the functional significance of these circuits? From the point of view of synaptic organization an interesting comparison can be made with the cerebellum. Wilson (1928) first pointed out that both of these regions project to the thalamus, and lesions in them produce chorioathetoid movements. Both have two distinct subdivisions, one a large receptive region (striatum and cerebellar cortex) that projects to a smaller region (globus pallidus and deep nuclei) whence proceeds the output to other parts of the nervous system. Kemp and Powell (1971e) have pursued this comparison, and pointed out certain similarities with respect to internal organization: the homogeneous structure throughout; the cells with high densities of dendritic spines; the considerable convergence and divergence of inputs; the presence of intrinsic circuits. They note that both striatum and cerebellum receive input from widespread areas of the cerebral cortex, but have projections limited to the motor cortical area. Against these similarities are marked differences: the lack of lamination and distinct neuronal types and input fibers in the striatum; the high frequency of resting and induced impulse activity in the cerebellum; the differing dopaminergic and noradrenergic inputs.

The point of such comparisons, of course, is not to insist that two regions are basically similar or basically different, but rather to attempt to gain insight into the functional significance of the similarities and differences. It is one of the steps toward identifying the unique contributions of the striatum and cerebellum as they "act in parallel to set up patterns of thalamo-cortical output necessary for the appropriate activation of cortico-spinal neurons" (Evarts and Thach, 1969).

SYNAPTIC ACTIONS

The three inputs—from cortex, thalamus, and substantia nigra—are the starting points for analysis of synaptic actions in the striatum. They are all central inputs, and, therefore, as in the case of the cerebellum, it is not possible to activate them selectively by natural stimuli. However, each can be electrically stimulated independently of the others, and without serious complications from antidromic activity.

Intracellular recordings by several laboratories (Purpura and Malliani, 1967; Buchwald et al., 1973; Kocsis, Sugimori, and Kitai, 1977) have been consistent in showing that, after a single shock to the cerebral cortex or the thalamus, the responses in caudate neurons consist of a synaptic depolarization, or a depolarizing-hyperpolarizing sequence. These are shown in Fig. 12.5 (A-a,b). The responses are graded with stimulus strength, and have the properties of EPSPs and IPSPs, respectively. The latencies of the EPSPs are brief, indicating monosynaptic input pathways. Responses to intralaminar thalamic input tend to be pure EPSPs. The EPSPs elicited from the cortex and thalamus summate, as expected if fibers from these regions converge onto the same caudate neuron. Dye-injection experiments show that many of the cells receiving monosynaptic inputs are medium-size spiny cells (Kocsis and Kitai, 1977). The monosynaptic EPSPs correlate with the anatomical description of type I synapses made by the input axons onto these cells. Thus, there is a rather close correlation between the physiological results and the anatomical studies cited earlier.

When an IPSP occurs, it either follows the EPSP, or, if appearing alone, begins at a longer latency. The IPSPs could be due to more slowly conducting input fibers, or to intrinsic circuits; the prevalence of type II synapses on the spines, cell bodies, and initial segments of the spiny cells may be recalled in this regard.

For the third type of input, from the substantia nigra, the story is similar, but also more complicated. As shown in Fig. 12.5 (B), there are

A   STIMULATE CORTEX, THALAMUS

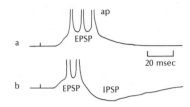

B   STIMULATE SUBSTANTIA NIGRA

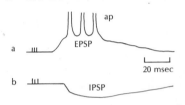

C   IONTOPHORESE DOPAMINE

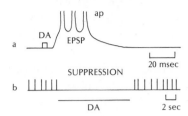

D   ABLATE SUBSTANTIA NIGRA

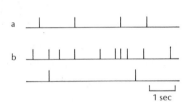

FIG. 12.5. Synaptic actions in the neostriatum. (A) Intracellular responses to single volleys from cortex or thalamus; long-duration EPSP (a) or EPSP-IPSP sequence (b). (B) Responses to repetitive volleys from substantia nigra. (C) Responses to iontophoresis of dopamine: (a) intracellular recording; (b) extracellular recording. (D) Striatal unit activity before (a) and after (b) ablation of substantia nigra. For references, see text.

pure EPSPs, EPSP-IPSP sequences, and pure IPSPs in response to a volley from the substantia nigra (see Purpura, 1976). The short-latency EPSPs indicate a monosynaptic excitatory input, which correlates with the type I synapses that these input axons are believed to make on caudate neurons. The conduction velocities are of the order of one meter per second, indicating rather thin fibers. Some of the cells receiving inputs from the substantia nigra are output cells which send their axons to the substantia nigra, as shown by the fact that they can be activated antidromically [Fig. 12.5 (B-c)]. Note in this record the absence of synaptic potentials associated with the antidromic impulse, suggesting a lack of axon collateral (or other types of feedback) pathways onto this cell, a point deserving further investigation.

The nature of the neurotransmitter for this input is of great interest, in view of the demonstration of dopaminergic fibers from the substantia

nigra to the striatum. Kitai, Sugimori, and Kocsis (1976) combined intracellular recordings with extracellular microiontophoresis, and found that
brief administration of dopamine causes a slow depolarization that gives
rise to action potentials, as shown in Fig. 12.5 (C-a). Some 30% of cells
tested were depolarized; none was hyperpolarized. The depolarization is
graded with the iontophoretic current, summates with the EPSPs elicited from the substantia nigra, and is blocked by chlorpromazine. All
these findings point to properties associated with synaptic transmission.
Procion dye injections indicated that the cells recorded from were medium size spiny cells.

The conclusion from this study was that dopamine excites the striatal
neurons that receive monosynaptic excitatory inputs from the substantia
nigra, implying that the dopaminergic fibers are excitatory. This of
course is consistent with previous electrophysiological studies and with
the type I synaptic terminals, as described above. However, it flies in
the face of a host of studies, beginning with Bloom, Costa, and Salmoiraghi (1965), reporting that the effect of dopamine on spontaneous extracellular unit activity in the striatum is inhibitory (cf. Bunney and
Aghajanian, 1976a). A typical recording is shown in Fig. 12.5 (C-b).
Furthermore, this evidence for an inhibitory action has seemed consistent with the results of biochemical studies of the substantia nigra and
striatum (see below).

At present it is not possible to reconcile these results, but one can
begin to identify the factors that need to be assessed more carefully (see
review by Moore and Bloom, 1978). One critical factor is the time course
of the effects. The excitatory responses to dopamine were obtained in
experiments in which the iontophoretic pulse was brief and intense, and
the response latency short, only a few msec. The inhibitory responses
were obtained with pulses lasting a minute or more; the latencies were
2–15 sec, and the responses often persisted for several minutes after the
current was turned off. Perhaps in these two situations one is seeing
dopamine acting in either a short-term neurotransmitter mode, or a long-
term neuromodulatory mode (see Chapter 4). Associated with this is the
possibility that there are two pathways from the substantia nigra which
mediate the rapid and slow actions. Another factor is the local circuit
environment in the striatum; it is possible that some actions of iontopho-
resed transmitters are on presynaptic terminals rather than on the neurons recorded from, in analogy with inferences that have been made in

the olfactory bulb (see Chapter 8). Additional factors include differences in species, anesthetics, iontophoretic techniques, and types of cells recorded from.

Although these disparities have brought despair to some hearts, it is perhaps as well to recognize that this is an extremely complex system, and that we are still at an early stage in experimental analysis and understanding.

An important physiological property of striatal cells remains to be noted, and that is the extremely low resting rates of impulse activity. Rates of about one impulse per second are common, and many cells show little or no impulse activity. This does not mean that these cells are inactive, for there may be considerable synaptic activity and integration in the dendritic trees of these cells that is not reflected in the extracellular recordings of spike activity at the cell body (see Dendritic Properties below). However, it does put important constraints on the type of output from the striatum, and provides a contrast in this respect with the high resting rates of impulse activity in another region closely involved in control of movement, the cerebellum.

STRIATAL OUTPUT   Some evidence is available regarding the synaptic actions of the output axons from the striatum (see Purpura, 1976). In the globus pallidus, intracellular recordings show EPSP-IPSP sequences, or pure IPSPs, in response to a single volley from the striatum. It has been suggested that the input to the globus pallidus may include both excitatory and inhibitory fibers.

In the substantia nigra, intracellular recordings show EPSP-IPSP sequences, and pure IPSPs. The IPSPs have either short or long onset latencies, suggesting two separate inhibitory input pathways. These could reflect the direct pathway from the striatum, or the indirect pathway through the globus pallidus (cf. Figs. 12.1 and 12.4).

From these studies it appears that the striatal output can produce both excitatory and inhibitory actions on its target cells. The functional significance of these inputs to the globus pallidus is not yet understood. The impulse firing frequencies of these inputs are very low, judging from the recordings from the striatal neurons. The inhibitory inputs to the substantia nigra and globus pallidus are believed to be the GABA-ergic fibers to these structures (see below).

NEUROTRANSMITTERS

Our understanding of the biochemistry of neurotransmitters in the striatum has been built in three major areas. First, the striatum has the highest concentrations of ACh and choline acetyltransferase in the brain, and a very high concentration of acetylcholinesterase. Second, there is, as we have already noted, a specific dopaminergic (DA) input from the substantia nigra. Numerous studies have been directed toward characterizing the dopamine receptor. Experiments paralleling those in sympathetic ganglia have provided evidence that the response to DA in the striatum is mediated by a dopamine-sensitive adenylate cyclase (Kebabian, Petzold, and Greengard, 1971; Siggins et al., 1976). The specific ligand binding sites for dopamine have been demonstrated (Burt, Creese, and Snyder, 1976). Third, the globus pallidus and substantia nigra have the highest concentrations of GABA and GAD in the brain, and these are also abundant in the striatum.

Based on these data, a model has emerged for correlating biochemical and neuropharmacological studies of the basal ganglia. As shown in Fig. 12.6, the main elements of the circuit consist of the dopaminergic input to the intrinsic neurons of the striatum, the cholinergic intrinsic connections within the striatum, and the GABAergic output from the striatum to the globus pallidus and substantia nigra. Thus there is a negative feedback loop from striatum to substantia nigra, such that increases in nigral activity lead to increased inhibition of the substantia nigra. This circuit evolved from an original suggestion by Carlsson and Lindquist (1963), and has been coherently articulated by Bunney and Aghajanian (1976a). It is supported by a variety of evidence. In particular, ^{3}H-GABA uptake has been demonstrated in cell bodies and terminals of the striatum and globus pallidus, and in terminals in the substantia nigra (Hattori et al., 1973); and GAD has been localized in the substantia nigra in terminals arising from the striatum (Fonnum et al., 1974; Ribak et al., 1976). In the striatum, the model presumes an inhibitory action of DA, based on extracellular unit recordings [cf. Fig. 12.5 (D)] and the effects of a large variety of pharmacological agents. We have noted previously that the action of DA is in fact a warmly debated suject. We have also noted the problem of identifying intrinsic and output neurons in the striatum. These inconsistencies must be resolved by future work.

Two refinements to the feedback circuit have been introduced by

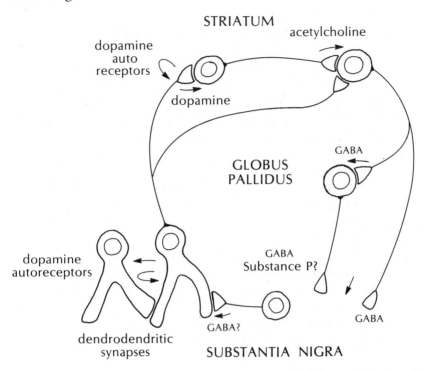

FIG. 12.6. Summary of putative neurotransmitters and their possible sites of action in the basal ganglia. Diagram is schematic and tentative.

recent work. One is that there is local feedback at the level of the axon terminals in the striatum. Biochemical studies have suggested that presynaptic receptors for DA may function to modulate transmitter synthesis (Carlsson et al., 1972). It has been hypothesized that these effects may be mediated by the gating of calcium entry into the terminal (Nowycky and Roth, 1978). These authors note that modulation of the axonal terminals could also occur by means of feedback through local synaptic circuits.

A second refinement extends these ideas to include local dendrodendritic interactions between the dopaminergic cells in the substantia nigra (Groves et al., 1975). This is supported by the finding of DA in the dendrites of nigral cells, using the sensitive glyoxylic acid method of histofluorescence (Bjorklund and Lindvall, 1975). The actions of DA may be extrasynaptic, on autoreceptors on the same dendrites or on receptors on neighboring dendrites, or they may be mediated by dendro-dendritic synaptic junctions (Wilson, Groves, and Fifkova, 1978).

DENDRITIC PROPERTIES

The dendrites of the spiny cells appear to provide the main substrate for synaptic integration in the striatum. Unfortunately, there are no data available on the membrane properties of these cells, nor have there been attempts at biophysical models of these cells and their dendritic trees. We must therefore rely on comparisons with other types of neurons.

The heavy investiture of spines is the outstanding aspect of the structure of spiny cell dendrites. The similarity in this respect with the cerebellar Purkinje cell has been noted, and one can also make a comparison with the granule cells of the dentate fascia and the small pyramidal cells of the olfactory cortex. In all these cases the spines are believed to be primarily postsynaptic in position. In the spiny cell, as elsewhere, the spines presumably provide for an elaboration of the synaptic surface of the dendrite in a specific manner, such that certain connections are made with the spines and others are made to the dendritic shafts. The high input resistance of the spine would produce large synaptic potentials within the spine, and there would be relatively effective spread through the short neck into the dendritic shaft. The effectiveness of spread to distant sites, including the axon hillock where impulse generation occurs, would be balanced against the electrical isolation of the spine from its neighbors, which would restrict the shunting effects between active spines. These and other aspects of spine function are discussed elsewhere in relation to the spines of olfactory granule cells (Chapter 8), Purkinje cells (Chapter 10), and cortical pyramidal cells (Chapter 15).

Apart from these general considerations there has been no evidence for more complicated dendritic or spine functions. For example, no fast prepotentials or small unitary spikes have been reported, indicative of impulse generation in dendritic branches or spines, as in the case of the Purkinje cell and hippocampal pyramidal cell. Nor is there evidence for the partial dendritic inhibition inferred from the action of stellate cells on Purkinje cells, though more needs to be known about intrinsic connections in the striatum before this can be adequately assessed. The possibility of dendrodendritic interactions requires further study, both anatomically and physiologically, particularly in view of the recent evidence in the substantia nigra.

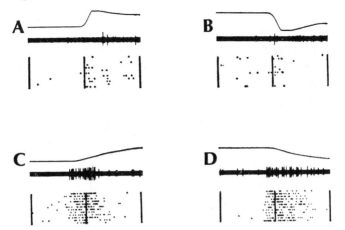

FIG. 12.7. Relation of striatal single-unit activity to movement in awake monkey. *Upper traces,* movement of lever; *lower traces,* unit activity. Note weak relation of unit activity to a rapid, ballistic movement (A and B), but strong relation to slow, ramp movement (C and D). (From Delong and Strick, 1974).

With respect to synaptic integration, the picture that emerges, though rather sketchy at present, is of a cell subjected, on the one hand, to powerful excitatory inputs to a great number of dendritic spines, and, on the other hand, controlled by potent inhibitory inputs, both extrinsic and intrinsic, onto the dendritic shafts, cell body, and initial segment. These aspects of synaptic organization are reminiscent of the cerebellar Purkinje cell, receiving excitatory inputs to its spines from parallel fibers and inhibitory inputs from stellate and basket cells to its dendrites, soma, and axon hillock. These similarities make all the more dramatic the differences in resting impulse frequencies—50–100 impulses/sec for the Purkinje cell, but less than 1/sec, and often silence, in the case of the striatal neuron. Here again the principle that structural similarities do not necessarily correlate with function seems evident; rather, function is determined by the dynamic interplay of structural components and their physiological properties.

The low level of impulse firing has several interesting implications. One is that a great deal of synaptic input and integration may occur out in the dendritic tree below the threshold for affecting impulse output. The input-output functions of the striatum are often characterized in terms of "impulse flow". However, behind this flow there appears to be a great deal of synaptic activity—"synaptic flow", one might say—that is not registered in immediate changes in impulse output. This would include not only the activity in dendrites, but also that involving autoreceptors on presynaptic terminals that has been postulated in the dopaminergic input pathway.

The differences between the striatum and cerebellum, in terms of dendritic properties and local synaptic actions, are likely to provide much of the basis for their differing roles in the control of movement. An attractive theory has been that the cerebellum is related primarily to the programming and initiation of rapid, "ballistic" movements, whereas the basal ganglia are primarily involved in the generation of slow, "ramp" movements (Kornhuber, 1974). Physiological recordings, in fact, give some support to this concept; as shown in Fig. 12.7, some single units show little change in activity in relation to a rapid movement in a trained, awake monkey, but a clear and prolonged discharge during the onset and termination of a slow movement. However, DeLong and Strick (1974) emphasize that there is considerable variation in these properties, and the specific relation of the neuronal activity to movement will require further information such as the topographical relations between the basal ganglia and the body musculature. Recent studies (cf. Hore et al., 1977) support a role for the basal ganglia in the central generation and programming of movement.

13

OLFACTORY CORTEX

We turn now to consider the synaptic organization of the cerebral cortex of vertebrates. From an evolutionary point of view, the olfactory cortex, defined as the part that receives the output fibers from the olfactory bulb, was the first to differentiate, becoming recognizable in the brains of primitive aquatic species. By virtue of this primal position, it is termed *palaeocortex;* later in the evolutionary sequence come the *archicortex* (hippocampus) and *neocortex* (the cerebral expansions of higher vertebrates). These three divisions will be the basis for our study. It is often stated that the olfactory cortex is the precursor or anlage from which the other types have been differentiated, but this is reading between the lines in the book of evolution, and the reader is referred to Herrick (1948) and Nauta and Karten (1970) for orientation to this question.

Of the three divisions, the olfactory cortex has been the least studied. One need not look far for the reasons. It is due, in part, to our persisting ignorance of the nature of the olfactory input. In part, it is the lesser role that olfaction plays in human behavior, compared with the auditory and visual systems. And, in part, it is a simple matter of the general inaccessibility of the olfactory structures, relegated as they have been to the antipodes of the brain by the overgrowth of the neocortex.

Despite its declining fortunes, the olfactory cortex is, in fact, the appropriate subject with which to begin the study of cortical organization. Not only is it phylogenetically the primordial cortex, it is, by virtue of that fact, the principal cortical region of most lower vertebrate species. Indeed, the entire telencephalon of most lower vertebrates is dominated by the olfactory system. And it also plays this dominant role in many higher vertebrates. Evidence is accumulating that, despite the overgrowth of the neocortex, the sexual and social behavior of most

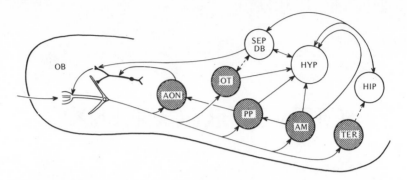

FIG. 13.1. Relations between olfactory and limbic parts of the brain. Primary olfactory areas, which receive input from mitral cells of the olfactory bulb (OB), are shown as shaded circles: anterior olfactory nucleus (AON); olfactory tubercle (OT); prepyriform cortex (PP); amygdaloid complex (AM); and transitional entorhinal cortex (TER). Limbic structures are shown as open circles: septum and diagonal band (SEP-DB); hypothalamus (HYP); and hippocampus (HIP). Note multiplicity of interconnections, including centrifugal pathways to granule cells of the olfactory bulb.

mammalian species is primarily mediated by olfactory substances and pheromonal agents acting through the olfactory system (see Whitten and Bronson, 1969).

To these considerations is added the fact that the olfactory cortex is the simplest of the cortical regions in terms of its intrinsic structure. Having stated this, we must indicate more precisely which regions we have in mind when we refer to the olfactory cortex. The commonly accepted definition is in terms of the projection of the olactory bulb (see Pribram and Kruger, 1954). Figure 13.1 shows this projection in schematic form; it can be seen that there are several sites that receive direct synaptic input from the bulb and qualify, thereby, as olfactory cortex. The largest site is the so-called *prepyriform cortex*, which is that region lying beneath and to either side of the lateral olfactory tract. This is usually regarded as the primary cortex in the olfactory pathway, and it will be the subject for our study.

NEURONAL ELEMENTS

The neuronal elements of the prepyriform cortex are shown in Fig. 13.2. We follow the descriptions of Calleja (1893), Cajal (1911; 1955), O'Leary (1937), Valverde (1965), Stevens (1969), and Price (1973).

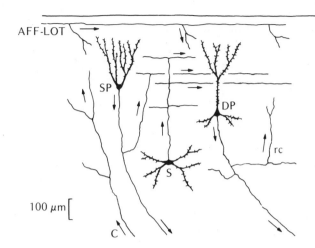

FIG. 13.2. Neuronal elements of the olfactory (prepyriform) cortex.

Inputs: mitral cell afferent axons in the lateral olfactory tract (AFF-LOT); fibers from central brain regions (C).

Principal neurons: superficial pyramidal neuron (SP); deep pyramidal neuron (DP); recurrent axon collateral (rc).

Intrinsic neuron: stellate cell (S).

INPUT The *afferent* input is from the olfactory bulb, through the mitral cell axons in the lateral olfactory tract (LOT). The LOT lies as a band of fibers on the surface of the cortex, from which numerous branches are given off to the underlying and surrounding cortex. The branches fan out over the surface and reach considerable lengths (several millimeters). The branches all terminate in the outer molecular layer of the cortex; none pass to the deeper layers. Thus, as in the olfactory bulb, the afferent fibers enter at the surface and terminate in a superficial layer. The situation is also similar to that in the hippocampus but differs from the cerebellum and neocortex, in which all inputs arrive from the cortical depths. The axons in the LOT are thinly myelinated and range in diameter from about 0.2–3 μm (Allison, 1953; Price and Sprich, 1975).

Another type of input is through fibers entering the depths of the cortex; following the convention we have used elsewhere, it may be termed the *central* input. These fibers terminate at various levels in the cortex, except the most superficial (see Fig. 13.2). Their sources have not been identified. Association fibers from neighboring olfactory regions will be described later.

PRINCIPAL NEURON   The output from the prepyriform cortex is carried in axons that arise from several types of neuron. The major type is usually termed a *superficial pyramidal cell*, although, as Cajal (1955) noted, the cell bodies take on a variety of forms that may be semilunar, mitral, triangular, or polymorphic. The cell bodies are 15–30 μm in diameter, of modest size for principal neurons in the brain. As shown in Fig. 13.2, they are arranged in a distinct sheet some 400 μm below the cortical surface. Each cell has several dendritic trunks (several microns in diameter) that are directed superficially and arborize and terminate in the superficial molecular layer. The branches are moderately invested with spines. These are usually termed *apical* dendrites. As such, they are regarded as analogous to the apical dendrites of neocortical pyramidal cells. However, a resemblance to the dendritic trees of granule cells in the dentate fascia has also been pointed out (O'Leary, 1937). The terms *pyramidal* and *apical*, like *granule* and many other terms we have encountered, must therefore not be taken to imply similar structures and functions when we compare neurons in different parts of the brain.

From some of these cells, one or more *basal* dendrites arise at the sides of the cell body; they branch sparingly and terminate within 100–200 μm of the cell body. They also are moderately invested with spines. Many of the superficial pyramidal neurons, however, do not have any clearly identifiable basal dendrites. This is noteworthy, since differentiation of the dendritic tree into apical and basal branches is a prominent feature of the pyramidal cells in the hippocampus and the neocortex. These prepyriform neurons are, therefore, distinctive in being cortical "pyramidal" neurons that lack basal dendrites.

The second, less numerous type of principal neuron is the *deep pyramidal neuron*. These neurons lie scattered in the zone just deep to the sheet of superficial pyramidal cells. The cell bodies are somewhat larger (20–40 μm in diameter). Each gives off a stout *apical dendrite* (3–6 μm in diameter) that ascends into the molecular layer and ramifies there. Each also gives rise to several *basal dendrites;* they have bushy arborizations that are often directed toward the depth of the cortex, giving them a brushlike appearance (see Fig. 13.2). Both apical and basal dendrites are liberally invested with spines. Many of these cells resemble the small pyramidal neurons of the neocortex. In both cases, it should be noted, the term *pyramidal* has no necessary significance beyond the geometrical form of the cell body imparted by the characteristic origins of the apical and basal dendritic trunks (see Price, 1973).

A third, infrequent type of principal neuron is described as *polymorphic* or fusiform; these neurons lie in the depths of the cortex (see Fig. 13.2). The cell bodies range in size from 15–40 μm in diameter. Each gives off several dendritic trunks, which have different orientations and which ramify and terminate within the cortical depths over distances of several hundred microns.

The fact that the principal neurons of the prepyriform cortex have these different forms and locations is a notable feature which is obviously significant for the synaptic organization of this region. It is probable, for example, from the above description, that the more superficial neurons are primarily related to the afferent input, whereas the deeper neurons are primarily related to the central input. For our purposes, we will consider the pyramidal neurons, both superficial and deep, as forming the main population of principal neurons.

The axons of the pyramidal cells give off several collaterals within the cortex. Some of these collaterals terminate within the deep layers, either immediately or after extending for variable distances in the lateral direction, whereas other collaterals recur to the molecular layer (see Fig. 13.2). The latter collaterals are analogous to association fibers of the hippocampus and neocortex; we will have more to say about their significance later. Some of the pyramidal cell axons do not leave the cortex; these cells qualify thereby as intrinsic neurons. The axons that do leave the cortex join the great mass of deep white matter and distribute to several regions. These include neighboring olfactory regions and parts of the hypothalamus and thalamus (Powell et al., 1965; Heimer, 1968; Price and Powell, 1971) (see Fig. 13.1). By these connections, the olfactory cortex is strategically placed to affect central brain structures that play crucial roles in many types of behavior.

INTRINSIC NEURONS Scattered throughout the cortex are cells whose axons do not leave the cortex; these cells qualify, therefore, as intrinsic neurons, by our general definition. The majority are polymorphic cells in the middle and deep layers. They are often referred to as *stellate cells* from the star-shaped form imparted to the cell body by the several dendritic trunks. The cell bodies are 10–20 μm in diameter, and the trunks are several microns in diameter. The latter arborize over fields of

100–300 μm and are lightly invested with spines. A thin axon (1–2 μm thick) is directed toward the depths, the surface, or laterally, as the case may be; branches and terminals are given off at all levels (except the most superficial). Some of the branches extend in the lateral direction for considerable distances (up to a millimeter or more). It has been reported (O'Leary, 1937) that some stellate axons terminate in baskets around the cell bodies of pyramidal cells.

Despite the often considerable length of their axons, these cells may be termed *short-axon cells*, by our previous definition, on the basis that the axon remains confined to the cortex within which it arises (see Chapter 8). But as we have already noted, the stellate cells are part of the population of polymorphic cells, and there is a gradation in lengths and destinations of axons within this population. Possibly, the axons that enter the white matter do not re-enter the prepyriform cortex, but evidence on this point is lacking. It is therefore premature to draw a hard and fast line between principal and intrinsic neuronal types in this region. We have already mentioned this problem in our discussion of the neurons of the spinal cord and we will encounter it again for the neuron types of the neocortex. The fact that some pyramidal cell axons do not leave the cortex should also be recalled in this regard.

CELL POPULATIONS Quantitative studies of prepyriform elements are almost completely lacking. Such studies are hampered by the fact that the output axons do not form a single tract that can be subjected to quantitative analysis. It would appear that there are more pyramidal cells in the prepyriform cortex than the 60,000 or so LOT axons that have been estimated (Allison, 1953; Price and Sprich, 1975), so that the input-output ratio appears rather low. The input side is raised considerably by the large number of branches of the LOT fibers, but the convergence ratio would still appear to be less than 10:1. Within the cortex, intrinsic elements (the stellate cells) are much less numerous than pyramidal cells, so the ratio I:P must be less than 1:1.

These very approximate figures are enough to suggest a low input-output convergence and low I:P ratio in the prepyriform cortex. This is similar to the case in the cerebellar cortex vis-à-vis the climbing fiber input, and also the neocortex. These regions stand in sharp contrast to the high convergence ratios and high I:P ratios in the olfactory bulb and retina. The ratios have significance for the kinds of signal processing

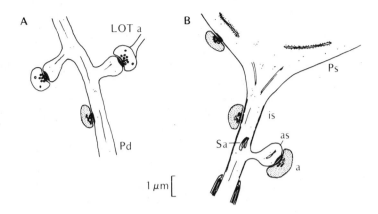

FIG. 13.3. Synaptic connections in the olfactory (prepyriform) cortex. (A) Axo-dendritic connections from LOT axons (LOT a) onto the spines of a pyramidal cell dendrite (Pd). (B) Axosomatic connections to the cell body of a pyramidal neuron; axoaxonic connections to the initial segment of an axon (is); and axoax-onic connection to an axonal spine (as) of the initial segment. Note also a spine apparatus (sa) in the initial segment. (After Westrum, 1970.)

carried out in these regions, as we will discuss below in connection with the basic circuit diagram for the prepyriform cortex.

SYNAPTIC CONNECTIONS

The main fact known about the synaptic connections in the prepyriform cortex is that the branches of the LOT fibers make exclusively axoden-dritic synapses onto the apical dendrites of the pryamidal cells. The synapses are made onto the dendritic shafts and spines in the superficial molecular layer; see Fig. 13.3 (A). Most of the synapses have round vesicles in the presynaptic terminal and asymmetric membrane thicken-ings, i.e., they are type I chemical synapses (Lund and Westrum, 1966; Westrum, 1966a,b, 1970). The LOT axons arise from mitral cells in the olfactory bulb, and it will be recalled that, in the bulb, the mitral cells make type I chemical synapses at all levels: dendrodendritic in the olfac-tory glomeruli, dendrodendritic in the EPL onto granule cells, and axo-dendritic through the axon collaterals (see Chapter 8). The fact that the mitral cell also appears to make the same type of synapse at its afferent axon terminal in the prepyriform cortex has been adduced as evidence of the morphological corollary of Dale's Law (see Chapter 4) that a neuron secretes the same transmitter substance at all its synapses (see also Neurotransmitters below). A few terminals in the superficial layer are type II; it has not been determined whether they arise from extrinsic or intrinsic sources.

In deeper layers, type II chemical synapses predominate onto the cell bodies of the pyramidal neurons [see Fig. 13.1 (B)]. Of particular interest is the finding of synapses onto the initial segments of the axons of these cells (Westrum, 1966b, 1970). These studies have also shown that there are spines arising from the initial segments, with a spine apparatus either within the spine or within the nearby initial segment. As shown in Fig. 13.3 (B), the synapses onto both initial segments and spines are type II; classified in terms of the pre- and postsynaptic structures, they are axo-axonal. It seems likely that they arise, at least in part, from the basket arborizations observed in the Golgi-stained material.

These findings demonstrate several principles. They show that a spine, together with a characteristic spine apparatus, may arise from an axon as well as from a dendrite. They show that an axonal process—initial segment or spine—may receive synaptic inputs. We have discussed instances of this in the cerebellum and striatum and similar synaptic arrangements have been observed in the neocortex. These findings are, of course, inconsistent with traditional views of synaptic orientations and reinforce the need to revise our concepts of the functional organization of neurons accordingly.

Apart from these observations, little is known about synaptic connections in the prepyriform cortex; no dendrodendritic synapses have been described, and the sources of intrinsic connections have not been identified. The specific connections between neuronal types, therefore, have had to be inferred from the Golgi preparations and from the electrophysiological analysis of synaptic actions (see below).

BASIC CIRCUIT

The organization of the prepyriform cortex is summarized in the basic circuit diagram of Fig. 13.4, which is derived from the accounts of Biedenbach and Stevens (1969) and Haberly and Shepherd (1973). In addition to subsuming the anatomical evidence just reviewed, the diagram anticipates the physiological evidence for synaptic actions that is presented in the following section.

To summarize briefly, the branches of the LOT axons make synapses onto the apical dendrites of superficial pyramidal cells and, probably, the

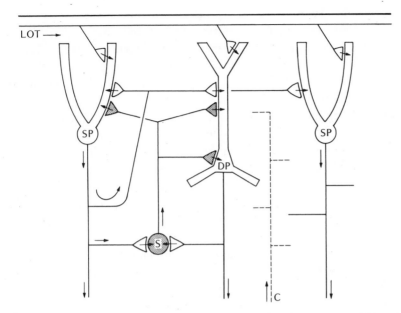

FIG. 13.4. Basic circuit diagram for the olfactory (prepyriform) cortex. Abbreviations as in Fig. 13.3.

deep pyramidal cells. Both types of pyramidal cell, through their deep axon collaterals, make synapses onto stellate cells. It is also probable that through their long axon collaterals, either deep or recurrent, the pyramidal cells make synapses back onto the apical dendrites of other pyramidal cells. The axons of the stellate cells also distribute to the apical dendrites of the pyramidal cells, again over both short and long distances. Finally, little is known with regard to the central inputs coming through the cortical depths, but it is probable that these fibers make connections onto both the pyramidal cells and the stellate cells.

Let us now consider some aspects of synaptic organization within this basic circuit in more detail. To begin with, the connections within the prepyriform cortex are made within a strongly horizontal and vertical framework, as is emphasized by the diagram. The afferent input in the LOT propagates as a strictly horizontal wave across the cortical surface, as rigidly horizontal as the parallel fiber input to the Purkinje cell dendrites in the cerebellum. Moreover, this sequence is unidirectional for the entire cortex, always proceeding from anterior to posterior, away from the olfactory bulb. In the cerebellum, by comparison, each granule cell axon bifurcates to give rise to two parallel fibers that run in opposite directions. This means that, in the prepyriform cortex, there is a temporal sequence of activation by the afferent input, which is possibly even more rigid than the cerebellar sequence. A similar rigid sequence is present in the hippocampus.

The afferent input to the prepyriform cortex is transferred synaptically to the ends of the apical dendrites of the principal neurons, similar to the way that the olfactory input is transferred to the terminal tufts of the mitral cells in the olfactory bulb. It seems highly significant that two successive relays of this same basic type (axodendritic, to distal dendritic terminals) should occur in succession. What the implication might be for information processing in the olfactory pathway, in contrast to other sensory pathways, is not immediately evident, but it can at least be concluded that vertical dispersion of inputs onto the principal neuron dendrites is one parameter of synaptic organization not used in this pathway.

It is further noteworthy that the afferent input through the LOT is transferred only to the principal neuron of the prepyriform cortex, the pyramidal cells. This may immediately be recognized as different from the close relation between the afferent, principal, and intrinsic elements of the synaptic triad we have seen in the olfactory bulb, retina, cerebellum, and thalamus. It is also different from the situation in the ventral horn and in the neocortex, in which the afferent fibers have direct access to intrinsic neurons. It is similar, however, to the case of the hippocampus. This would appear to be an important aspect of the olfactory relay in the prepyriform cortex. The central inputs, on the other hand, arriving through the cortical depths, have access to both the deep stellate cells and the pyramidal cells, so that the patterns of connections established over this route may involve the triad of synaptic elements. The two inputs—afferent and central—thus can make quite different use of the prepyriform neuronal circuits. It should be noted that this over-all picture is modified by the extent to which pyramidal neurons have axons that do not leave the cortex, and stellate cells have axons that do leave the cortex, as has been discussed previously.

The diagram of Fig. 13.4 indicates that there are two major types of intrinsic pathway within the prepyriform cortex. One consists of the circuit from axon collaterals of principal neurons through inhibitory intrinsic neurons back onto the principal neurons. There is an obvious similarity to the Renshaw circuit in the ventral horn, in that this provides for inhibitory feedback of responses to afferent inputs. In relation to central inputs, on the other hand, the intrinsic neurons can provide a feedforward as well as feedback pathway. As is shown in Fig. 13.4, the deep position of most of the intrinsic neurons and their inaccessibility to direct LOT activation ensure their different use by these two inputs.

The other type of intrinsic pathway is by way of the long axon collaterals of the pyramidal cells. We have already suggested that because of their length they may be regarded as analogous to the association fibers of the hippocampus and neocortex. Recent studies have provided evidence that these collaterals make direct connections, of an excitatory nature, onto the pyramidal cells themselves. The evidence, both anatomical and physiological, will be discussed in later sections; here, it may simply be recalled that such *recurrent re-excitatory pathways*, formed by axon collaterals of principal neurons onto other principal neurons, have been conspicuously absent in the regions of the brain thus far considered in this book. We will encounter this type of pathway in the hippocampus, and we will discuss the evidence for such pathways in the neocortex. In the cerebellum, the axon collaterals of Purkinje cells also connect to other Purkinje cells, but the connections are inhibitory. We note for now the possibility that re-excitatory circuits may be an important constituent of the organization of cerebral cortical regions.

SYNAPTIC ACTIONS

The LOT is a clearly defined bundle of axons that can be discretely stimulated with an electric shock. This, and the fact that the axons all make their synapses onto the distal dendrites of the pyramidal neurons, has permitted an electrophysiological analysis of synaptic actions over this route.

The single unit responses are illustrated in Fig. 13.5 (A). Here an intracellular recording from a pyramidal neuron shows an initial depolarization lasting 10–20 msec; at threshold amplitude, it leads to the generation of an impulse. This is followed by a wave of hyperpolarization that cuts short the initial excitation and lasts for several hundred milliseconds if the volley is strong. It has been concluded that this sequence represents an initial EPSP followed by an IPSP (Biedenbach and Stevens, 1969; Haberly, 1973a). Observe that the sequence is very similar to that

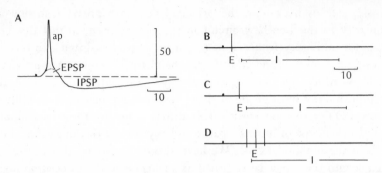

FIG. 13.5. Synaptic actions in the olfactory (prepyriform) cortex. (A) Intracellular recording of the response in a pyramidal neuron to a volley in the lateral olfactory tract. (After Beidenbach and Stevens, 1969; Haberly, 1973a.) (B) Extracellular unit recordings of the response of a superficial pyramidal cell to a LOT volley. Periods of excitation and inhibition, as revealed by a second test volley, are indicated by E and I, respectively. (C) Response of a deep pyramidal neuron. (D) Response of a deep stellate cell. [(B)-(D) after Haberly, 1973a.]

which we have seen in the principal neurons of other brain regions subjected to a single afferent volley.

Intracellular recordings from prepyriform neurons are difficult to obtain, and a comparison between the responses of the different neuronal types has therefore been carried out using extracellular unit recordings (Haberly, 1973a). In Fig. 13.5 (B) is shown an extracellular recording of a superficial pyramidal neuron undergoing the same response as in (A). The horizontal bar indicates the time during which the response to a second testing volley is suppressed; note that this coincides with the time during which the cell is undergoing the IPSP, as shown in (A).

For comparison, the response of a deep pyramidal neuron is shown in Fig. 13.5 (C). The synaptic action is similar, consisting of an initial excitation followed by a long period of unresponsiveness. The latency of the initial impulse is longer, however, allowing for a synaptic relay in the pathway of activation. The obvious candidate for this pathway is through the axon collaterals of the superficial pyramidal neurons. The physiological experiments have shown that there is indeed a wave of activity that spreads at a slow rate (0.8 m/sec) throughout the cortex after the initial LOT input, which is presumably due to impulses traveling through the long collaterals of the pyramidal axons. It has been concluded (Haberly, 1973b) that most deep pyramidal neurons respond to afferent input by this relay. A direct route cannot be ruled out for some deep pyramidal neurons; this connection is, therefore, shown by the dotted line in Fig. 13.4. The axon collaterals provide the pathways for re-excitatory circuits within the prepyriform cortex, as discussed later in relation to dendritic properties.

RECURRENT INHIBITION   The intrinsic neurons (stellate cells) also respond to an LOT volley. As shown in Fig. 13.5 (D), the responses have relatively long latencies, indicating at least one relay through the pyramidal neurons. Also, these deeply situated cells tend to fire several impulses in response to a single volley. The excitatory phase is followed by a period of unresponsiveness to testing volleys, as shown in Fig. 13.5 (D).

It has been concluded that the inhibition that is present in all three types of prepyriform neuron is mediated by the stellate cells acting as inhibitory neurons (Biedenbach and Stevens, 1969; Haberly, 1973a; Haberly and Shepherd, 1973). As indicated in the basic circuit diagram of FIg. 13.4, the stellate cell axons are directed laterally and superficially to make synapses onto both the superficial and deep pyramidal neurons. As already noted, the circuits thus formed are analogous to the Renshaw pathway in the ventral horn (Chapter 7). By inhibiting the pyramidal neurons, the stellate cells also cut off their excitatory input from the pyramidal neurons, as is shown by the unresponsiveness of the stellate neurons to a testing volley after their initial excitation [Fig. 13.5 (D)]. The unresponsiveness is therefore not due to a direct IPSP onto the stellate cells themselves but rather an indirect action; it is, in fact, a variety of presynaptic inhibition of the excitatory pathway onto the stellate cells. This does not rule out the possibility that some stellate cells may also receive direct inhibition, through connections between each other.

RHYTHMIC ACTIVITY   The prepyriform cortex is notable for the prominent rhythmic potentials that can be recorded from it by electroencephalography, and the mechanism for the generation of these potentials was the subject of some of the earliest electrophysiological studies of this region (Freeman, 1959). The point of departure for these studies was the interesting fact that, with very weak shocks to the LOT, the threshold response of the prepyriform cortex takes the form of a low-amplitude oscillating field potential. Analysis showed that the response in the depths of the cortex was of similar form but opposite polarity to that recorded at the surface, indicating a potential dipole across the cortex. Using a systems engineering approach, Freeman (1962) developed a model for the oscillations, based on an excitatory input with intrinsic negative feedback. The negative feedback performed a gating function that gave rise to the rhythmic activity.

It may be recognized that such a model is formally similar to that proposed for the generation of rhythmic potentials in the olfactory bulb, thalamus, and neocortex. Indeed, stripped to its essentials, the model is applicable in some form or other to almost any rhythmic system, neural or non-neural. This qualifies its use as an analytical tool but, nonetheless, suggests that the prepyriform cortex shares certain properties of rhythmic potential generation with other regions of the brain.

Freeman (1968) further demonstrated that removal of the bulbar input eliminates the oscillations recorded from the prepyriform area; the effect appears to be due to the removal of a steady excitatory input from the olfactory bulb through the LOT axons. This is in accord with the model, which requires an excitatory background as the continous input that is then subjected to inhibitory gating. Unit recordings have shown that the pyramidal cells fire impulses in synchrony with the rhythmic waves.

NEUROTRANSMITTERS

The olfactory cortex contains relatively high concentrations of amino acid transmitters. After olfactory bulb ablation the concentration of aspartate is substantially reduced, suggesting that it may be a transmitter at the synapses of lateral olfactory tract terminals onto pyramidal cell dendrites in the cortex (Graham and Aprison, 1975). This is intriguing, in view of the evidence for aspartate as an excitatory transmitter of mitral cells in the olfactory bulb (cf. Fig. 8.9). Thus, it has been hypothesized that aspartate might be the transmitter at both the dendrodendritic and axodendritic synapses of the mitral cells. We have already noted that the mitral cell synapses all appear to be type I. However, there are also other transmitter candidates, as discussed in Chapter 8.

The olfactory tubercle not only receives input from the olfactory bulb; it is also a projection site of the mesolimbic dopaminergic system from the brainstem. Histofluorescence studies show the presence of dopamine-containing fibers throughout this region (cf. Ungerstedt, 1971). In analogy with sympathetic ganglia and with the nigrostriatal pathway, the synaptic responses to this input are believed to be mediated by a dopamine-sensitive adenylate cyclase (Kebabian et al., 1971; Greengard, 1976). Laminar analysis has shown that the adenylate cylcase is mainly present in the molecular layer of the olfactory tubercle, which is consistent with the postulate that it is localized in the dendrites of the pyramidal cells (Krieger et al., 1977). This synaptic input is of special interest because of the implication of the mesolimbic dopaminergic system in certain types of behavioral disorders. It is of interest that GABA and GAD have a different localization, being present mainly in the deeper cellular layers of the tubercle (Krieger and Heller, 1978).

DENDRITIC PROPERTIES

Our interest naturally focuses on the apical dendrites of the pyramidal neurons. All the evidence to date indicates that these dendrites are exclusively postsynaptic in position. Although this does not rule out the possibility that dendrodendritic synapses may, in fact, be present, it does provide a starting point for assessing the properties of the apical dendrites in relation to local integration of synaptic inputs and transfer of signals to the axon hillock.

An electrotonic model is not available for the assessment of these functions, but the geometry of the pyramidal neurons is sufficiently stereotyped that the essence of a model can be sketched in outline. Such a model is depicted in Fig. 13.6. The upper diagram reproduces a Golgi-stained pyramidal cell; noted again the relatively small size of this cell as a type of principal neuron. Combining the apical dendrites yields an equivalent cylinder, as shown in the middle of the figure. There is no direct evidence concerning the electrotonic length of the cylinder, but if the electrical paramenters for other neurons are used, a value of about one is obtained, as shown.

Let us consider first the simplest case of a synchronous synaptic input through the LOT. This input activates excitatory synapses onto the peripheral branches of the apical dendrites, giving rise to an EPSP. The electrotonic spread of this EPSP to the cell body and axon hillock, to trigger an action potential which propagates into the axon, is depicted in the lower diagram in Fig. 13.6. Note that because of the relatively short electrotonic length of the apical dendrite, this spread is very effective by passive means alone. The reader will realize that the diagram gives the spatial distribution for the EPSP and the action potential at the instant of

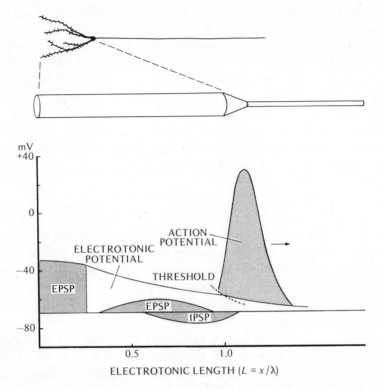

FIG. 13.6. Electrotonic model for a superficial pyramidal neuron of the olfactory (prepyriform) cortex, to show distribution of potentials for the case of an afferent input through LOT axons to superficial dendrites of the pyramidal neuron. Distribution of EPSP and IPSP due to intrinsic pathways is also shown.

impulse generation shown in the recording of Fig. 13.5. There is no evidence for fast prepotentials or other forms of active properties, in addition to the passive potentials depicted in Fig. 13.6.

Subsequent to this initial synaptic excitation is the recurrent inhibition through the stellate cells, as shown in Fig. 13.5. The electrotonic model illustrates particularly vividly how this inhibition is not only located close to the cell body, to exert direct control over impulse generation there, but also is sited between the distal dendrites and the cell body, the more effectively to gate, as it were, the transfer of the afferent EPSP to the axon hillock. This may be taken as yet another example of the strategic siting of inhibitory input relative to the site of excitatory synaptic input. Under some conditions, the nearness of the inhibitory site to the axon hillock may, in fact, not be sufficient for control over impulse initiation there; experiments have shown, for example, that inhibition cannot prevent an impulse from invading the cell body antidromically from the axon (Haberly, 1973a).

The second major excitatory input to the apical dendrites is through the axon collaterals of the pyramidal cells. This has come to light in the course of recent work, in which anatomical studies have demonstrated the presence of the collaterals (Heimer, 1968; Price, 1973) and physiological studies have independently demonstrated their synaptic actions (Haberly, 1973a,b; Haberly and Shepherd, 1973). The anatomical studies have shown that the collaterals from the pyramidal cells extend throughout the prepyriform cortex, terminating preferentially at the level of the proximal shafts of the apical dendrites, as has been shown in the basic circuit diagram of Fig. 13.4, and is indicated in Fig. 13.6. We have seen that this level is near one of the sites of inhibitory input from the stellate cells. Thus, the inhibitory input is sited in close proximity to the excitatory input from the long-axon collaterals. As in the case of the overlapping inputs to the motoneuron, this provides for direct competition between excitatory and inhibitory conductance changes in the control of pyramidal cell output.

Under natural conditions of asynchronous afferent inputs, there must be a delicate balance between the intrinsic inhibition and the two types of excitatory input. Physiological recordings have, in fact, revealed both inhibitory and excitatory responses of prepyriform cells when the nose is stimulated with odors (Haberly, 1968; see Fig. 13.7). These results have suggested the possibility that there are sequences of processing in the olfactory cortex equivalent to those that have been identified in the sensory areas of the neocortex.

CORTICAL ORGANIZATION We conclude by noting that some years ago Lorente de Nó (1938) stated that "the primary olfactory cortex is in fact a subcortical center comparable to the geniculate bodies, etc." This is a useful point to discuss because it challenges us to define more precisely what is meant by the term *cortex*. By cortex, some authorities mean only the neocortex; some mean a region with a certain number of layers of cell bodies and nerve fibers; and some mean any part of the pallium or covering layer of the brain. As with so many other terms, there are too

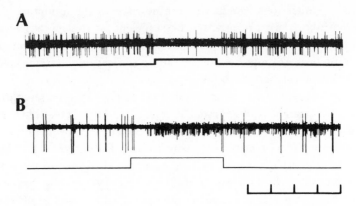

FIG. 13.7. Unit activity in olfactory cortex in relation to olfactory stimulation. (A) Suppression of activity. (B) Suppression of large unit and long-latency activation of small unit. Time bars, 1 sec divisions. (From Haberly, 1969.)

many exceptions to any of these definitions; and, although the worker on the neocortex may be satisfied to use the term only as he defines it, this is no help to the student who is interested in comparing the organization of the neocortex with other parts of the nervous system.

In previous chapters (e.g., Chapter 8), it is been indicated that the study of synaptic organization may provide a basis for distinguishing between cortical and noncortical types of regions in the brain. Following this approach, we may note certain features of the prepyriform cortex that are distinctive in its synaptic organization: (1) there is a parallel orientation of apical dendritic trees of the principal neurons; (2) there is a nonrepeating sequence of layers in relation to the vertical extent of the principal neurons; (3) the principal neurons are graded in terms of vertical extent and dendritic geometry; (4) the principal axon collaterals give rise to internal feedback circuits that are widespread and excitatory to principal as well as intrinsic neurons; and (5) inhibitory actions by intrinsic neurons onto principal neurons are profound and long lasting. A columnar organization is a prominent characteristic of the neocortex; whether there is a similar or analogous organization of prepyriform cortex is still a matter of conjecture (Stevens, 1969; Haberly, 1969).

The features enumerated above are shared by the prepyriform cortex with other parts of the cerebral cortex—the hippocampus and the neocortex—and are absent, to a greater or lesser extent, in subcortical regions; we may cite as examples the spinal cord and the thalamus. On the other hand, the prepyriform cortex shares with many subcortical regions the following features; (1) the principal neurons are small; (2) some principal neurons lack differentiation of the dendritic tree into apical and basal dendrites; and (3) the principal neurons receive afferent input that has not passed through the thalamus. It may be best to recognize, therefore, that the olfactory cortex combines features of both cortical and subcortical regions.

From these considerations, it is suggested that the study of synaptic organization provides a basis for distinguishing certain characteristics of local organization that may be termed cortical. That such a distinction may lead to the recognition that some regions with the anatomical label of nucleus may have an organization that has cortical characteristics, and that some cortical regions may have parts with a nuclear type of organization, is not inconsistent with this use of terms. What is significant is the extent to which otherwise diverse regions share such aspects of synaptic organization as the features mentioned above. It implies that certain modes of information processing are possible with a cortical type of organization that are not possible with the other, noncortical, type. This may be regarded as only a tentative proposal toward a rethinking of this problem, which now must be incorporated into the traditional views of the distinctions between cortical and nuclear regions.

14

HIPPOCAMPUS

The hippocampus is designated the archicortex, intermediate in evolutionary development between the olfactory palaeocortex and the neocortex. It is closely associated with a neighboring region, the *dentate fascia;* together they form an S-shaped structure (see Fig. 14.1), which reminded the early histologists of a sea horse (hippocampus) or a ram's horn (Ammon's horn).

In lower vertebrates, the hippocampus lies in a dorsal position in the brain, near the septal and hypothalamic regions. In the evolution of higher vertebrates the hippocampus is dragged, as it were, in a long arc through the brain, coming to lie in a ventral position within the cerebral hemispheres. A large bundle of fibers, the *fornix,* containing the connections to the septal and hypothalamic regions, traces the path of this migration. These relations were indicated diagrammatically in Fig. 13.1.

In its position within the cerebral hemispheres, the hippocampus lies close to the olfactory cortex, as shown in Fig. 13.1. Traditionally, therefore, the hippocampus was considered an olfactory structure. This concept has been modified by the discoveries that there are no direct olfactory bulb fibers to the hippocampus (Brodal, 1947) and that the hippocampus is well developed in such animals as the dolphin which lack olfactory bulbs altogether. These discoveries had the useful effect of removing the term *rhinencephalon* from the literature as a catch-all term for those various and sundry nether parts of the brain that were not obviously related to other systems. But any field abhors a terminological vacuum, and the term *limbic system* has come to be used generally for these erstwhile rhinencephlic domains. These developments have had the effect of denying any olfactory function whatsoever to the hippocampus, which seems, in the light of recent studies, to be too extreme a

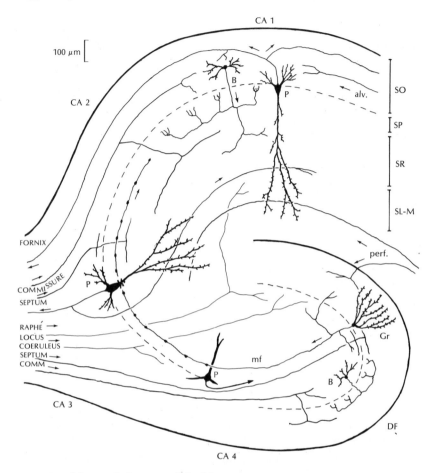

FIG. 14.1. Neuronal elements of the hippocampus.

Inputs: right, fibers in the perforant (perf) and alvear (alv) pathways; *left,* fibers arriving through the fornix (f); *below,* mossy fibers (mf) from dentate fascia.

Principal neuron: pyramidal neuron (P); recurrent Schaffer collateral (Sc).

Intrinsic neuron: basket cell (B).

The hippocampal regions are indicated by CA 1–4.

The layers are indicated on the right: SO, stratum oriens; SP, stratum pyramidale; SR, stratum radiatum; SL-M, stratum lacunosum-moleculare. Another layer, stratum lucidum, occurs at the level of mossy fibers (mf) in CA 3.

Neuronal elements of the dentate fascia are shown at DF.

Inputs: from the right, perforant (perf) pathway; from the left, fibers arriving through the fornix (f).

Principal neuron: granule cell (Gr) gives rise to mossy fibers (mf).

Intrinsic neuron: basket cell (B).

position. Recent work indicates that the hippocampus receives input from several sensory modalities: visual, auditory, somatic, and, when present, olfactory.

The anatomical position of the hippocampus makes it a key structure, a head-ganglion, of the limbic system. The primordial connections to the hypothalamus indicate a close involvement in such functions as endocrine control and the expression of emotional states. There has also been much interest in the role of the hippocampus in memory and learning. Finally the proclivity of the hippocampus to generate rhythmic activity may be mentioned, and its involvement, thereby, in certain seizure states of clinical importance. The reader is referred for orientation to standard textbooks and to Isaacson and Pribram (1975).

Apart from its relevance to these aspects of behavior, the hippocampus has been of interest to neuroanatomists and electrophysiologists because of its remarkably stereotyped internal structure. For this reason alone, it warrants an important place in the study of principles of synaptic organization in the brain. As we shall see, the results of recent studies provide useful comparisons with other regions of the brain. In addition, they provide the initial steps toward an understanding of the neural basis of the behavioral functions of the hippocampus.

NEURONAL ELEMENTS

The hippocampus forms a long cylinder, opened at one side; in cross section it has a C-shape as shown in Fig. 14.1. The dentate fascia has a similar form, its open face abutting onto the lower lip of the hippocampal cortex. Within the hippocampus, there are gradations of internal structure along the longitudinal axis. Also, as one passes along the circumference of the C, the structure varies in important respects. In one terminology (Lorente de Nó, 1934), there is a sequence of CA 1, 2, 3, and 4, as shown in Fig. 14.1. In another terminology (Cajal, 1911), there is a regio superior (roughly CA 1) and regio inferior (CA 2 and 3).

It can be gathered from these remarks that the internal structure of the hippocampus, although stereotyped, is by no means simple. The complicated geometry and the gradations of internal structure require than any description be based on an oversimplification, particularly if variations of species are further borne in mind. For the purpose of accurately describing the neuronal elements, we will at least retain as much of the geom-

etry as possible. This is done in Fig. 14.1; the diagram is adapted from
Cajal (1911), Lorente de Nó (1934), and more recent work (see Swanson
and Cowan, 1977; Storm-Mathisen, 1977); it is drawn to the same scale
as the diagrams of other brain regions.

It should be noted that because of the migratory contortions of the
hippocampus, the deep layers abut on the surface of the lateral ventricle,
whereas the superficial layers are covered by the infolding of the dentate
fascia. The student must not be deceived by these appearances; the
former are analogous to the deep layers, and the latter to the superficial
layers, of other cortical regions.

INPUTS One of the main inputs to the hippocampus comes from the
entorhinal cortex. As shown in Fig. 13.1, this is a nearby cortical region
of the temporal lobe. It is itself a complicated region, receiving as it does
inputs from several sensory modalities (van Housen, Pandya, and Butters, 1972) and from certain regions of the brain, the cingulum in particular. The fibers mediating these inputs may be regarded as *afferents* in
the sensory sense of the term.

The fibers from the entorhinal cortex enter the hippocampus by two
pathways. One of these is the so-called *perforant* pathway. These fibers
pass through ("perforate") intervening regions (the subiculum) en route;
as shown in Fig. 14.1, they enter the most superficial layer of the hippocampus, pass through region CA 1, and terminate in region CA 3
(Hjorth-Simonsen and Jeune, 1972). The other part of the entorhinal
input arrives through the so-called *alvear* pathway; these fibers pass into
the ventricular (alvear) layer and terminate in region CA 1.

The second main source of input fibers is the septal region, just anterior to the hypothalamus. These fibers distribute in thin layers just
superficial and just deep to the pyramidal cell bodies, mainly in the regio
inferior. This is perhaps analogous to the *central* inputs of other regions
we have considered.

There are substantial commissural connections, through the fimbria,
between the two hippocampi. These fibers distribute superficially and
deep to the pyramidal cell bodies in all regions.

The input to the hippocampus from the dentate fascia arrives through
the so-called *mossy fibers*, which are distributed in a thin sheet within the
hippocampus (see Fig. 14.1). They will be further described in our
discussion of the dentate fascia.

This completes the description of the classical anatomical pathways to the hippocampus. In addition, recent work with histofluorescence techniques has shown that noradrenergic fibers from the locus coeruleus distribute to pyramidal and dentate granule cells (Pickel, Segal, and Bloom, 1974). Similarly, serotonin-containing neurons of the midbrain raphé nucleus project to the hippocampus (stratum lacunosum of CA 1) and dentate fascia (infragranular layer) (Moore and Halaris, 1975). These inputs are also included in Fig. 14.1.

PRINCIPAL NEURON The output from the hippocampus is carried in axons that arise from one type of cell, the *pyramidal neuron*. The cell bodies of the pyramidal neurons are arranged in a thin sheet about 300 μm below the ventricular surface. As the name implies, the cell bodies have a pyramidal shape, imparted to them by their apical and basal dendritic trunks. The cell bodies vary in size, being 20–40 μm across the base and 40–60 μm in height. Each has a stout apical dendrite, 5–10 μm in diameter, at its origin. As shown in Fig. 14.1, these dendrites are directed in radial array toward the "surface" (see preceding discussion) of the cortex; they reach lengths of 500–1000 μm. The apical dendrite gives off several side branches and typically divides into two or more terminal branches within the most superficial layer (stratum lacunosum-moleculare).

It is notable that there is a gradation of cell body size and apical dendrite configuration as one goes from region CA 1 to CA 3; as can be seen in Fig. 14.1, the cell bodies become larger, and the apical dendrites become rather shorter, stouter, and more irregular and profuse in their branching patterns. The largest neurons of CA 3 are, in fact, referred to as *giant pyramidal cells*. Thus, although the hippocampus has one type of output neuron, there is a distinct regional variation within that type; this is in contrast to the cerebellum and olfactory bulb but similar to the regional variation in the retina and the cerebral cortex.

The basal dendrites arise as several trunks, 3–6 μm in diameter. They are oriented toward the ventricular surface and arborize extensively over a field some 200–300 μm in diameter. A striking feature of both basal and apical dendrites is their liberal investiture with *spines*.

The axons of the pyramidal neurons are directed toward the ventricular surface, where they form the *alveus*, whence they pass medially to form a sheet, the *fimbria* (see Fig. 14.1). Within this ambit, they give off several types of collateral. Some collaterals are short and local in character, simply recurring to the immediate vicinity. A special type is the so-called *Schaffer collateral*, which arises principally from the pyramidal neurons in regio inferior. They arise a short distance (several hundred microns) from the origin of the axon as a thick myelinated branch. According to the Golgi studies (Schaffer, 1892; Cajal, 1911; Lorente de Nó, 1934), these collaterals pass across the hippocampus within the same *axial* segment into the apical dendritic layer of regio superior, as is shown in Fig. 14.1. These collaterals terminate within the middle layer (stratum radiatum) of the regio superior. Another specific type of collateral from the axons of regio inferior neurons is oriented along the *longitudinal* axis of the hippocampus to terminate in the middle layer of the regio inferior. These were termed *longitudinal association fibers* by Lorente de Nó (1934). The question of whether the Schaffer collaterals and the longitudinal association fibers form two distinct types, or are at two extremes of a continuum, has been discussed by Hjorth-Simonsen (1973).

From the fimbria, the pyramidal axons gather to form the *fornix*, through which they pass in a long arc anteriorly and then ventrally. The axons are divided into two groups, depending on whether they pass rostral or caudal to the anterior commissure. The *pre*commissural fibers, arising from CA 1–CA 3 pyramidal cells, distribute to the lateral septal region. This is the only subcortical projection of the hippocampus. The pyramidal cells of CA 1 also send fibers to the subiculum (Hjorth-Simonsen,, 1973; Andersen, Bland, and Dudar, 1973). The pyramidal cells of CA 4 project bilaterally to the dentate fascia.

It may be noted that the *post*commissural fibers in the fornix distribute to the mamillary bodies and ventromedial nucleus of the hypothalamus. It used to be believed that these fibers also arise from the hippocampus, but recently it has been discovered that they arise instead from the subiculum (Swanson and Cowan, 1977). The older degeneration experiments had involved lesions in the hippocampus which interrupted the fibers of passage from the subiculum. The subiculum also sends pre- and postcommissural fibers to the lateral septum and several other ventral forebrain structures. The classical projection through the postcommissural fornix to the anterior thalamus is now believed to arise from the parasubiculum. The paper of Swanson and Cowan should be consulted for a thorough discussion of these revisions in our knowledge of hippocampal projections.

INTRINSIC NEURONS   There is a variety of neurons whose axons remain within the hippocampus. By this token, they may be regarded as *short-axon cells;* on the basis of the irregular shapes of their cell bodies and dendrites, they are referred to as *polymorphic cells.* An example of this type is shown in Fig. 14.1 (B); its cell body is located in stratum oriens. The cell bodies range in diameter from 15–30 μm; each gives rise to several relatively stout dendrites, 3–6 μm in diameter. The dendrites are notable in that they branch sparingly and have very irregular orientations; the dendritic surface, although knobbly, has few spines. The dendrites attain lengths of several hundred microns. Thus, as intrinsic neurons go, they are rather large.

As Fig. 14.1 shows, the axon of this cell type follows a complicated course. It first ascends through the pyramidal cell body layer to the middle layer (stratum radiatum), where it undergoes several divisions. Some of the branches terminate within the middle and superficial layers, whereas others recur to the layer of pyramidal cell bodies. Here they ramify extensively, forming clusters of terminals around individual pyramidal cell bodies and dendrites. There is a resemblance in outward form to the terminations of basket cells in the cerebellum; this resemblance extends also to the basket terminations in the neocortex.

Other types of intrinsic neuron are found at other levels in the hippocampal cortex. The shapes of the cell bodies and dendritic fields of these intrinsic neurons appear to reflect the orientations of surrounding structures. For example, near the ventricular surface (alveus) and at the other surface (stratum lacunosum-moleculare), there is a horizontal orientation, whereas in the middle layer (stratum radiatum), there is a vertical orientation. In general, the axon of a superficially located cell distributes deeper in the cortex, and vice versa. It is interesting to note that Cajal (1911) mentioned an intrinsic neuron that lacks an axon, in the stratum lacunosum-moleculare. These and other varieties of intrinsic neuron are not included in Fig. 14.1 for the sake of simplicity.

CELL POPULATIONS   Counts of the number of fibers in the fornix on one side have yielded estimates of 500,000 in monkey (Daitz and Powell, 1954), 1,200,000 in man (Powell, Guillery, and Cowan, 1957; see also Brodal, 1970). These, however, can no longer be used to estimate numbers of pyramidal cells, in view of the contribution of the subiculum to the fornix. Swanson and Cowan (1977) estimate that there are approximately 300,000 pyramidal cells in CA 1 and 150,000 in CA 3, and that the commissural and association projections from these regions are much greater than the septal projections. It may be noted that this is a relatively large population of principal neurons, larger than that of the olfactory bulb (50,000) or the entire ventral horn (200,000), slightly smaller than that of the retina and the pyramidal tract from the cerebral cortex, and much smaller than that of the cerebellum (7,000,000). No figures are available for the numbers of input fibers to the hippocampus, so no estimate can be made of the input-output ratio; one can guess that, in view of the large number of output neurons, the ratio might be relatively low. Similarly, no estimates are available for the numbers of intrinsic neurons. It is stated (Cajal, 1911) that they are much fewer in number than the pyramidal cells. This is offset by the very large divergence from one basket cell onto the pyramidal cells. It has been estimated that one basket cell in the hippocampus establishes contact with 200–500 pyramidal cells (see Eccles, 1969). This is more than an order of magnitude greater than the comparable estimate for the basket cells in the cerebellum. The overall I:P ratio might be estimated very roughly to be of the order of 1–10:1.

DENTATE FASCIA   The main *input* to the dentate fascia is through the fibers of the *perforant pathway* (see Fig. 14.1); most of these fibers, in fact, terminate in the dentate. It is especially notable that the entorhinal cortex projects to both the hippocampus and the dentate fascia over this pathway. Other inputs come from collaterals of pyramidal neurons in regio inferior of the hippocampus on the same and opposite sides, and from septal nuclei through fibers in the fornix. Fibers from the septum distribute just superficial and just deep to the granule cell bodies, similar to their pattern in the hippocampus. A recently described input is from the pyramidal cells in CA 4 of both sides. These and other commissural fibers terminate in the deep third of the molecular layer. Finally, the fibers from the locus coeruleus and raphé nucleus in the brainstem distribute to the hilar region.

The *output* from the dentate fascia is through the axons of so-called *granule cells*. As shown in Fig. 14.1, their cell bodies are arranged in a thin sheet about 200 μm below the surface. The cell bodies are only about 10 μm in diameter. From the superficial aspect of the cell body arise several dendritic trunks (each several microns in diameter); these trunks course through the superficial (molecular) layer and branch and terminate near the surface. The dendrites are richly invested with spines. In outward form these cells are not unlike smaller versions of cerebellar Purkinje cells. This gives us the opportunity to once again point out that the term *granule* has no necessary significance, either anatomical or physiological, in comparing neurons of different regions. These granule cells are not of the same morphological type as their namesakes in either the olfactory bulb or the cerebellum.

The axons of the granule cells give off several collaterals within the dentate fascia. They then gather to form a band (or, more correctly, a sheet) of fibers that come to lie within the hippocampus just superficial to the layer of pyramidal cell bodies (see Fig. 14.1). Along their lengths these axons have large varicosities, and they end in bulbous swellings; this has earned them the name of *mossy fibers*. Again, there is no relationship to the mossy fibers of the cerebellum.

The *intrinsic* neurons of the dentate fascia include various kinds of *short-axon cells*. They are found at all levels and have shapes and sizes not unlike many of the polymorphic cells of the hippocampus. The main type has a cell body situated in the deep layer; as can be seen in Fig. 14.1, the axon ascends to the superficial layer and then recurs to the layer of granule cell bodies, where it ramifies and terminates in clusters of terminals. These cells have been regarded as analogous to the basket cells of the hippocampus (cf. Eccles, 1969), although this is a comparison Cajal (1911) did not himself make. It is interesting to note that, here and there, are found neurons that have a pyramidal form, with apical and basal dendrites, but whose axons ramify locally (Cajal, 1911). The fact that such a neuron is, by definition, a short-axon cell, is a reminder that the term *pyramidal* is descriptive of outward form only.

No estimates are available for the numbers of input fibers or of principal neurons in the dentate fascia. It seems safe to guess that the number of principal neurons is rather high. Similarly, there are no estimates of the population of intrinsic neurons, but they are certainly less numerous than the principal neurons.

SYNAPTIC CONNECTIONS

By virtue of the lamination of fibers in the hippocampus and dentate fascia, it has been possible to obtain reliable evidence in both regions for the identification of connections made by different types of synaptic

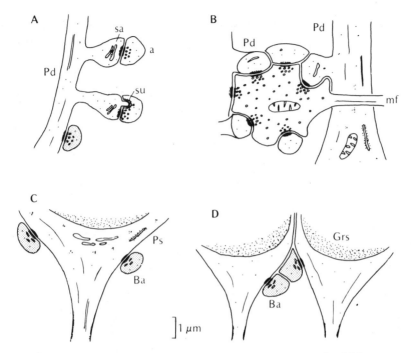

FIG. 14.2. Synaptic connections in the hippocampus. (A) Axodendritic connections onto a pyramidal cell dendrite (Pd); note the spine apparatus (sa) and
spinule (su). (B) Axodendritic connections from a mossy fiber terminal (mf) onto
the proximal dendritic shafts and spines of pyramidal cells (Pd). (C) Axosomatic
connections onto the cell body of a pyramidal neuron (Ps) from basket cell axons
(Ba). [(A)-(C) after Hamlyn, 1963; Westrum and Blackstad, 1962; Blackstad,
1967; Gottlieb and Cowan, 1971.]

Synaptic connections in the dentate fascia. (D) Axosomatic connections from
basket cell axons (Ba) onto cell bodies of granule cells (Grs). (After Laatsch and
Cowan, 1966.)

terminal (see Hamlyn, 1963; Blackstad, 1967; Nafstad, 1967; Gottlieb
and Cowan, 1971). The main types are illustrated in Fig. 14.2.

The input fibers in the perforant pathway make axodendritic synapses
onto the spines of the apical dendrites of the pyramidal cells. As shown
in Fig. 14.2 (A), these are mainly type I chemical synapses, with asymmetrical membrane thickenings and round vesicles. The spines are rather
small, with diameters of about 1 μm or less; the larger ones contain a
spine apparatus. Many of the spines have a "spinule" protruding into the
presynaptic terminal, as shown in Fig. 14.2 (A).

Next to be described are the input connections made by the dentate granule cells onto the pyramidal cells. As already mentioned, these are by way of the mossy fibers and terminals. As shown in Fig. 14.2 (B), the terminals are some 3–6 μm in diameter, in contrast to the thin axons (less than 0.5 μm) from which they arise. The terminals have tortuous shapes, with many protrusions and invaginations, which accommodate the shafts and spines of the apical dendrites near their origin from the pyramidal cell bodies. It is particularly striking that a terminal may entirely surround a dendrite, as shown in Fig. 14.2 (B). Each mossy terminal has synaptic connections onto numerous dendrites and spines. The contacts are type I chemical synapses. In addition to these large terminals, the mossy fiber has numerous swellings along its course; these swellings are the sites of *en passant* type I synapses onto the pyramidal cells. The swellings, like the terminals, are packed with vesicles ranging in size up to 2000 Å (0.2 μm) diameter, some of which contain dense cores [see Fig. 14.2 (B)].

A third type of connection within the hippocampus has been identified within the layer of pyramidal bodies. Here are found terminals with contacts onto the cell bodies; these axosomatic synapses are type II chemical contacts [see Fig. 14.2 (C)]. It is believed that these synapses are made by the axon terminals of the basket cells. The majority of synapses onto the somata of pyramidal cells have been reported to be of this type (Gottlieb and Cowan, 1971). These contacts are not numerous; Gottlieb and Cowan have estimated that they occupy less than 5% of the surface area of the pyramidal cell bodies. These terminals, and their synaptic contacts, contrast with the highly specialized terminal complex made by a basket cell axon around the cell body and initial segment of a Purkinje cell in the cerebellum.

We have thus far described three of the main types of synaptic connection within the hippocampus. There are many more. Among them should be mentioned the connections made by the Schaffer collaterals from the pyramidal cell axons; these are made within the middle layer (stratum radiatum) and have been reported to be mostly type I axodendritic synapses made onto the branches and spines of the apical dendrites. Elsewhere in this layer, most of the synapses are type I onto the dendritic spines; these synapses come from the afferent fibers from the septum and from commissural fibers from the opposite hippocampus. A small number of type II chemical synapses have been found onto the apical dendrites in the "superficial" zones. In "deeper" layers, type I synapses are present on the basal dendrites of the pyramidal cells; type I synapses are also presumed to arise from fibers from the septum and commissure. For the sake of simplicity we will not depict these and other connections here.

In the *dentate fascia,* we have already noted that the perforant fibers make type I synapses onto the spines of the granule cells (Laatsch and Cowan, 1966). These connections resemble rather closely their counterparts in the hippocampus—the spines are small (0.5–1 μm in diameter); many spines have a spinule protruding into the presynaptic terminal, similar to what is seen in the hippocampus. Most of these connections from the perforant pathway are made onto the spines of intermediate and distal branches of the granule cell dendrites. Proximally, connections onto large dendritic branches and onto stubby spines come from association, commissural, and septal fibers; these are also type I chemical synapses.

On the granule cell bodies are found terminals that make type II synapses, as is shown in Fig. 14.2 (D). Electron-microscope studies have, in addition, revealed several unusual features of the granule cell bodies. These include the fact that there is only a thin rim of cytoplasm around the nucleus, that there are no distinct Nissl bodies, and that the cell bodies are packed so tightly that much of the surface membrane of a cell is directly apposed to that of its neighbor. These features are indicated only very sketchily in Fig. 14.2 (D). In addition to these findings regarding the cell bodies, it has also been found that the mossy axons arising from them form bundles or sheets within which their surface membranes are also directly apposed, a situation not unlike that of the unmyelinated olfactory nerve fibers and the parallel fibers of the cerebellum. The obvious possibility for 'ephatic" interactions through the appositions of the cell bodies and the axons of the granule cells has been noted (Laatsch and Cowan, 1966) (cf. Chapter 2).

BASIC CIRCUIT

The organization of the hippocampus, together with that of the dentate fascia, is summarized in the basic circuit diagram of Fig. 14.3. It is well perhaps to begin by acknowledging the problem of simplifying the geometry of the hippocampus to fit with the conventions used in the diagrams for other parts of the brain. The diagram follows the usual practice in the literature, of reducing the hippocampus to its two main

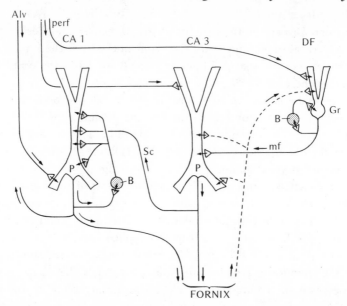

FIG. 14.3. Basic circuit diagram for the hippocampus and dentate fascia. Abbreviations as in Fig. 14.2.

regions, regio superior and inferior, and placing by its side a single representation of the dentate region (see, for example, Hamlyn, 1963; Gottlieb and Cowan, 1973). As in most diagrams in this book, the main afferent input arrives from above and the output of the region is below. It is to be hoped that we have not, like Procrustes, mutilated the traveler by fitting him to this bed.

By way of brief summary, the perforant pathway connects to the distal dendrites of the hippocampal pyramidal cells in regio inferior. The alvear pathway connects to the basal dendrites of cells in regio superior. The third main input pathway, from the septum, distributes just above and below the pyramidal cell bodies, as indicated by the dotted line. Commissural fibers, not shown for the sake of clarity, have a wider distribution at these two levels.

Within the hippocampus, two main circuits are organized in relation to the recurrent collaterals of the pyramidal neurons in the two main regions. One is formed by the Schaffer collaterals from the pyramidal neurons of regio inferior to regio superior. The other is formed by the collaterals of regio superior neurons to basket cells, which feed back to the cell bodies and the dendrites of the pyramidal neurons in that same region, as is shown in Fig. 14.3.

The dentate fascia receives its main input from the perforant pathway, as shown in Fig. 14.3; other inputs come from the pyramidal cells of CA 4, the septum, commissural fibers, and the brainstem (not shown). Within the dentate is postulated a feedback circuit from granule cell axon collaterals to basket cells and back onto the granule cell bodies. The output from the dentate fascia, through the mossy fibers of the granule cells, is directed to the pyramidal neurons of regio inferior of the hippocampus.

In assessing these organizational patterns, the first fact to be noted is that, although the three elements of the synaptic triad are all present, most of the inputs appear to make their connections onto the principal elements (pyramidal cells) and not the intrinsic cells (basket cells). The basket cells are possible targets for septal fibers in the stratum oriens, but this has not been established. Be that as it may, there are few intrinsic cells in a position to receive inputs from the perforant pathway, the mossy fibers, and the septal terminals in the deeper layers. This means that these several, different, presumably excitatory, inputs impinge directly onto the pyramidal cell dendritic tree. There is no softening of the blows, no stage of input processing through intrinsic neurons to provide for integration, dispersion, or commutation of these actions or modalities.

The intrinsic circuits are organized mainly in relation to internal sequencing (see below) and control of output. The major role of intrinsic neurons thus is at the output stage, to provide for control of activity sent to the various projection sites.

In addition to these internal sequencing circuits, there is a short-range feedback circuit from the CA 4 pyramidal cells to the dentate fascia, and, of course, much longer extrinsic circuits from projection sites in the hypothalamus, thalamus, and cortex.

Most of these characteristics of hippocampal organization have counterparts in the olfactory cortex. They stand in contrast to olfactory bulb and retina, in which dendrodendritic synapses are prominent, synaptic triads are well defined, and principal neurons feed back onto intrinsic neurons but not onto each other. The reader may further study the points of similarity and difference with other regions.

The diagram in Fig. 14.3 emphasizes that a horizontal and vertical framework provides the main scaffolding for the connections in the hippocampus. In this respect, the framework is similar to that of other

cortical and laminated regions of the brain. The recognition of this
framework is important, since certain implications immediately follow
for the functional organization of the hippocampus.

In the *horizontal* plane, there are clearly different regions as one moves
around the circumference of the hippocampus, and this means that these
regions form narrow strips or segments in the longitudinal axis of the
hippocampus. These regions grade into each other much more gradually
than the diagram of Fig. 14.3 indicates; there are gradations in the longitudinal axis as well. It is important to note that there are *multiple bases for
regional parcellation;* there are specific inputs to different regions, specific
intrinsic circuits within and between different regions, and specific projection sites from different regions; these are all illustrated in Fig. 14.3.

In this respect, the hippocampus is more complicated than most other
regions of the brain. In the olfactory bulb, for example, there is no
evidence for parcellation on any of these bases. In the cerebellum, different parts have different input and output connections, but the intrinsic
circuits, basically, appear similar, and there are no obvious sequences
from one part of the cerebellum to another. The neocortex, of course, is
characterized by multiple parcellation on all these bases; we need only
mention, as an example, the differences between the motor cortex and
the visual cortex. By way of speculation, one may ask whether it is
possible that the regions of the hippocampus are analogous to motor and
sensory areas of the neocortex? Or must we conceive of entirely different
central or behavioral "modalities"? In reply to such questions, the hippocampus only grins back like a Cheshire cat.

In the horizontal plane there is at any rate a clear implication of a
sequencing of activity in several of the circuits. Prominent among these are
(1) the mossy fiber input from dentate fascia to regio inferior and (2) the
Schaffer collaterals from regio inferior to regio superior. This sequencing
of activity in the horizontal plane is similar to, though more rigid than,
that in the olfactory cortex. It is also similar to that in the cerebellum,
with the qualification that, in the cerebellum, the sequencing through
the parallel fibers is bidirectional, not unidirectional as in olfactory and
hippocampal cortex.

The circuits that have been described above are notable in being oriented transversely across the longitudinal axis of the hippocampus. In
recent experiments, these circuits have been mapped by anatomical
(Blackstad, 1967; Hjorth-Simonsen and Jeune, 1972), histochemical

(Storm-Mathisen and Blackstad, 1964), and physiological means (Anderson, Bliss, and Skrede, 1971). From these studies, it has been concluded that the hippocampus is organized into parallel transverse lamellae. The diagram of Fig. 14.3 may, therefore, be taken to represent the organization of one lamella.

In the *vertical* axis, there is a layering, or lamination, of inputs to the output neuron (pyramidal neuron). The attempt has been made in Fig. 14.3 to indicate the vertical locus of various inputs onto the dendritic trees of the hippocampal (and dentate) neurons. This lamination has traditionally been regarded as the outstanding feature of hippocampal organization (cf. Lorente de Nó, 1934), more distinct than in any other region of the brain. We have already noted, however, the lamination of inputs to the dendrites of granule cells in the olfactory bulb and the olfactory cortex. It should be clear that, in one form or other, this is a common feature in the organization of most regions of the brain. We will discuss its significance for neocortical organization in Chapters 15 and 16. The interpretation of the functional significance of the inputs at different vertical levels in the hippocampus is dependent, as elsewhere, on a knowledge of the dendritic properties of the pyramidal cells, which will be discussed later in this chapter.

Let us finally discuss briefly the dentate fascia. As the diagram of Fig. 14.3 indicates, this region consists essentially of an input-output relay with an intrinsic feedback circuit. The diagram also indicates the special position of this region with regard to its input and output. The essence of this position was recognized long ago by Cajal (1911), and we can do no better than to quote from him:

> The granules . . . are not long-axon neurons . . . but rather special corpuscles, of which the semi-long axon is charged . . . with carrying to the bodies and the protoplasmic shafts [i.e., dendrites] of the large pyramidal cells the olfactory excitations that they receive from the temporoammonic pathway.

We see, therefore, that the granule cells provide a special relay along the entorhinal input pathway to the large hippocampal pyramidal cells. They also receive a short-range feedback from CA 4 pyramidal cells. The dentate may be analogous to the thalamus and to the granule cells of the cerebellum, in that all three of these regions perform some special function of staging or preprocessing of an input to a specific cortical region.

SYNAPTIC ACTIONS

Even more so than the cerebellum, the hippocampus is at a remove from the major sensory input pathways in the brain, as well as from the final outflow through the motoneurons. The neurophysiologist is, therefore, faced with a region in which there are few obvious or identifiable characteristics of the inputs or outputs that would provide starting points for the analysis of synaptic actions. Indeed, in such a situation, the problem gets stood on its head, and the analysis of synaptic actions becomes part of the evidence for what those characteristics might be. At any rate, the input and output pathways are clearly separated, so that electrophysiological analysis of synaptic actions can be carried out as effectively as in the spinal cord and the olfactory bulb (see Kandel, Spencer, and Brinley, 1961; Andersen, Blackstad, and Lømo, 1966a; Andersen, Holmquist, and Voorhoeve, 1966b). Recent *in vitro* studies of hippocampal slices (Skrede and Westgaard, 1971; Schwartzkroin, 1977) have confirmed and extended many of the results obtained *in vivo* (see below). This type of preparation holds great promise for analysis of local circuit organization in the hippocampus and in other regions.

The responses of the hippocampal pyramidal neurons to single volleys in the different input pathways are illustrated in Fig. 14.4. In (A) there is an intracellular recording of the response to a volley originating in the olfactory bulb. It consists of a long-latency, slow-depolarizing wave, which has been ascribed to an EPSP elicited over a polysynaptic pathway from the bulb. Presumably this route passes from the olfactory bulb to the entorhinal cortex (refer to Fig. 13.1), thence, through one or more synaptic relays, to the hippocampus via the perforant pathway. A notable feature of the response is that it does not lead to impulse firing; the synaptic potential remains subthreshold for impulse initiation in the pyramidal neuron. This has been interpreted as indicating that the EPSP is set up in the distal branches of the apical dendrites where the fibers of the perforant pathway terminate (Yokota, Reeves, and MacLean, 1970). These findings indicate that there is in fact an olfactory input to the hippocampus, but that its synaptic action appears to be limited to subthreshold effects. The suggestion has been made that these synaptic actions are comparable to conditional stimuli that might have a role in memory and learning (MacLean, 1972).

A single volley from the septal region elicits in a pyramidal neuron the

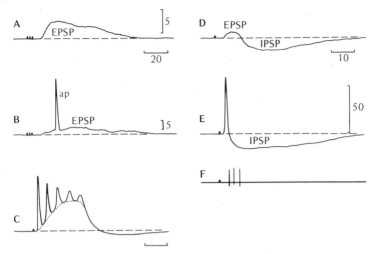

FIG. 14.4. Synaptic actions in the hippocampus. (A) Intracellular response of a pyramidal cell to a volley from the olfactory bulb. (After MacLean et al., 1970.) (B) Response to a volley from the septum, through fibers in the fornix (MacLean et al). (C) Response to a strong volley in the perforant pathway. (After Kandel and Spencer, 1961.) (D) Response to a volley in the fornix. (After Kandel et al., 1961.) (E) Antidromic response to a volley in the de-afferented fornix (Kandel et al.). (F) Extracellular unit recording of a presumed basket cell response to a volley in the fornix. (After Andersen et al., 1964.)

response shown in Fig. 14.4 (B). The long-lasting, low-amplitude depolarizing wave has been ascribed to an EPSP and is associated with the discharge of one or two impulses (Yokota et al., 1970; see also Andersen et al., 1966a,b). MacLean (1972) has pointed out that, through the septum, the hippocampus receives input from the hypothalamus, which is involved in aversive, appetitive, visceral, and humoral reactions of an unconditional nature. In his view, the septal inputs are comparable to unconditional stimuli, insofar as they are themselves capable of causing pyramidal impulse discharge. Whatever the interpretation, the fact that synaptic excitation is so effective over this route, in contrast to the inability of large amplitude EPSP's to elicit spikes over the route from the olfactory bulb (described above), appears to be an important aspect of synaptic integration in the hippocampus.

A distinctive type of discharge in the pyramidal neuron is seen in response to a strong volley in the perforant or the septal (fornix) pathways. This consists of a rapid discharge of several spikes that arise from an intense depolarizing wave [Fig. 14.4 (C)]. As the wave builds up, the spikes decrease in amplitude, until the discharge is terminated. This has been termed an *inactivation burst* (Kandel and Spencer, 1961), in analogy with the similar discharges (complex spikes) of Purkinje cells in the cerebellum. In the hippocampal neuron, it seems that the spikes are generated in response to the prolonged membrane depolarization and that the termination of the spike discharge is directly determined by the amount of excessive depolarization, which gradually "inactivates" the spike-generating mechanism. In the hippocampal slice preparation there is evidence that the depolarizing wave is due to the turning on of a slow calcium conductance in the apical dendrites of the pyramidal cell (Schwartzkroin and Slawsky, 1977); we shall discuss this further in the next section. The tendency to discharge in bursts has been taken to reflect the highly excitable nature of the pyramidal neurons, a property that is important for the generation of rhythmic activity in the hippocampus (see below).

INHIBITORY PATHWAYS   The analyses of synaptic actions and synaptic morphology are consistent, as far as is known, with the view that all the external inputs to the hippocampus are excitatory; in addition, there is an internal pathway for re-excitation through the Schaffer collaterals. Against these numerous excitatory inputs is a rather small population of intrinsic neurons for inhibitory actions. Despite this, electrophysiological experiments give ample evidence of strong inhibitory actions within the hippocampus in response to activation over any of the input pathways. A typical recording is shown in Fig. 14.4 (D), in which the response of a pyramidal neuron to a volley in the fornix is shown. The response consists of an initial depolarization followed by a long-lasting hyperpolarization, which have been interpreted as an EPSP and IPSP, respectively (Kandel et al. 1961). This is another example of the excitatory-inhibitory sequence that is characteristic of synaptic actions engendered by an input volley in the principal neurons of many regions of the brain (see Purpura, 1967). The inhibitory period is often followed by a rebound excitation, similar to that in neurons in the thalamus.

That the EPSP is due to connections of the input fibers [septal afferents in the case of Fig. 14.4 (D)] has been shown by chronic transection of the fornix, which causes these fibers to degenerate. This leaves only the pyramidal axons in the fornix, and the response to a volley in these axons is simply an antidromic spike followed by the IPSP, as shown in Fig. 14.4 (E).

The pathway for the IPSP has been deduced from experiments analogous to those carried out in the spinal cord. Microelectrode recordings from small units in the superficial layer of the hippocampus have revealed responses characterized by a repetitive discharge that begins within a millisecond or so of the antidromic spike, and that continues into the time period of the IPSP. An example of an extracellular recording from such a unit is illustrated in Fig. 14.4 (F). In analogy with the Renshaw circuit in the spinal cord, it has been concluded that these units are basket cells and that there is a pathway from pyramidal axon collaterals to basket cells back onto the pyramidal cells (Andersen, Eccles and Løyning, 1964; Eccles, 1969). The sites of inhibitory input by the basket cells to the cell body and the apical dendrites of the pyramidal neurons have been indicated in the basic circuit diagram of Fig. 14.3.

In sum, the intrinsic (basket) neurons appear to provide for inhibitory control, at the level of pyramidal neuron output, that is powerful, long-lasting, diffuse, and largely of a feedback nature. It may well be that these are the properties necessary to oppose the powerful excitatory pressure of the hippocampal inputs. Note that the basket cell axons ramify in the transverse plane (Fig. 14.1), so that they also reflect a lamellar organization. The inhibitory field established within a lamella is reminiscent of the compartment of inhibition established by the widely ramifying axon of a Golgi cell in the cerebellum.

RHYTHMIC ACTIVITY The hippocampus is notable for the prominent rhythmic potentials it generates. It might be thought, and indeed it was thought by the early workers, that the hippocampus would provide a model system for studying the generation of rhythmic activity. The subject, however, has become quite complicated, for it encompasses not only the problem of interpretation of summed extracellular potentials but also the tendency of the hippocampus to develop paroxysmal discharges and, finally, the relation of these discharges to epileptic seizure states. Our interest must be restricted to certain aspects relevant to synaptic organization.

The resting activity of the hippocampus takes the form of relatively slow waves (3–8/sec), the *theta rhythm*. The sequence of excitation-inhibition-rebound excitation in hippocampal pyramidal cells (Fig. 14.4) appeared to be an obvious mechanism for the generation of the theta rhythm, in analogy with the inhibitory phasing of activity in the thalamus. The experimental evidence thus far, however, is not entirely consistent with this mechanism, and the subject requires much more investigation (see Green, 1964; Spencer and Kandel, 1968). In behavioral experiments there is much interest in the relation of patterns of theta-wave activity to specific aspects of exploratory and consummatory motor behavior (Isaacson and Pribram, 1975).

If rhythmic activity is forced on the hippocampus by repetitive stimulation (e.g., of the fornix), some remarkable properties of the synaptic actions onto pyramidal neurons are revealed (Purpura, 1967; Spencer and Kandel, 1968). These properties take the form of sustained shifts of the membrane potential, potentiation of EPSPs to large amplitudes, depression of IPSPs, and a long-lasting period in the aftermath of stimulation during which evoked EPSPs are much larger than normal. These findings may be taken to reflect a remarkable lability in the potency of excitatory and inhibitory synapses in the hippocampus, also notable for its long-lasting time course. These are, of course, the kinds of properties that are suspected of being crucial for learning and memory, as has already been discussed (Chapters 4 and 10). However, the task of proving that these mechanisms are operative in the hippocampus has barely begun. We have previously noted changes in potency of certain synapses onto motoneurons, but the effects in the hippocampus are much more prominent and complex. Similar effects have been found in the neocortex.

An increase in the level of excitability of hippocampal neurons, either occurring naturally or under artificial conditions of electrical stimulation in an irritative focus, produces an unstable situation, which rapidly gives way to uncontrolled activity. This can take various forms; a common form consists of a large depolarizing wave in a pyramidal neuron of 30–40 mV, which generates a burst of impulses not unlike the burst response already described (Fig. 14.4). This is followed by a prolonged plateau of depolarization and discharge of impulses, which constitute the period of the epileptic seizure. The initial wave is termed a *paroxysmal depolarizing shift* (PDS) (Matsumoto and Ajmone-Marsan, 1964) and is currently under intensive investigation for the insight it can give into the mechanism that triggers a seizure. In one view, the PDS and subsequent discharge are due primarily to altered excitability of neuronal membrane (the "epileptic neuron"); in another view, they are due to abnormal activity circulating through the synaptic circuits (the "epileptic aggregate"). An excellent summary of recent research in this problem has been provided by Ayala et al. (1973). The analysis of the mechanism of this neurological problem—epileptic seizure—is being carried out precisely at the level of synaptic organization. Similar problems are currently under investigation in the neocortex.

DENTATE FASCIA   In the dentate fascia, a volley in the perforant pathway (the main input) elicits in the granule cells an EPSP-IPSP sequence similar to that in the hippocampal pyramidal cells. Unit recordings deep to the granule cells have provided evidence that the basket cells there respond with a discharge similar to that of the basket cells in the hippocampus. It has therefore been concluded that there is a feedback circuit from granule cell axon collaterals through basket cells back onto granule cells, as in the similar circuit in the hippocampus, and in analogy with the Renshaw circuit in the spinal cord (Andersen et all, 1966a). Note that the inhibitory interneuron (basket cell) is not directly accessible to the afferent input in the perforant pathway; the dentate fascia and the hippocampus are similar in this respect.

Recently it has been found that the granule cells respond to repetitive stimulation in much the same way as do the hippocampal pyramidal cells, that is, with a potentiation of EPSPs, depression of IPSPs, and a long-lasting aftermath of potentiation; according to Bliss and Gardner-Medwin (1973), the potentiation may be detectable over periods of hours or even days. This is long enough to be implicated as a possible mechanism for information storage, but "whether or not the intact animal makes use in real life of a property which has been revealed by synchronous, repetitive volleys . . . is", as Bliss and Lømo (1973) wisely caution, "another matter." The mechanism of this potentiation will be discussed below.

NEUROTRANSMITTERS

The hippocampus has served as a model system for the identification of neurotransmitters in a central region. We summarize briefly, in relation to the diagram of Fig. 14.5.

Perhaps the best documented transmitter is acetylcholine in the input fibers from the septum. There is heavy staining for acetylcholinesterase in narrow bands just above and below the pyramidal and granule cell

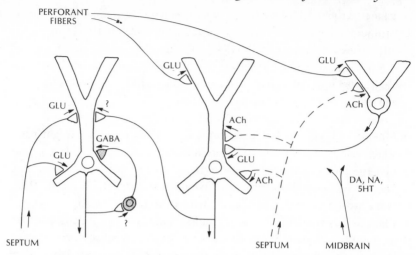

FIG. 14.5. Summary of putative neurotransmitters and their sites of action in the hippocampus and dentate fascia.

body layer, and choline acetyltransferase has a similar distribution (Storm-Mathisen, 1977). After lesions in the entorhinal areas in very young rats, there is evidence that the septal fibers undergo compensatory sprouting and spread from their normal terminal zones in the inner third of the molecular layer of the dentate fascia to occupy the outer two-thirds vacated by the degenerated terminals of the perforant pathway (Nadler, Cotman, and Lynch, 1973). Microiontophoresis of ACh usually produces slow excitation of hippocampal pyramidal cells (Salmoiraghi and Stefanis, 1965). This is antagonized by atropine, indicating a muscarinic receptor. After lesions in the septum, the pyramidal cells become supersensitive to ACh (Bird and Aghajanian, 1975). Dentate granule cells respond more briskly to applied ACh (Bland, Kostopoulos, and Phillis, 1974).

Glutamate uptake has been demonstrated by combined autoradiography and electron microscopy in the terminals of three input pathways: perforant, mossy, and commissural (cf. Storm-Mathisen, 1977). These of course are all characterized by type I synapses and excitatory synaptic actions. In the hippocampal slice preparation, glutamate-sensitive spots in the dendritic layer can be demonstrated by microiontophoresis during recordings from pyramidal cell bodies (Schwartzkroin and Andersen, 1975).

The synthesizing enzyme for GABA, GAD, was early localized to the stratum moleculare and layer of pyramidal cell bodies (Albers and Brady, 1959). It has been confirmed by immunocytochemistry (Barber and Saito, 1976). GABA uptake occurs in terminals around the pyramidal cell bodies (Hökfelt and Llungdahl, 1972; Iversen and Bloom, 1972). GAD and GABA are unaffected by deafferentation procedures, indicating that they are in terminals of intrinsic cells. Iontophoresis of GABA inhibits pyramidal cells (Curtis, Felix, and McLennan, 1970), an action blocked by bicuculline. The sensitivity is highest in the pyramidal cell body layer (Schwartzkroin and Andersen, 1975). All of these findings are consistent with the interpretation that GABA is the transmitter for basket cell inhibition of pyramidal and granule cells.

The inputs from the brainstem include all the major transmitter systems: noradrenaline (NA) (from locus coeruleus), dopamine (DA) (from ventral tegmental nucleus), serotonin (5HT) (from raphe nucleus), and histamine. For a review of the extensive histochemical and biochemical studies of these systems the reader is referred to Storm-Mathisen (1977). Iontophoretic studies indicate that NA, DA, and 5HT all have inhibitory actions on hippocampal and dentate cells.

It remains to note that the hippocampus is of additional interest biochemically because of its high content of metals, particularly zinc, but also copper and lead. The zinc is especially concentrated in the mossy fibers; special stains show that it is present throughout the mossy fibers and within the granule cells of the dentate fascia from which the fibers arise (von Euler, 1962; McLardy, 1962). Within the mossy terminals it has been reported to be present in the vesicles (Ibata and Otsuka, 1969). These intriguing findings are little understood; it has been speculated that the zinc could be involved in storage of transmitter, by forming a complex; associated with a protein or enzyme; or released to act as a transmitter or modulator, possibly inhibiting transmitter synthesizing enzymes in other terminals (see Storm-Mathisen, 1977).

DENDRITIC PROPERTIES

The hippocampal pyramidal neuron is dominated by its apical and basal dendritic trees. The evidence indicates that the dendrites are only postsynaptic in position, similar to the dendrites of neurons in the ventral horn, cerebellum, and prepyriform cortex, and in contrast to the olfactory bulb, retina, and thalamic neurons. We confine our attention therefore to local postsynaptic integration within the apical dendritic branches and transfer through the trunk to the axon hillock.

ELECTROTONIC MODEL It has been reported that the total resistance (R_N) of a pyramidal neuron is in the range of 10 MΩ (Spencer and Kandel, 1961a). This is larger by a factor of five to ten than the value for motoneurons; this has been taken to reflect the smaller size of the hippo-campal neuron and a higher specific membrane resistance (R_m) of the neuronal membrane.

In response to an intracellular current pulse the membrane potential changes with an overall time constant (τ_N) of about 10 msec. This is several times longer than that for the motoneuron. Spencer and Kandel (1961a, 1968) suggested that the longer time constant reflects a funda-mental difference in the nature of the dendritic membranes, in that it provides a greater opportunity for temporal summation of synaptic po-tentials than does a short time constant. We will see that neocortical pyramidal cells share this property.

Similar results for whole neuron properties have been obtained in the isolated hippocampal slice by Schwartzkroin (1977). Using these data, Traub and Llinás (1978) have constructed an electrotonic model of the hippocampal cell. The model is based on the compartmental representa-tion of dendritic geometry and electrical properties according to Rall, and the Hodgkin-Huxley equations for the impulse, as adapted for the computer by Dodge and Cooley (1973) (see Chapter 5). The model helps to understand two important properties of the pyramidal cells, the fast prepotentials and the inactivating bursts.

FAST PREPOTENTIALS The synapses of perforant fibers onto the termi-nal branches of the pyramidal-cell apical dendrites pose the problem of how the postsynaptic response is transferred to the axon hillock, in the face of what appears to be a considerable electrotonic decrement if the transfer is by passive means alone.

The answer to this problem seems to be provided by the fact that in recordings from pyramidal neurons it is sometimes observed that the large spike arises from a small spike (see Fig. 14.6). These small spikes are seen during spontaneous firing and also in response to volleys in the input pathways, but they never precede an antidromic spike invading from the pyramidal cell axon. These small spikes are termed *fast prepoten-*

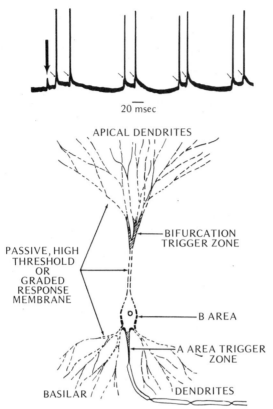

FIG. 14.6. Properties of hippocampal pyramidal cell dendrites. *Above*, intracellular recording from a pyramidal cell body of spontaneous action potentials. Large arrow, fast prepotential (FPP) in isolation; small arrows, inflections that indicate FPPs preceding large action potentials. *Below*, diagram to illustrate site of generation of FPPs in the bifurcation trigger zone of a dendritic tree. (From Spencer and Kandel, 1961b.)

tials. It is believed that they register a spike generated at an isolated patch of membrane somewhere in the apical dendritic tree.

The original model developed by Spencer and Kandel (1961b) to explain the sequence of events is shown in Fig. 14.6. It envisages a patch of excitable membrane at the juncture of the peripheral branches with the dendritic trunk. Synaptic potentials spreading through the peripheral branches trigger the active membrane in the bifurcation zone to generate an all-or-nothing response analogous to, or identical with, an action potential. The action potential then spreads over the passive trunk membrane to the axon hillock to trigger the active membrane there. The sequence is somewhat similar to that in saltatory conduction (see Chapter 3) but without the intervening myelin. The dendritic trigger zone thus acts as a booster for transmitting peripheral dendritic input to axonal output. The model is similar to that for spike activity in the dendrites of chromatolytic motoneurons and cerebellar Purkinje cells.

This conceptual model has been made explicit in the computational model of Traub and Llinás (1978). They found that they could reproduce the fast prepotentials with local "hot spots" of high Na conductance situated in small branches on either the apical or basal dendrites, at least 0.3λ from the cell body. Their results are discussed further below.

The capacity for active dendritic properties has several implications for synaptic organization. It makes a distal input much more effective vis-à-vis the axon hillock, indeed, possibly more effective than proximal inputs whose responses spread only by passive means. It provides a more effective mechanism for overcoming inhibition along the proximal dendrites or at the cell body. It possibly increases the computational complexity of the dendritic tree, in line with Rall's comment (Chapter 10). Finally, it digitalizes the input, in contrast to the graded nature of synaptic responses spreading by passive means. The significance of these factors for the input-output functions of the hippocampus remains for further investigation.

DEPOLARIZING BURSTS The bursts of impulses arising from a large depolarizing wave were reproduced by the electrotonic model of Traub and Llinás, as shown in Fig. 14.7. In this computational experiment, each dendritic compartment had a Ca conductance and a slow calcium-controlled K conductance (middle diagram). The cell body had impulse-generating properties, and there was a Na "hot spot" in one apical dendritic branch (right diagram). Orthodromic synaptic input was to the apical dendrites at the locations indicated by the arrows.

The response to the orthodromic input is shown on the left. The turning on of the slow Ca conductance causes a slow depolarization that gives rise to a burst of impulses. At the soma, the slow wave is relatively small but the impulses are large, this being the site where impulses are generated. In the dendrites the slow wave is large, this being its site of generation, and the spikes spreading from the soma are small because of

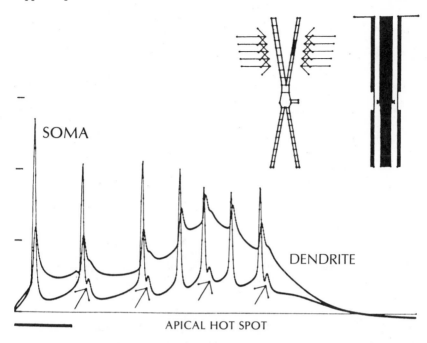

FIG. 14.7. Electrotonic compartmental model of hippocampal pyramidal cell. *Middle*, model showing sites of input (arrows) and "hot spot" (filled compartment). *Right*, distribution of slow K^+ density (left) and Ca^{2+} density (right) in model. *Left*, responses generated by 12-msec duration input, in soma and dendrites. Note large slow Ca^{2+} depolarization with small superimposed spikes in dendrites, and large spikes and after-bumps at soma (see text). (From Traub and Llinás, 1979.)

passive electrotonic decrement. The active dendritic site is fired by these soma spikes, giving rise to the "afterbumps" on the spikes recorded at the soma (arrows).

From these results it has been suggested that pyramidal cell activity is controlled by the interplay of a Ca conductance distributed rather widely throughout the dendritic tree, and local Na sites in the dendrites. Bursting appears to be controlled especially by the apical dendrite. It has been concluded that the bursts that underlie epileptogenesis may be brought about either by altered electrical properties of the apical dendrites, or by abnormal synaptic input, or by both acting together. The question of the epileptic neuron or the epileptic aggregate, mentioned previously, thus remains unresolved.

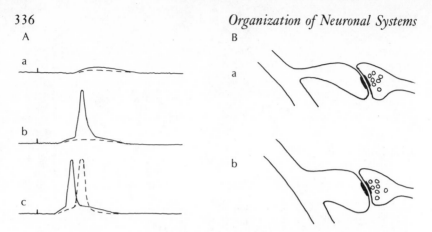

FIG. 14.8. Plasticity in the hippocampus. (A) Intracellular recordings from CA 1 pyramidal cells in hippocampal slice. (a) Response to weak volleys in radiatum fibers before (dotted trace) and after (solid trace) tetanization of radiatum fibers. (b,c) Same, stronger volleys. (After Andersen et al., 1977). (B) Schematic representation of dendritic spine size in dentate fascia before (a) and after (b) tetanization of perforant pathway. (After Fifkova and van Harreveld, 1977.)

POTENTIATION AND PLASTICITY The physiological evidence for long-lasting potentiation of synaptic responses in the hippocampus and dentate fascia has been of great interest for its possible relation to the critical role of the hippocampus in learning processes. Bliss and Lømo (1973) suggested several possible mechanisms for the potentiation: (1) increase in size of the afferent volley; (2) increased transmitter release by individual synapses; (3) increased postsynaptic response; (4) increased excitability of postsynaptic cells; (5) increased synchrony of firing.

Analysis of these factors has recently begun in the isolated hippocampal slice (Andersen, Sundberg, Sveen and Wigstöm, 1977). Intracellular responses of CA 1 pyramidal cells before and after tetanic stimulation of the stratum radiatum fibers are shown in Fig. 14.8 (A). It can be seen that after the tetani, the responses to single volleys gave larger EPSPs with shorter latencies, and were more effective in eliciting an impulse. The membrane potential did not change, nor did the spike threshold, and the effects were not dependent on the size of the input volley. These results indicate that the effect is input-specific, and most likely caused by an increase in transmitter release. Other experiments in the slice preparation (Lynch, Dunwiddie, and Gribkoff, 1977) have suggested that a potentiation of inputs to the apical dendrites is associated with depression of the pyramidal cell responses to inputs to the basal dendrites.

An attractive hypothesis is that morphological changes underlie the response potentiations, and this has been tested by Fifkova and van Harreveld (1977). They compared the morphology of dendritic spines of the granule cells in the dentate fascia before and after tetanization of the perforant pathway. Their findings are summarized in Fig. 14.8 (B). The main result of the tetanization was an increase in the size of granule dendritic spines in the outer molecular layer, where the perforant fibers terminate. Such changes were not found in the inner part of the layer. The axon terminals initially decreased in size and vesicle content, within the first hour, and then returned to their normal condition. It was postulated that the spine swelling might be induced by glutamate, liberated synaptically or perhaps nonsynaptically, by the axon terminals. Fifkova and van Harreveld noted that the increased size of the spine and spine stem could provide for more effective spread of synaptic currents (Rall and Rinzel, 1973), and more effective movement of substances from and into the spines (see Chapter 15 below), thus providing a basis for the physiological potentiation of responses in the postsynaptic cells.

15

NEOCORTEX:
SENSORY AREA

The term neocortex refers to the "new pallium", the most recent of the cortical regions to differentiate in vertebrate evolution. It is a remarkable fact that throughout phylogeny most regions of the central nervous system are either clearly present (i.e., spinal cord, olfactory bulb, retina, cerebellum) or else have obvious counterparts (i.e., thalamus and other brain-stem regions). This is also true of the palaeocortex (olfactory cortex) and, to a certain extent, of the archicortex (hippocampus). Some regions (i.e., retina) may even be more elaborately developed in lower than in higher forms.

The neocortex, however, and to some extent the associated basal ganglia, stands out as an exception. It is barely discernible in the brains of fishes and but ill-defined in amphibians and reptiles, and even in birds. As a specific and well-differentiated area it is, in fact, virtually specific for mammals. Once established in the mammalian brain, it has evolved to such an extent as to account for the major part of the brain substance. It should be remarked, however, that the neocortex is not the only region to evince this capacity for overgrowth; the cerebellum achieves a similar overwhelming dominance in the brains of certain electric fish, as discussed in Chapter 10. Like the cerebellum, the neocortex has increased its volume not only by expanding outwards, but also be developing deep convolutions that greatly increase the surface-to-volume ratio; in fact two-thirds of the human cortex lies within the fissures of the convolutions. The olfactory cortex and hippocampus, in contrast, have retained their smooth surfaces.

Although the neocortex has a basically similar layered structure

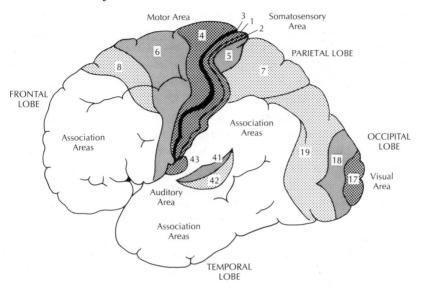

FIG. 15.1. Neocortex of the human brain and its main anatomical and functional areas. (Adapted from Brodmann, in Fulton, 1938.)

throughout its extent, different regions vary not only in their connections with different subcortical regions, but also in certain aspects of their cellular constituents and internal organization. This was recognized in the earliest histological investigations around the turn of the century. On this basis the areas of the cortex which are parts of the main sensory and motor systems were identified, and maps constructed such as that illustrated in Fig. 15.1.

It is generally agreed that the capabilities that set man apart from other mammals, and mammals from other vertebrates, have their basis in the large and diversified population of cortical neurons, the multiplicity of connections with other parts of the brain, and the complexity of interactions within the cortex itself. These factors lead directly to the study of synaptic organization as the necessary basis for understanding the particular contribution of the cortex to mammalian and human behavior.

Having said this, we must face the fact that few regions of the brain seem more designed to frustrate the analysis of synaptic organization. Two obvious problems can immediately be mentioned. One is that the fibers carrying the inputs and outputs are intermingled in the cortex. Because they do not form separate and discrete bundles (as in most of the

other regions we have studied) selective degeneration and electrophysiological methods are very difficult. The other problem is that, with the
exception of those parts of the cortex that receive direct input from specific sensory pathways, the types of information entering and leaving the
cortex are difficult to characterize. Consider, finally, the areas not frankly
motor or sensory, the so-called association areas. It is obvious from the
palaeontological record that these parts of the neocortex have evolved most
briskly in primate evolution and are presumably most responsible for
those capabilities that characterize human behavior—speech, thought,
memory, etc. Yet it is precisely these areas that are the most difficult to
analyze in terms of inputs, outputs, and intrinsic organization.

One approach to understanding the cortex is in terms of an abstract
synthesis incorporating general properties common to all regions. However, this does injustice to myriads of details, some of which reflect distinctive properties of different regions. The strategy adopted here will be
to build from the particular to the general. We shall start with the simplest
and most readily accessible type of cortex, the primary sensory areas
receiving direct input from specific relay nuclei in the thalamus. Our
focus will be on the visual area, thus providing continuity with the previous accounts of the retina and the lateral geniculate nucleus. Comparisons
will be made with the somatosensory cortex. It is fair to say that most of
the principles of synaptic organization of the cortex, as we understand
them at present, have been built on work in these two areas, and much of
the present-day excitement is related to the application of new methods to
them. The motor cortex will be considered in Chapter 16.

NEURONAL ELEMENTS

By virtue of the outward expansion of the neocortex, the fibers to it
arrive through the depths, and the fibers from it also leave through the
depths. The neocortex is therefore doubled back on itself, as it were, like
the cerebellum. As with the cerebellum and the thalamus, we will depict
the neuronal elements in their actual relations.

The neuronal elements of the visual cortex are illustrated in Fig. 15.2.
The description is taken from the accounts of Cajal (1911) and Lorente de
Nó (1938), together with more recent work of Garey (1971), Valverde
(1971), Szentagóthai (1973), and Lund (1973) using the Golgi method.
One can get the impression from reading the voluminous literature that
there are as many types of neuronal elements as there are cells and investi-

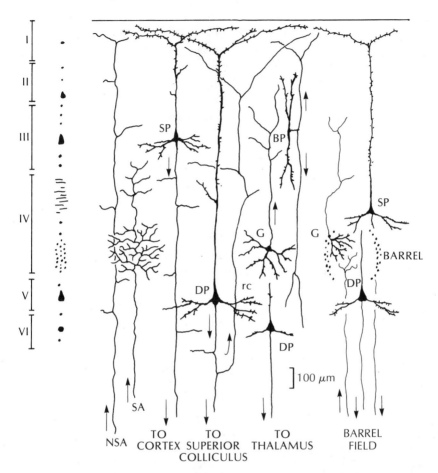

FIG. 15.2. Neuronal elements of visual cortex (somatosensory barrel field shown at right for comparison).

Inputs: specific sensory afferents (SA); nonspecific sensory afferents (NSA).

Principal neurons: superficial pyramidal neurons (SP); deep pyramidal neurons (DP); recurrent axon collaterals (rc).

Intrinsic neurons: granule cell (G); bipolar cell (BP).

Histological layers from I to VI are shown at left, together with a diagrammatic representation of cell types and densities in the layers.

gators; the following account is greatly simplified. Results with new methods such as HRP tracing are just becoming available; they will be described briefly here and in the following section on Synaptic Connections.

INPUTS The specific afferent fibers arise from the principal neurons of the lateral geniculate nucleus, which have been described in Chapter 11. The fibers are several microns in diameter and myelinated. They enter through the cortical depths and terminate with an extensive and dense arborization. As shown in Fig. 15.2, the field of arborization extends 100–400 μm in both vertical and horizontal planes. It is so placed as to be about in the middle of the cortical thickness, in a layer usually designated as layer IV (see Fig. 15.2); a few branches are often described as reaching layer III above, and, in some species, layers I and VI. There are two types of fiber, thick and thin, which come from the large and medium-to-small cells, respectively, of the lateral geniculate nucleus (Garey and Powell, 1971).

In contrast to this specific sensory input is a type of fiber that may be referred to collectively as a nonspecific afferent (NSA in Fig. 15.2). This fiber meanders upward through the cortex, giving off single branches at several levels, including the most superficial. In area 17 these fibers are relatively sparse, and are mostly fibers from nonspecific reticular nuclei of the thalamus. Also present, but not shown in the diagram, are fibers of the diffuse noradrenergic projection system arising in the locus coeruleus in the brainstem.

Most regions of the cortex have a rich supply of association and commissural fibers. Area 17 is distinctive in receiving few association fibers from neighboring areas, and few if any commissural fibers from its contralateral counterpart.

PRINCIPAL NEURON Traditionally the pyramidal cell has been regarded as the output neuron of the cortex. Like pyramidal cells of the cortical regions, it derives its name from the shape of the cell body, which is imparted by the characteristic apical and basal dendritic trunks. There are, in general, two groups of pyramidal cells, depending on whether the cell bodies are located superficial or deep to layer IV. The superficial group is located in layers II and III (SP). There is a size continuum in these layers, with the smallest and more superficial cells about 15×30 μm, and the largest and deeper cells up to 25×30 μm. The other group is in layer V and layer VI, where the cell bodies, as seen in visual cortex, may reach dimensions of about 40×80 μm.

The single, long *apical dendrite* ascends vertically through the cortex to branch and terminate in the most superficial (molecular) layer. The length of this apical dendrite thus depends on the depth of the cell body from which it arises. As can be seen in Fig. 15.2, this varies considerably, from a minimum of perhaps 200 μm (cell body in layer II) to a maximum of approximately 1600 μm (cell body in layer V). The superficial branches reach a radius of 200–400 μm. The apical dendritic trunk ranges in diameter from about 5 to 10 μm. It is therefore among the thickest, as well as longest, of dendrites in the nervous system. In the motor cortex, as we shall see, it is even bigger. A prominent feature is the numerous *spines*, particularly on the most superficial branches; we will discuss these in greater detail later.

The pyramidal cell also gives off several *basal dendrites*. The trunks vary up to 6 to 8 μm in diameter. They branch somewhat sparingly to an extent of 200 to 400 μm from the cell body. They also bear spines but not as many as the apical dendrites.

The axon leaves the deep aspect of the cell body or a large dendrite. Many axons give off *collaterals* while still within the cortex. These are of two main types. Some are short *horizontal collaterals*, given off to various layers during the descent of the axon (as shown for the SP cell in Fig. 15.2). Others are *recurrent collaterals*, which ascend through the cortex, varying greatly with respect to the level they reach, the number of branches, and the lateral extent of the branching. Variation in these collaterals appears to be a special characteristic of pyramidal cells. An example of a recurrent collateral with limited branching and lateral extent is shown for the DP cell of Fig. 15.2. According to the Scheibels (1970), the greatest lateral extent for the branching field of collaterals from a single axon is of the order of 3000 μm (3 mm). To what extent such collaterals are part of the strictly local circuits in the cortex, and to what extent they represent intra- and intercortical association pathways, is a matter of definition.

This description summarizes the main aspects of the principal neuron as it applies to its geometry within the cortex. But one of the problems with the neocortex is that there seem to be exceptions to any rule. For example, some pyramidal cells have axons that do not leave the cortex; these appear, therefore, to be intrinsic neurons rather than principal neurons. On the other hand, some fusiform cells of the deep layers have axons that leave the cortex, and must, therefore, be included as principal neurons. There are even reports that some stellate cells (next section) may give rise to projection fibers. It is best to recognize this overlap of cell types as one of the characteristics of the neocortex. There is not such a rigid correlation between dendritic branching pattern and axonal projection pattern as there is for cells in other parts of the nervous system.

The axons of the principal neurons have several destinations, which fall into two main groups. Some axons remain at the cortical level and serve to connect to other parts of the cortex; they are *association fibers*. In visual cortex they arise from superficial pyramidal cells, and connect to areas 17 and 18. The other group of axons carries the cortical output to subcortical regions; these are termed *projection fibers*. There are two types. The deep pyramidal cells of layer V project to the superior colliculus; the cells of layer VI project to the lateral geniculate. The localization of different output cells in different laminae has been established with electrophysiological techniques (see Toyama et al., 1974) and demonstrated particularly clearly by HRP tracing (Gilbert and Kelly, 1975; Lund et al., 1975). These different types of principal neuron are an important feature of the neocortex.

INTRINSIC NEURONS   Distinct from the pyramidal cell is a second main type, the stellate cell. In primary sensory areas, such as the visual, there is a heavy concentration of these in layer IV. By virtue of the relatively small size of their cell bodies (10–20 μm diameter) compared with the pyramidal cells, they are often called *granule cells*. We note, as we have noted before, that this term does not imply any similarity of structure or function with the granule cells of the olfactory bulb, cerebellum, or dentate fascia. Their numbers and density give a characteristic grainy appearance to Nissl-stained histological sections of sensory cortex and have become, thereby, the basis for distinguishing between sensory cortex (granular) and nonsensory, or motor, cortex (agranular).

The stellate cells are multipolar neurons, sending out several dendritic trunks at apparently random orientations. The trunks are several microns thick, and they ramify to a modest degree through a field of 200–400 μm. The dendrites are described as having a modest investiture of spines or none at all (Colonnier, 1968), and on this basis one distinguishes between spiny stellate and nonspiny stellate cells (see next section). The axon is thin (several microns in diameter) and thinly myelinated. It generally is oriented vertically and ascends in the cortex to ramify largely in layer III, among the pyramidal and stellate cells there (see Fig. 15.2). The vertical extent of the axon may reach 500 μm or so.

Another type of stellate cell has, in contrast, an exclusively vertical orientation, as illustrated (BP) in Fig. 15.2. As can be seen, it is, in fact, a *bipolar cell*, with superficial and deep dendritic fields. Its axon bifurcates into ascending and descending branches, which presumably carry the output of this cell to the most superficial and deep layers of the cortex.

There are a number of other types of neuron. Among them may be mentioned a stellate cell with an axon which sends basket terminations to neighboring pyramidal cells, resembling thus the basket cells of the cerebellum. This cell is scarce or absent in visual cortex (Lund, 1973) but numerous in motor cortex (see next Chapter). Other stellate cells have axons which branch and terminate locally, or course deeper or horizontally. Another type of cell is the fusiform or polymorphic cell situated in the deeper layers of the cortex.

In defining the intrinsic neurons of the cortex, one can with certainty include the several types of stellate cells whose axons remain within the same region of cortex, even though their axons may extend through several laminae. However, by this criterion we must also include the pyramidal cells mentioned above which have axons that do not leave the cortex. We must also recognize reports (Szentágothai, 1973) of stellate cells with axons that enter the white matter; these would be classified as principal neurons. For practical purposes, most workers consider pyramidal cells as principal neurons and stellate cells as intrinsic neurons, and this is a satisfactory *modus operandi* if one remembers that there are exceptions.

COLUMNAR ORGANIZATION An aspect of cytoarchitecture that has particular relevance for synaptic organization is the strong element of vertical orientation that cuts across the cortical layers. This is a reflection of the vertically oriented axons and apical dendrites (Fig. 15.2). The possibility that the cortex might be organized into vertical columns of interconnected cells that extend across all the layers was recognized by Lorente de Nó (1938), and it has taken on special significance in view of the variety of anatomical and physiological evidence for functional columns within the cortex; we will review the evidence later. The diameters of the anatomical columns and the physiological columns both fall within the range of 50–500 μm.

A particularly clear manifestation of columnar organization is to be found in the islands of neuropil within layer IV of the somatosensory area of the rat cortex. Lorente de Nó (1922) first described them and showed that they are regions containing the terminal arborizations of afferent fibers and the dendrites of cortical neurons. He termed them "glomeruli" in analogy with the glomeruli of the olfactory bulb. They were rediscovered and studied in detail by Woolsey and van der Loos (1969), who have shown that they measure from 100–500 μm in diameter and 100 μm in depth (i.e., the thickness of layer IV). The cell types have been described recently by Woolsey, Dierker, and Wann (1975) and White (1978); see Fig. 15.2.

Woolsey and van der Loos have characterized such a region as a "multicellular cytoarchitectonic unit", and have introduced the term "barrel" for it, citing an illustration of a barrel from the earlier work of Breughel (fl. 1560). One need intend no disrespect for such august authority if one notes that insofar as this is a circumscribed region providing for synaptic interconnections of afferent fibers and cortical neurons, it probably falls within the definition of macroglomerulus as discussed in Chapter 11. There is, indeed, a close similarity to the glomerulus of the olfactory bulb, in terms of position at the site of afferent input, dimensions, and in its being a region of synaptic processes surrounded by cell bodies. There is evidence that a cortical glomerulus receives the input from one vibrissa in the rat's snout and that within this input are several different sensory submodalities (see below).

OVERVIEW In summary, what seems to stand out most clearly in viewing the neuronal elements of the cortex is their great variety. There are many different inputs and outputs; a wide variety, and overlap, within the types of principal and intrinsic neuron populations; and a multiplicity of intrinsic interrelations. The variety in all these categories is much greater than that present in other regions; conversely, there is little of a stereotyped nature in the elements, as is obvious in many of the other regions. An important point is the fact that cells with the same dendritic pattern may have different axonal projections; conversely, cells with different dendritic patterns may be in the principal or intrinsic neuron categories. From these considerations one can surmise that the cortex is concerned with a minimum of fixed or obligatory functions; it provides rather a neuronal substrate that is generalized, possibly flexible, and presumably open and utilizable in a maximum number of different ways.

CELL POPULATIONS

It is a commonplace to cite an estimate of 10 billion neurons contained within the human neocortex as evidence for the fantastic overgrowth and therewith unprecedented capabilities for complex functions of this region. Those who cite this figure invariably fail to recall that the number of granule cells in the cerebellum is probably several times this number (i.e., 20–40 billion); hence, it is not the large population of neurons *per se* that accounts for the special capabilities of the neocortex. The complexity of synaptic interactions within the cortex, and with other brain regions, are as already indicated the crucial factors.

There is of course a dramatic increase in the population of cortical neurons as one ascends the vertebrate series. Among mammals with a well-developed cortex, there are also large differences according to size. Associated with this are differences in the density of neuron packing, with, in general, a relatively high density in a small brain and a low density in a large brain. The density also varies in different parts of the brain, being higher in the visual area than the motor area, for example, by a factor of about 3:1. In man the over-all packing density of cortical cells is about $10/0.001$ mm^3; the density in the visual area is about $70/0.001$ mm^3. By comparison the packing density of granule cells in the cerebellum is about $2400/0.001$ mm^3. These and other quantitative data have been summarized and discussed by Sholl (1957) (see also Mountcastle, 1978).

There is, thus far, little evidence regarding the populations of principal and intrinsic neurons. One can only estimate that the principal neurons are quite numerous, and the I:P ratio must, therefore, be relatively modest, particularly if the stellate cells of lamina IV are regarded as local relay cells (see below).

SYNAPTIC CONNECTIONS

The first systematic study of cortical synapses with the electron microscope was by Gray in 1959. He reported that cortical synapses fall into two main groups, one (type I) characterized by extensive areas of contact and asymmetrical membrane thickenings, the other (type II) by smaller areas of contact and symmetrical thickenings. As noted in Chapter 2 and in subsequent chapters, these two types have been found in many parts of the brain and have served as a useful tool in identifying the synaptic connections made by a given class of neuron.

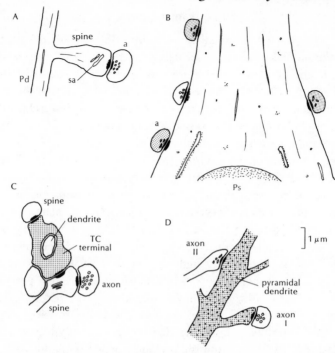

FIG. 15.3. Synaptic connections in visual cortex. (A) Axodendritic synapses from
axon terminals (a) onto dendritic (d) spine; sa, spine apparatus. (B) Axosomatic
connections onto pyramidal cell. (After Gray, 1959; Colonnier, 1968.) (C) Synaptic connections of a degenerating thalamocortical (TC) terminal. (After Peters
and Feldman, 1977.) (D) Synaptic connections onto basal dendrite of a Golgi-impregnated pyramidal cell. (After Fairén et al., 1977.)

Type I synapses are mostly axodendritic, from axon terminals onto
dendritic spines; examples are shown in Fig. 15.3 (A). Gray was the first
to describe in detail the *dendritic spine:* an elongated knob-like protuberance, 2–4 μm in length and 1–2 μm in diameter. These spines typically
contain a collection of flattened sacs, or cisternae, as shown in Fig. 15.3
(A). This was given the name of *spine apparatus,* rather for want of a better
term. For a time, it was assumed that a spine needed a spine apparatus to
qualify as a spine, but it has developed that few of the spines in other parts
of the brain contain organelles of this nature; since they are spinelike in
appearance, they may also be referred to as spines, as we have done.

Type II synapses were reported by Gray to be preferentially located
on the cell bodies of cortical neurons [Fig. 15.3 (B)]. A subsequent study

has provided evidence that the type I and II synapses within the cortex are extremes of a continuum that grades from the one into the other (Colonnier, 1968). In this study, the synapses onto pyramidal neurons were distinguished from those onto stellate neurons. Most synapses onto pyramidal neurons were onto the dendritic spines and fell into the category of type I. Synapses onto the pyramidal cell bodies were relatively few, and of type II. Stellate cells, on the other hand, were reported to have an intermingling of type I and II synapses onto both the dendrites and the cell bodies.

In the difficult task of sorting out the cortical neuropil, it has been commonly assumed that a presynaptic terminal is an axon and a postsynaptic terminal is a dendrite. That this assumption, based on classical notions, is now obsolete has been amply documented in the course of this book. The first evidence that this might also be true of the neocortex was provided by van der Loos (1959), who reported that, in Golgi-stained material, dendrites from two neighboring neurons could be seen crossing each other and making a synaptic contact. He called these dendrodendritic synapses, the first use of that term in the central nervous system. In the absence of electron-microscopic confirmation, however, this report has remained unsubstantiated (see next chapter).

Several other types of synaptic connection have been noted in recent work. One of these is a connection from an axon collateral back onto the dendrite of the pyramidal neuron from which the axon arose; this has been termed an *autapse* by van der Loos and Glaser (1971). The evidence was obtained from Golgi-stained material and awaits confirmation with the electron microscope. There is the implication that the collateral might also connect to other pyramidal neurons. We have seen an example of this type of connection between output neurons among sympathetic ganglion cells, Purkinje cells in the cerebellum (where the connections are inhibitory), and between pyramidal neurons in the olfactory cortex and hippocampus (where the connections are excitatory).

Among the other types of connection may be mentioned axoaxonic synapses onto initial segments arising from pyramidal cell bodies (Peters, Proskauer, and Kaiserman-Abramof, 1968); the basal ganglia, olfactory cortex and hippocampus have similar connections, as already mentioned.

INPUT CONNECTIONS The essential step for understanding cortical organization is to identify the connections of the input fibers, because this permits one to specify the synaptic triad at the first integrative level in the cortex. A consensus on this point has been elusive (see Garey and Powell, 1971; LeVay, 1973; Szentágothai, 1978) largely because in single electronmicrographs the dendritic processes and spines of pyramidal and nonpyramidal cells are too much alike. Several studies have shown that degenerating afferent terminals, induced by lesions in the lateral geniculate nucleus, make contacts on dendritic shafts and spines in layers III, IV, and V; an example is shown in Fig. 15.3 (C). Note that a terminal may contact more than one spine, and a spine may receive inputs from more than one terminal, each of a different type.

An important technical advance has been to identify Golgi-impregnated cells, and then de-impregnate them in order to visualize synaptic morphology. A de-impregnation procedure was introduced by Blackstad (1975) and further refined and applied to the cortex by Fairén, Peters, and Saldanha (1977). A schematic representation of one of their results is shown in Fig. 15.3 (D). Here one sees a basal dendrite of a pyramidal cell receiving a type I synapse on a spine and a type II synapse on its shaft.

Obviously, the next step is to bring together the two methods, degeneration and de-impregnation, so that both pre- and postsynaptic processes can be identified. Thus far this has been reported only for the barrel field of somatosensory cortex (see below). Pending this evidence in visual cortex, we may summarize the situation at present with the following observations:

> . . . every component of layer IV capable of forming asymmetric junctions is a potential recipient for the thalamic input. (Peters and Feldman, 1977)

> Results to date do not preclude the possibility that any cell type in any layer may receive specific thalamic inputs. (Christensen and Ebner, 1978).

These statements are not as negative as they may seem, and we shall discuss their implications in the next section.

BARREL FIELD   Studies of synaptic connections in somatosensory cortex, and particularly the barrel field of the rodent, have provided interesting parallels with those on visual cortex. In somatosensory cortex there has been evidence that the majority of synapses made by afferent fibers are on to dendritic spines in layer IV (Jones and Powell, 1970a; Jones, 1975).

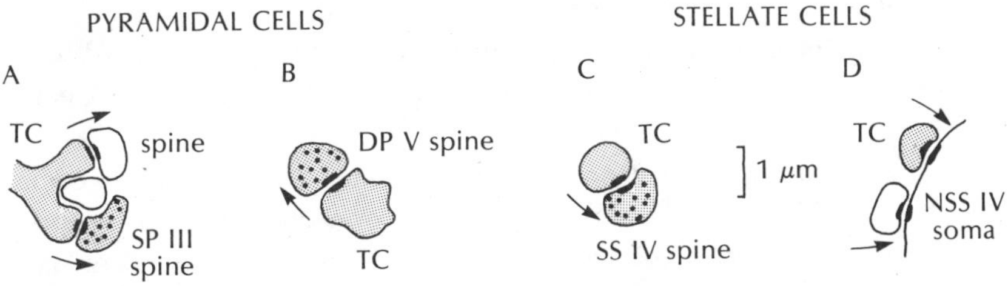

PYRAMIDAL CELLS   STELLATE CELLS

A   B   C   D

FIG. 15.4. Synaptic connections in somatosensory barrel field of the mouse. Shaded profiles, degenerating thalamocortical (TC) terminals; speckled profiles, Golgi-impregnated cortical cells. SP III, superficial pyramidal cell of layer III; DP V, deep pyramidal cell of layer V; SS IV spiny stellate cell of layer IV; NSS IV, nonspiny stellate cell of layer IV. (After White, 1978.)

Very recently, two new methods have been introduced. Christensen and Ebner (1978) have recorded intracellularly from somatosensory cells activated monosynaptically from the thalamus, filled them with Procion Brown or HRP, and identified them under the electron microscope. Most of the labeled cells were superficial pyramidal cells in layer III; surprisingly, no cells in layer IV were found, but this could be due to several factors, including the small size of the cells.

The second method has been to combine degeneration with de-impregnation, as mentioned above. White (1978) has recently achieved this in the barrel field of the rat. Representative results are illustrated in Fig. 15.4, summarizing the main types of afferent connections thus far identified: onto the dendritic spines of either superficial (A) or deep (B) pyramidal cells, and onto the two main types of stellate cell, spiny (C) and nonspiny (D). Note the multiple synapses of a single terminal onto two different spines (A). All of these synapses made by the afferent fibers are type I. This study unequivocally confirms that thalamocortical fibers make synapses onto all of the main cell types that have processes in layer IV: superficial and deep pyramidal cells; and spiny, nonspiny, and fusiform stellate cells. The discretion expressed in the statements of the preceding section was well founded.

BASIC CIRCUIT

In most of the regions of the brain considered in this book, it has been possible to assimilate the information about neuronal elements and their main synaptic connections into a summary diagram. In those regions, the connections and pathways illustrated by the diagram are either obvious consequences of the internal architecture, or they represent a broad consensus drawn from mutually supportive evidence from many workers.

In the neocortex the evidence is obviously much more difficult to come by. Nonetheless, from the work on synaptic connections and on synaptic actions (next section) a coherent picture is in fact beginning to emerge. The two key questions are the identity of the synaptic triad and the organization of intrinsic circuits. Before summarizing the present state of our knowledge it will be useful to sketch in a little historical background.

Our concepts about both of the questions mentioned above have their origins in a historic chapter on the cerebral cortex written in 1938 by Lorente de Nó for Fulton's textbook on the *Physiology of the Nervous System*. Drawing largely on his own Golgi material and that of Cajal, under whom he had trained, Lorente de Nó provided not only a masterful survey of what was then known about the neuronal elements of the cortex, but also a hypothesis of their organization. The diagram summarizing his views is shown in Fig. 15.5.

First, with regard to afferent connections, he noted as follows:

> . . . there are cells which establish synaptic connections with the afferent fibre and cells which make no such connections; the latter cells, of course, will be stimulated only as a result of cortical activity. Save for layers I and II, all cortical layers contain cells having synaptic contacts with the specific afferents, so that it would be improper to call any one layer "receptor". On the other hand, every layer except I has axons reaching the white matter, and therefore no layer may be called "effector".

Second, with regard to intrinsic connections, Lorente de Nó proposed that the cortex is composed of vertical cylinders of cells, each cylinder having a specific afferent fiber as an axis:

> All the elements of the cortex are represented in it, and therefore it may be called an *elementary unit*, in which, theoretically, the whole process of transmission of impulses from the afferent fiber to the efferent axon may be accomplished.

The cells within the vertical cylinder were assumed to be connected together in loops and chains, as shown in the simplified schema at the

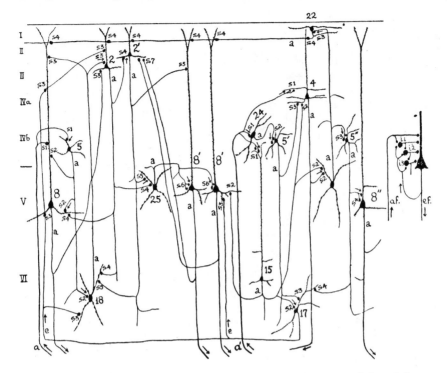

FIG. 15.5. Diagram of some intracortical neuronal pathways, as inferred from Golgi-impregnated neurons. Summary diagram of internuncial chains shown on the right. (From Lorente de Nó, 1938.)

right of Fig. 15.5. Cajal (1911) had suggested that axon collaterals provide for rapid dispersion of activity to larger populations of cells, a process he termed *avalanche conduction*. In the cortex this was incorporated into the evidence for closed loops, suggesting the presence of multiple chains of neurons and reverberating circuits.

It will be recognized that in these passages Lorente de Nó dealt with the nature of the synaptic triad and laid the basis for the modern concept of the cortical column. Many details have been added since then to our picture of neuronal elements, but the hypotheses still stand, all the more remarkable in view of the fact that they were made in the complete absence of any data regarding synaptic connections or synaptic actions.

The basic circuit diagram of Fig. 15.6 may be regarded as a simplified and updated version of its predecessor. The specific afferents are shown

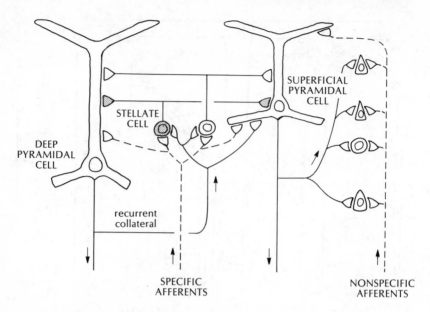

FIG. 15.6. Basic circuit diagram of visual cortex.

providing input to all the main targets thus far identified: deep and superficial pyramidal cells, spiny and nonspiny stellate cells. The pyramidal cells are considered to be principal neurons, and the stellate cells to be intrinsic neurons. Thus, the diagram indicates the *possibility* that the synaptic triad at the first integrative stage in the cortex can involve input to both principal and intrinsic elements. This is a common pattern, as we have seen in many other parts of the nervous system. However, it must be stressed that the triad will vary in different sensory areas and different species, in terms of subtypes of neurons and relative proportions, or in some cases, absence, of connections to each subtype.

Similar considerations apply to the intrinsic circuits. These are constituted of two elements: the axon collaterals of the principal neurons and the axons of the intrinsic neurons. Note in Fig. 15.6 that the intrinsic circuits make connections onto the same elements receiving afferent input, i.e., deep and superficial pyramidal cells, and the intrinsic stellate cells themselves. The pyramidal cell axon collaterals may be excitatory, providing for spread of excitation to both intrinsic cells and to other pyramidal cells. The latter action was envisaged by Lorente de Nó, and would be similar to the re-excitation previously discussed in the olfactory cortex and hippocampus. The spiny and nonspiny subpopulations of intrinsic cells are assumed to be associated with the excitatory and inhibitory actions, respectively. The interplay of feedback and feedforward inhibition with the re-excitatory circuits appears to be the basis for much of the complex processing that takes place in the cortex. All of these circuits have their primary orientation vertically within a column, and are horizontally grouped with respect to the input fibers supplying the column.

These remarks apply only to the main elements thus far identified as contributing to the synaptic organization of the visual cortex. Additional details, such as further subgroups of cells, or types of interactions such as axoaxonic or dendrodendritic, can be added as the evidence becomes sufficient. The same applies to other sensory areas; in the barrel field, for example, the groupings of cells in relation to a column are evident in layer IV. Many of these same principles apply also to the motor cortex, which is considered in the next chapter.

SYNAPTIC ACTIONS

SENSORY PROCESSING   In the analysis of sensory regions of the cortex, the main impetus for concepts of functional organization has come from the use of carefully controlled sensory stimuli, as in the retina. In the temporal domain, this has meant the use of pulses and steps of sensory stimuli; in the spatial domain, it has meant the use of stimulus spots, points, annuli, edges, arcs, etc.

The application of these methods, in conjunction with micro-electrode recordings, to the analysis of intracortical organization was introduced by Mountcastle (1957) in his studies of somatosensory cortex, which receives its input from peripheral receptors via the dorsal column nuclei (Fig. 1.1) and the ventrobasal complex in the thalamus. We will follow Mountcastle's (1974) account in summarizing the essence of the results.

When microelectrode penetrations are made vertically through the cortex, all the neurons encountered are of the same modality and approximately the same peripheral receptive field. The cells of the middle layers (III and IV) are activated earliest by an afferent input; those of the deeper layers have longer latencies. Thus, within a few milliseconds, allowing for only a few synaptic relays within the cortex, the activity arriving through the input is "translated", to use Mountcastle's phrase, or processed, vertically through the superficial pyramidal neurons to yield an output through the deep pyramidal neurons. From these findings, it is deduced that the *elementary functional unit* of the cortex is a vertically oriented column of cells that composes an input-output linkage. The physiological evidence thus supports and extends the inferences of Lorente de Nó drawn from the vertical orientation of the neuronal elements (see above). The columns for different modalities are sharply demarcated from each other, and there is evidence (e.g., Mountcastle and Powell, 1959) that activation of one column produces a surround inhibition of neurons in neighboring columns.

The organization into columns has been found in visual and auditory as well as somatosensory cortex. The results in visual cortex have been especially clear, because of the nature of the stimulus control and the fact that the sequence of intracortical processing has been followed through several integrative stages. As is well known, this work is associated with the names of Hubel and Wiesel (1962, 1968). We may recall that in the simple retina of the primate the ganglion cells are organized in terms of centers and surrounds of light, and that this holds also for the relay through the lateral geniculate nucleus. However, in the visual cortex, to which the lateral geniculate nucleus projects, the simplest responses are to bars or edges of light, shone on a part of the retina with a particular orientation; the cells giving these responses are termed *simple cells* [Fig. 15.7 (A)]. More complex responses are to a bar or an edge moving over the retina in a particular direction; the cells giving these responses are termed *complex cells*. Typical responses of a cell of this type are illustrated in Fig. 15.7 (C). The most complex responses (of *hypercomplex cells*) are to bars or edges, moving with particular orientations, with various critical dimensions, and with antagonistic regions within their peripheral fields.

From these responses, Hubel and Wiesel deduced that there is a hierarchical sequence of processing within the cortex, through the simple cells to the highest orders of hypercomplex cells and beyond. The sequence takes place within a column of cells, as shown by the fact that all the cells encountered in a vertical microelectrode penetration have the same orientation to their receptive fields. The sequence from the retina to simple cells is illustrated in Fig. 15.7 (B), in terms of convergent excitatory synaptic connections. The convergence of simple cells onto complex cells is illustrated in Fig. 15.7 (D).

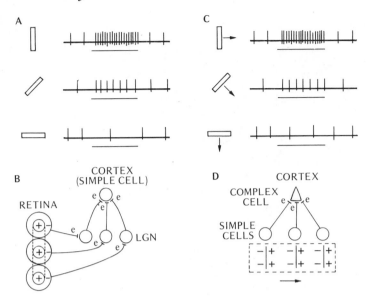

FIG. 15.7. Responses of neurons in the visual cortex to stimulation of the retina with light. (A) Extracellular recordings of unit spikes. Responses of a "simple cell" are shown to stimulation of the retina with a bar of light with three orientations; time of stimulation shown by the horizontal bar beneath the recording trace. (B) Schematic diagram to illustrate possible synaptic connections mediating the responses in (A). (C) Responses of a "complex cell" to a bar of light, moving as indicated by arrows. (D) Schematic diagram to illustrate possible synaptic connections mediating the responses in (C). (After Hubel and Wiesel, 1962; Michael, 1969.)

The cortical cells tuned to a given orientation are arranged in a narrow column (approximately 50 μm in diameter), and the columns for the sequence of all orientations are grouped into larger ocular dominance columns (approximately 500 μm in diameter) according to the dominant imput from one or the other eye. A schematic diagram of the arrangement is shown in Fig. 15.8. Two ocular dominance columns, containing input from either eye and all orientation columns, define a *hypercolumn*. In fact, the columns are not discrete cylinders, as originally envisaged, but rather continuous sheets, or slabs, as indicated in the diagram. This has been shown by several anatomical methods, and particularly clearly by the 2-deoxyglucose method (see Fig. 4.10 in Chapter 4).

The sequence within a column is presumably mediated by vertical circuits providing for excitation, re-excitation, and excitatory-inhibitory

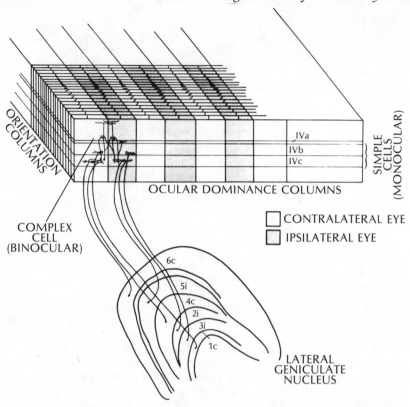

FIG. 15.8. Idealized relation between ocular dominance columns (slabs) and orientation columns (slabs) in visual cortex. Also shown are connections from lateral geniculate nucleus to simple cells, and from latter to complex cells, as proposed in hierarchical scheme. The columns are less rigidly orthogonal to each other than shown here. (From Hubel and Wiesel, 1972.)

interactions, as discussed previously in relation to the diagram of Fig. 15.6. The important point about these sequences is that, rather than providing for a wider dissemination of the input, they provide for a narrowing of responsiveness, a finer tuning, to more specific aspects of the input. Thus, whereas a retinal ganglion cell responds to diffuse light falling on the entire retina, a hypercomplex cell in the cortex responds not at all to this nonspecific stimulus, but discharges vigorously when a specific pattern falls in a specific part of the retina with a specific orientation and rate of movement. This is thought to be the basis for the abstraction and generalization of patterns in the visual world (see below).

SYNAPTIC PATHWAYS In parallel with anatomical studies of afferent connections, electrophysiological studies have been concerned with identifying the cortical cells receiving monosynaptic inputs. The early intracellular studies showed that an afferent volley characteristically elicits a brief EPSP followed by a long-lasting IPSP (Watanabe, Konishi, and Creutzfeldt, 1966; Toyoma et al., 1974). This is similar to the response sequence elicited by an input volley in many of the other systems we have reviewed earlier. The EPSP latency is short, and consistent with a monosynaptic pathway. The intracellular recordings also show slow depolarizations underlying the sustained impulse discharge in response to light stimuli (Creutzfeldt and Ito, 1968).

It will be recalled that the afferent input from the lateral geniculate nucleus is not homogeneous, but is divided into thick fibers (from large Y cells) and thin fibers (from smaller X cells). Hoffman and Stone (1971) asked whether the two types project onto separate cortical neurons or converge onto the same cells. They recorded from visual cortical cells, classified their responses to light stimuli, and then examined their responses to thalamic volleys. Surprisingly, the shortest latency responses were found in complex rather than simple cells. The data were consistent with monosynaptic activation of complex cells by rapidly conducting Y axons, and monosynaptic activation of simple cells by slowly conducting X axons. This suggested that simple and complex cell properties might arise by parallel rather than serial processing. An attractive aspect of this idea is that it matches the sustained responses of X cells with the preference of simple cells for stationary or slowly moving bars of light, and the transient responses of Y cells with the preference of complex cells for moving stimuli. A number of subsequent studies have given support to this idea, though with varying degrees of overlap between the pathways (Movshon, 1975; Singer, Tretter, and Cynader, 1975; Leventhal and Hirsch, 1978).

The cells giving rise to different types of responses were first identified with intracellular stains by Kelly and van Essen (1974). They reported that in the cat most (but not all) simple cells were stellate cells in layer IV; most (but not all) complex cells were pyramidal cells, located in both superficial and deep layers; and most (but not all) hypercomplex cells were pyramidal cells located in superficial layers. This was taken as generally supportive of the hierarchical processing model, with the simple cells receiving the afferent input in layer IV. However, the exceptions are of interest, indicating as they do that there is not a complete correlation of functional properties with morphological type.

The response types bear an interesting relation to the laminar sources of output fibers discussed earlier in this chapter. Gilbert (1977) noted that the superficial layers contain complex and hypercomplex cells, and project to other cortical regions; layer V contains complex cells and projects to the colliculus; layer VI contains simple and complex cells, and projects to the lateral geniculate nucleus.

Despite the differences to be expected when different investigators classify response types, there seems to be a consensus that simple cells have low spontaneous activity, small receptive fields, and respond best to stationary or slowly moving bars of light (see Movshon, 1975; Gilbert, 1977; Rose, 1977; Leventhal and Hirsch, 1978). Complex cells, in comparison, have high spontaneous activity, large receptive fields, and respond best to rapidly moving bars of light. Both types are orientation specific. Also, both may have the hypercomplex property of being sensitive to the length of a bar of light. The effect of increasing bar length may be either inhibitory or facilitatory, and there seems to be a grading of these effects in different cells (Rose, 1977).

SERIAL AND PARALLEL PROCESSING   From the foregoing account it can be seen that the identification of synaptic pathways in the cortex has turned out to be every bit as difficult as expected. At this point it is probably fair to say that the issue of serial *versus* parallel pathways for the processing of visual information is resolving itself into one of serial *and* parallel pathways, and the task at hand is to determine the relative contributions of straight-through routes and lateral interactions, just as in other regions of the nervous system. In a similar vein, it seems that the distinctions between response types are softening. This is reflected, for example, in the observation of Rose (1977) that area 17 neurons appear to fall into two broad families, simple and complex, and that "within each family we may look for gradual changes in properties between cells driven mainly by LGN inputs . . . and those driven by other cortical cells." The terms *simple* and *complex* need to be qualified to reflect these graded properties. It may be helpful in this respect for the student to think of response types in terms of a dominant physiological property, for example, simple cells are static edge detectors, whereas complex cells are dynamic edge detectors. One can then recognize that there may be gradations in the amount of static or dynamic properties, and one can incorporate other properties such as orientation tuning or length specificity, as the case may be.

In conclusion, the columnar organization of the cortex is clearly established, and a correlation of synaptic organization with mechanisms of visual processing is still in progress. The present state of affairs is perhaps best summarized by Kuffler and Nicholls (1976):

> The hierarchical scheme is not complete, correct in detail, or the only explanation. Rather it represents a useful hypothesis and an effective way of describing how the complex behavior of cells in the visual system could be brought about. While there remain huge gaps in knowledge, the description of receptive fields has supplied for the first time an inkling of how such concepts as verticality, length, thickness, depth, and squareness can be derived from properties and connections of individual cortical neurons.

NEUROTRANSMITTERS

Work on transmitters in the cortex has become voluminous, and the early studies have been comprehensively reviewed by Phillis (1970) and Krnjevic (1974). It appears that there is at least some evidence for most of the major types of transmitter substances.

The problem limiting the interpretation of all these studies is the still primitive state of our knowledge of the specific synaptic connections between identified cells, as discussed earlier in the chapter. An extensive account of the relation between neurochemical studies and synaptic circuits is therefore not yet warranted. Thus, the cortex is heterogeneous with respect to transmitters, and also putative neuromodulators. This heterogeneity applies at the cellular level and also at higher levels, as for example the association of dopamine with the frontal lobe (see Emson and Lindvall, 1979, for a recent review).

The role of GABA has perhaps the best support. Iontophoresis of GABA produces a hyperpolarizing IPSP in cortical cells associated with an increase in membrane conductance to Cl^-. A variety of biochemical studies has demonstrated the presence, uptake, and release of GABA in the cortex (see Krnjevic, 1974). Bicuculline opposes the action of GABA (Curtis and Felix, 1971). Recently, Sillito (1977) has shown that iontophoresis of bicuculline onto single cells in visual cortex has marked and specific effects on simple, complex, and hypercomplex response properties. Directional selectivity, in particular, apears to be mediated by

GABA, and there may be more than one type of inhibitory circuit involved in the generation of these response types. The identification of the cells in these circuits has just begun; Ribak (1978) reports that GAD is localized by immunocytochemical methods to nonpyramidal cells in the visual cortex, particularly to the aspiny and sparsely spiny stellate cells; he suggests that these local circuit neurons mediate the GABAergic inhibition in the cortex.

In addition to specific cortical circuits, the diffuse noradrenergic projection from the locus coeruleus in the brainstem has also been characterized (Pickel, Segal, and Bloom, 1974; Descarries, Watkins, and Lapierre, 1977; Levitt and Moore, 1978). The most common action of noradrenalin on cortical cells is inhibitory; there is evidence that the mechanism is similar to that in the spinal cord and cerebellum, though other properties may also be involved (see Krnjevic, 1974; Bloom, 1975).

DENDRITIC PROPERTIES

In our studies of other regions of the brain, we have seen that an understanding of synaptic organization requires knowledge of dendritic properties. This is also true for the neocortex, where the apical dendrites of the pyramidal neurons constitute the main vertical elements of the cortical framework and the major substrate for synaptic connections. Studies of the electrotonic properties of pyramidal cell dendrites will be considered in the next chapter; here, we confine our attention to the properties of dendritic spines.

DENDRITIC SPINES The presence of numerous spines is commonly regarded as one of the outstanding characteristics of pyramidal cell dendrites. The pyramidal cells are by no means unique in this respect; we have seen that spines are also outstanding characteristics of olfactory granule cells, cerebellar Purkinje cells, thalamic relay neurons, and the pyramidal cells of olfactory cortex and the hippocampus. The reader may wish to review the discussions of the properties of spines in these other neurons, for possible relevance to the case of cortical spines (see also Diamond, Gray, and Yasargil, 1970).

As in other parts of the brain, cortical spines do not appear to be a means simply for increasing the synaptic surface of a dendrite; where spines are present, synapses are located preferentially on them and not on the intervening parts of the branch.

Cortical spines have traditionally been regarded as entirely post-synaptic in position and, hence, receptive in function. The recent evidence for dendrodendritic synapses, in motor cortex, however (see next chapter), suggests that some cortical spines may occupy presynaptic positions and have output functions as well.

If the spine provides a specific synaptic site, what is the specific function of that site? Much attention has recently been focused on the possibility that the cortical spine provides a synaptic site that is especially subject to modification by use, i.e., by sensory input or learning experience. In kittens, deprivation of visual input in the early weeks of life has been reported to lead to deformation (Globus and Scheibel, 1967) and loss (Valverde, 1967) of spines. The spines affected are on the proximal shafts of apical dendrites in layer IV, i.e., in the layer in which the specific afferent terminals from the lateral geniculate nuclei are located. It has been suggested that these changes reflect the sensitivity of the immature developing cortex to changes in the external environment. Physiological experiments have shown that the functional properties of cortical neurons depend on early sensory input (e.g., Blakemore and Cooper, 1970). Thorough reviews of the interrelations between genetic and behavioral factors in controlling specific synaptic connections in the cortex are found in Lund (1978) and Rakić (1978).

If spines provide a modifiable synaptic substrate, it must be asked what kind of modification is involved? This brings us back to an assessment of electrotonic properties. Rall and Rinzel (1971) have pointed out the spine stem is the critical site for the control of the electrotonic relation between the spine head (the synaptic site) and the branch to which it is connected. The common variations in the morphology of this relation are illustrated in Fig. 15.9. In (A) is a very stubby spine, which is characteristic of spines found on the large-diameter apical shaft and dendritic branches. An intermediate case is shown in (B). In (C), a spine with a long thin stem arises from a distal dendritic branch of small caliber.

The amount of spread of a synaptic potential from the spine to the branch is governed by the ratio of the spine stem resistance to the input resistance of the branch. Rall and Rinzel (1971, 1973) have shown that, when this ratio is very large or very small, changes in spine stem caliber (and, hence, resistance) have little effect on synaptic potential spread to the branch. In the middle range, however, when the ratio is near one, a

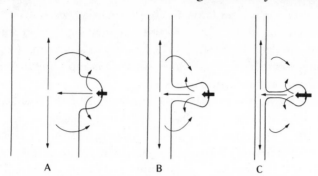

FIG. 15.9. Diagrams to illustrate electrotonic current flows generated by synaptic inputs to different types of dendritic spines. (A) Stubby spine arising from a thick branch; (B) Moderately elongated spine from a medium-size branch; (C) Elongated spine with a thin stem arising from a thin branch. (After Rall and Rinzel, 1971.)

small change in the spine stem resistance has a relatively large effect on this spread. "Over this favorable range . . . fine adjustments of the stem resistances of many spines, as well as changes in dendritic caliber . . . could provide an organism with a way to adjust the relative weights of the many synaptic inputs received by such neurons; this could contribute to plasticity and learning of a nervous system" (Rall and Rinzel, 1971). Preliminary study suggests that the cortical spines and branches have dimensions that are, in fact, what would be expected to provide optimal conditions for these mechanisms to occur (see Fig. 15.9; see also Rall and Rinzel, 1973).

It is of interest to note that the above considerations of electrotonic current spread are also relevant to the diffusion of substances through a solute; the equations for the two cases are exactly equivalent. Adjustments in spine stem caliber may, therefore, be postulated to have a critical effect on the movement of substances into and out of the spine, through which long-term control over metabolic processes in the spine could be exerted. From this point of view, the spine appears not only as a relatively independent input-output locus, but also as a device for creating a microenvironment, whose internal composition is subject to maximal effect by a synaptic action and to control through adjustments of the stem that links it to the metabolic sources of its parent neuron. The possibility that this may apply to the modifications of synaptic responses in hippocampal dendritic spines has been noted (see Chapter 14).

16

NEOCORTEX:
MOTOR AREA

The investigation of cortical motor function has one of the longest traditions in the history of brain physiology, originating in the studies of movements elicited by electrical stimulation of the cortex by Fritsch and Hitzig in 1870. The movements take the form of simple muscle twitches, from which it has been inferred that, during normal functioning, populations of cortical cells in the area stimulated control the spinal motoneurons that, in turn, innervate those muscles. There is an orderly representation of the body musculature, with the leg, arm, and face areas lying in a progression as one proceeds laterally along the motor strip (see Fig. 15.1). The areas vary in size depending on the density of innervation and precision of movements; the reader is referred to standard textbooks for further details of these aspects of the motor map.

These physiological experiments define the motor cortex in terms of the "electrically excitable" area which, when electrically stimulated, gives rise to discrete muscle movements. This is limited to an extent of cortex essentially identical with area 4 as defined anatomically by its cytoarchitecture (cf. Fig. 15.1). However, one may also define the motor area anatomically as that which gives rise to the fibers which connect directly, or even indirectly, as the case may be, to motoneurons. If this is done for the direct corticospinal fibers, one finds that only about one-third of them arise from area 4. Another third arise from the premotor area 6 (which causes more generalized movements when stimulated), and a final third arises from the classical somatosensory areas 3, 1, and 2 (see Fig. 15.1) which yield no movements at all.

Further ambiguities are encountered in defining the cortical motor out-

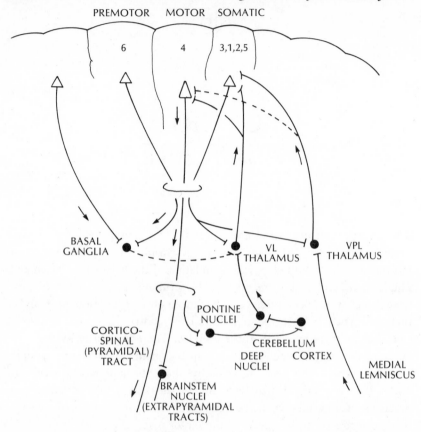

PREMOTOR   MOTOR   SOMATIC

6   4   3,1,2,5

BASAL
GANGLIA   VL   VPL
                                 THALAMUS   THALAMUS

PONTINE
NUCLEI

CORTICO-
SPINAL
(PYRAMIDAL)   CEREBELLUM
TRACT   DEEP   CORTEX
                        NUCLEI   MEDIAL
                                        LEMNISCUS

BRAINSTEM
NUCLEI
(EXTRAPYRAMIDAL
TRACTS)

FIG. 16.1. Schematic diagram of main connections established by motor outflow of the cortex, and the main sources of afferents to the motor cortex. (Modified from Phillips and Porter, 1977.)

put. One traditionally begins with the fibers that connect directly to the spinal cord. These are termed corticospinal fibers; because they gather in the medulla to form the medullary pyramids, they are also referred to as pyramidal tract fibers. However, these fibers give off many collaterals as they descend through the brainstem, to both sensory and motor nuclei, so one cannot consider them as exclusively corticospinal, nor exclusively motor, either, for that matter. Furthermore, the brainstem contains nuclear groups (i.e., red nucleus, vestibular nucleus, reticular nucleus) that have their own peripheral connections or descending tracts to the spinal cord. These various possibilities are all indicated in Fig. 16.1. The diagram also includes some of the relations of corticomotor pathways to the basal ganglia, cerebellum, and spinal cord, and to the afferent inflow from the thalamus. The reader may wish to refer to the relevant diagrams in earlier chapters to correlate the various pathways.

These considerations show that the definition of what is motor cortex is a relative matter, depending on how direct or indirect the connection between a given part of cortex and a given set of motoneurons. Thus, in making the traditional distinction between pyramidal and extrapyramidal motor systems, one must realize that the two systems overlap extensively. These problems of defining the motor cortex may seem frustrating, even sterile. But they give expression to one of the essential features of motor control by the brain: the control is not mediated by discrete central pathways. Rather, the functions of motor systems are to collect all relevant information and funnel it into the motoneurons, at the same time keeping the rest of the brain informed of what they have instructed the motoneurons to do. Thus, the Sherringtonian concept of the final common path, together with the requirement of corollary discharge (see Evarts, 1971), makes more understandable the necessity for the multiplicity of overlapping pathways that characterize motor systems.

Within this context, area 4 is that part of the cortex which, as a matter of degree, is most closely and predominately concerned with control of motorneurons. The reader may consult the recent monograph of Phillips and Porter (1977) on *Corticospinal Neurones* for a definitive account of this area as it relates to the control of movement.

NEURONAL ELEMENTS

Motor cortex shares with sensory cortex a laminar structure, but with certain differences. As indicated by Fig. 16.2, it is much thicker, as much as 3–4 mm in man, compared with 1.5–2.0 mm in the case of visual cortex. Most significantly, layer IV, with its large population of granule cells, is absent; as noted previously, this is the basis for use of the term *agranular* in referring to motor areas. We shall have occasion to assess the implications of this difference for motor as distinct from sensory functions. Apart from this, the differences between motor and sensory cortex are largely matters of degree. There has, in fact, been relatively little study of the neuronal elements in comparison with work in sensory areas; general accounts are available in Lorente de Nó (1938) and Szentágothai (1978).

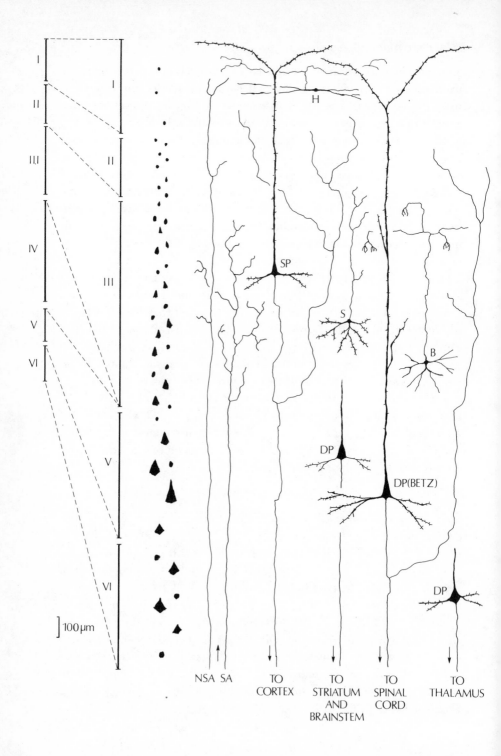

I

II

III

IV

V

VI

]100 μm

I

II

III

V

VI

H

SP

S

B

DP

DP(BETZ)

DP

NSA SA

TO
CORTEX

TO
STRIATUM
AND
BRAINSTEM

TO
SPINAL
CORD

TO
THALAMUS

INPUT There are no discrete sensory or other types of tracts or pathways to motor cortex. The main source of specific thalamic input is from the ventrolateral (VL) nucleus, which in turn receives input from the cerebellum and the basal ganglia (see relevant chapters). The VL axons are the counterparts to the specific afferents (SA) of sensory cortical areas. They ascend in the cortex and branch and terminate mostly in layer III (Asanuma et al., 1974; Jones, 1975). The ramifications are not as dense as those of the thalamic terminals in layer IV of sensory cortex.

The other main type of input fiber has traditionally been termed nonspecific afferent (NSA in Fig. 16.2). These fibers may give off branches in several layers, like their counterparts in sensory cortex. They arise either from reticular thalamic nuclei, or, at the cortical level, from other parts of the same or opposite hemisphere.

PRINCIPAL NEURON The main type of principal neuron, and the one considered quintessentially motor, is the large pyramidal cell of layer V. These cells have apical dendrites with lengths, in human cortex, of up to 4 mm (4000 μm); an example is shown in Fig. 16.2. These are probably the longest dendrites in the central nervous system. The cell bodies that give rise to these apical dendrites are also among the largest in the central nervous system. The largest measure up to 60 $\times$ 120 μm, and are called the *giant pyramidal cells of Betz.* For many years it was thought that these giant cells perform some ultimate "command" role in controlling movement, but it now appears that their size is correlated with the lengths of their axons to the spinal cord (see Walshe, 1947). This is a useful illustration of the fact that in the vertebrate brain the size of a neuron has no direct relation to complexity of function. If anything, the relation appears to be inverse; this, at least, was Cajal's belief in ascribing delicacy of function to the small (intrinsic) cells of the cortex.

Recent studies using HRP injections have verified that the corticospinal tract to the lumbar spinal cord arises from the large pyramidal cells of layer V (Coulter, Ewing, and Carter, 1976). Interestingly, the fibers to the neostriatum arise from a population of small pyramidal cells in

FIG. 16.2. Neuronal elements of the motor cortex.
Inputs: specific afferents (SA); nonspecific afferents (NSA).
Principal neurons: superficial pyramidal neurons (SP); deep pyramidal (DP).
Intrinsic neurons: stellate cells (S); basket cells (B); horizontal cells (H).
Histological layers shown at left, together with scale for layers in visual cortex for comparison (far left). Note absence of layer IV in motor cortex.

that same layer (Jones, Coulter, Burton and Porter, 1977). There is evidence that corticothalamic fibers rise from layer VI, association fibers from layers II and III, and commissural fibers from the deeper part of layer III (Jones and Wise, 1977). These axons all arise from pyramidal cells, and the laminar sites correspond closely to those for sensory cortex (see previous chapter). This subdivision of principal neurons, even within a layer, on the basis of size and projection site, recalls similar differences between retinal ganglion cells, alpha and gamma motoneurons, and mitral and tufted cells of the olfactory bulb. It is obviously a key aspect of synaptic organization in the cortex.

INTRINSIC NEURONS   The absence of the granule cells of layer IV has already been mentioned. The remaining varieties of intrinsic neuron include scattered stellate cells, with multipolar or bipolar dendritic trees and vertically ascending or descending axons, much like their counterparts in sensory cortex. Another type of stellate cell is the basket cell (B in Fig. 16.2). The cell body is 15–20 μm in diameter. Its dendritic arborization is multipolar, extending over a radius of several hundred microns, and flattened in one plane of section running in the long axis of the motor strip (Marin-Padilla, 1974). The axon distributes mainly in a horizontal direction. The field of distribution is of the order of 300–600 μm. The axonal branches of this type of cell end in a characteristic tuft that forms a nest around a pyramidal cell body. In this respect this type of cell resembles the basket ends of the cerebellum. This type is scarce or absent in visual cortex (Lund, 1973), but prominent in motor cortex (Marin-Padilla, 1974).

Another type of intrinsic neuron is the horizontal cell (H) of layer I. In his first description of the cortex (Cajal, 1890), Cajal reported that some of these neurons have more than one axon, each arising from a separate part of the cell body or dendritic tree; he termed them "cells with double axon." He later retracted this (Cajal, 1911), stating that, on re-investigation, one of the axons could always be identified as a dendrite. The rule that a neuron, if it has an axon, has only one, is so ingrained in our thinking that it might be of interest to restudy these cells from that point of view.

COLUMNAR ORGANIZATION   The retrograde HRP labeling method has not only provided the means to identify cells giving rise to projections from different laminae, but has also given evidence of their spatial distribution. Following injections into the spinal cord, the labeled pyramidal cells in layer V are often seen grouped in "clusters" (Coulter et al.,

1976). When serial sections are compared, it becomes evident that the clusters are arranged in strips that run along the mediolateral extent of area 4 and the adjoining areas that are sources of the corticospinal tract (Jones et al., 1977). The strips are 0.5–1.0 mm in width.

This arrangement is of course strongly reminiscent of the columns and slabs demonstrated both anatomically and functionally in sensory cortex. We shall discuss the functional evidence and the significance of the columnar organization of motor cortex later in this chapter. Strips are also found in motor cortex after injections in the medulla (labelling corticobulbar cells), red nucleus (corticorubral cells), and pons (corticopontine cells). At the cortical level, strips are found within area 4 after injections into neighboring parts of area 4 itself (short association cells) and after injections into the opposite hemisphere (commissural cells). They have not been clearly seen, however, after injections in the neostriatum.

SYNAPTIC CONNECTIONS

There have been relatively few studies of motor cortex aimed at systematic investigation of synaptic connections at the electron-microscope level. The information that is available suggests that many aspects appear to be similar to those we have discussed in the previous chapter. For example, it is believed that pyramidal cells receive type I synapses on dendritic spines, type II synapses on their cell bodies, and both types on dendritic shafts (cf. Strick and Sterling, 1974; Asanuma et al., 1974). Stellate cells also receive type I synapses on dendritic spines, and both types on cell bodies and dendritic shafts. Synapses are also present on the axonal initial segments and axonal spines of pyramidal cells.

The specific thalamic input from the ventrolateral thalamic nucleus has been studied by Strick and Sterling (1974). Most of the VL terminals are in layer III, with small proportions in layers I and VI. Most of the synapses are onto spines; some of the spines appear to arise from stellate cells in layer III, others from apical dendrites of pyramidal cells in layer V [see Fig. 16.3 (A)]. Thus, this input from the thalamus appears to connect to both intrinsic and principal neurons in the cortex.

With regard to intracortical connections, there is little direct information. However, there is an intriguing report of synapses between dendrites by Sloper (1971) as illustrated in Fig. 16.3 (B). It can be seen that one of the dendrites (InD) has a synapse onto the spine of dendrite PD; InD is also presynaptic to another profile and postsynaptic to several

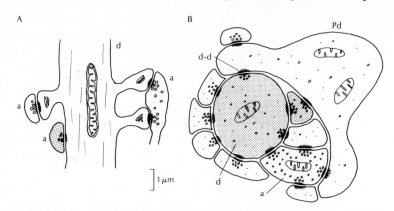

FIG. 16.3. Synaptic connections of the motor cortex. (A) Synapses made by axon (a) terminals onto shaft and spines of cortical dendrite (d) (After Strick and Sterling, 1974). (B) Complex arrangements of synapses in primate motor cortex, including dendrodendritic connections (d-d). (After Sloper, 1971.)

terminals. In addition, numerous axodendritic synapses can be seen. This report awaits more extensive confirmation. Meanwhile, its significance rests in the demonstration of dendrodendritic synapses at the cortical level in the primate brain, and in a motor region.

BASIC CIRCUIT

All of the problems discussed in relation to constructing a basic circuit for sensory cortex apply with even more force in motor cortex. Nonetheless, certain points seem reasonably well established, and certain similarities and differences between motor and sensory cortex can be identified, using the diagram of Fig. 16.4 as a summary.

The most outstanding difference between the two areas is the lack of lamina IV, with its large and densely packed population of granule cells, in motor cortex. Despite this, the triad of synaptic elements is still present and recognizable, though shifted in laminar position and modified in cellular detail. The specific thalamic inputs terminate instead in layer III, apparently on both stellate cells and the dendrites of pyramidal cells in that layer. These connections are shown in Fig. 16.4. By comparing with Fig. 15.5, it can be seen that the elements making up the synaptic triad are essentially the same as in sensory cortex, except for the shift in lamina and a marked reduction in the numbers of stellate cells.

With regard to intrinsic circuits, very little anatomical evidence has

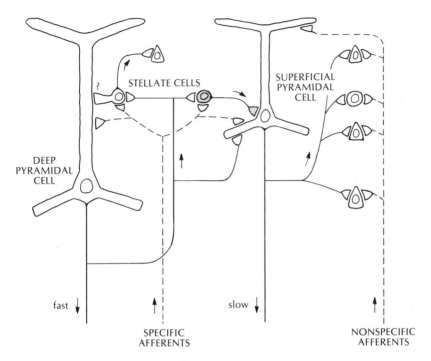

FIG. 16.4. Basic circuit diagram of motor cortex.

actually been added to the speculations of Lorente de Nó (1938). Thus, it seems likely that pyramidal cell axon collaterals connect to other pyramidal cells and to stellate cells, and that the stellate cells act as excitatory or inhibitory interneurons within the cortex. We shall note the physiological evidence for these actions in the next section. The basket cell is an especially prominent type of intrinsic neuron, and it is tempting to speculate that it provides for a specific type of inhibition by means of the terminals around the cell bodies and initial axon segments of the pyramidal cells. There is an obvious analogy in this respect to the basket cells of the cerebellum.

On the efferent side there is a laminar fractionation of outputs that is very similar to that in sensory cortex. The anatomical evidence has been summarized with respect to the neuronal elements in Fig. 16.2. Physiological studies have emphasized that the corticospinal output is mediated by both fast-conducting and slow-conducting pyramidal tract fibers, arising from large and medium-size pyramidal cells, respectively. These are indicated in the basic circuit diagram of Fig. 16.4.

The basic circuit gives only a hint of the multiple overlapping circuits related to the control of outputs from the pyramidal cells at each level of the cortex. The minimum number of such circuits necessary to perform the essential input-output functions at all levels defines the elementary functional unit of the motor cortex. This unit has much in common with the column of sensory cortex. We shall discuss the nature of this organization in the next section.

SYNAPTIC ACTIONS

The considerable overlap of neuronal elements and synaptic connections within the neocortex has presented electrophysiologists with problems not unlike those that arise in studies of the spinal cord, but without the redeeming feature of separate input and output pathways that have been the basis for the analysis of spinal organization (Chapter 7). There is one discrete pathway, however, and that is the *corticospinal tract*. It is represented in Fig. 1.1. It is particularly prominent in primates; as described in Chapter 7, it provides an important input to the motoneurons that control the hand (Phillips, 1971).

The importance of this tract to electrophysiologists is that it enables them to identify a pyramidal cell from which they are recording by the ability to backfire it (antidromically) through its axon; this is the same method used to identify motoneurons and the principal neurons in other parts of the brain. The first intracellular recordings in the brain, following the pioneering work on the spinal cord, were obtained from cortical neurons identified in this way (Phillips, 1956).

AFFERENT EXCITATORY AND INHIBITORY ACTIONS In analyzing synaptic actions on cortical cells, we first ask questions that concern the site of afferent input and the nature of that input; these questions parallel those asked by anatomists, as previously discussed. This has been investigated by recording the responses of cortical neurons to volleys in the sensory input pathways (Towe, Patton, and Kennedy, 1964; Amassian and Weiner, 1966; Watanabe, Konishi and Creutzfeldt, 1966; Oscarsson, Rosén, and Sulg, 1966; Swett and Bourassa, 1967). Representative results are illustrated in Fig. 16.5 (A), for the case of a volley set up by a single shock to a peripheral nerve that carries fibers mainly from muscle spindles in the arm (deep radial nerve). The response consists of a short-latency EPSP, which leads to the discharge of one or two impulses. Note the brief duration of the EPSP (similar to that in a motoneuron).

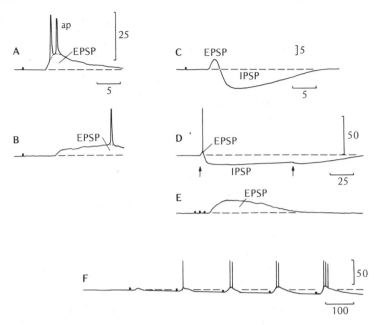

FIG. 16.5. Synaptic actions in the neocortex. (A) Intracellular response of a cortical neuron to a volley in the deep radial nerve. (B) Response to a volley in the superficial radial nerve. (C) Response to a volley in the dorsal column of the spinal cord. [(A)-(C) after Oscarsson et al., 1966.] (D) Prolonged antidromic stimulation (between arrows) showing an EPSP-IPSP sequence. (After Phillips, 1959.) (E) EPSP response to antidromic volleys (Phillips). (F) Intracellular response to slowly repeated volleys from the nonspecific thalamic nuclei. (After Purpura et al., 1964.)

The short latency has been interpreted as indicating that the pathway from the nerve to the cortex has a minimum of synaptic relays; as can be seen by tracing the connections in Fig. 1.1, this means three relays, in the dorsal column nuclei, the thalamus, and, finally, the cortex. This means, in particular, that there is a monosynaptic input from the thalamocortical relay axon to the cortical neuron. By comparison, a volley in a peripheral nerve that contains mostly fibers from the skin (superficial radial nerve) gives rise to a response, in the same cortical neuron, which consists of a long-latency EPSP with a much slower time course [Fig. 16.5 (B)]. This demonstrates that there is at least one additional synaptic relay at the cortical level—a disynaptic or polysynaptic input, in the terminology used for the spinal cord.

The monosynaptic responses are located preferentially in the middle cortical layers where the afferent fibers terminate. What is the identity of the cortical neurons giving these responses? One study reports that they are pyramidal tract neurons (Swett and Bourassa, 1967); another reports that they are non-pyramidal tract neurons (Oscarsson et al., 1966). This point, therefore, remains in doubt.

Inhibitory actions are also present in the responses of cortical neurons to a peripheral volley; an example is shown in Fig. 16.5 (C). It can be seen that the response consists of an initial depolarization followed by a long-lasting hyperpolarization. There is an obvious similarity to the excitation-inhibition sequences that we have seen in the responses of principal neurons in many parts of the brain to a volley in an input pathway (see Purpura, 1967).

In summary, these and other studies have shown that a cortical neuron may receive both monosynaptic and polysynaptic inputs from the periphery and that there is a convergence of different modalities onto the same neuron. They have shown that there are different patterns of spatial convergence, some neurons having wide peripheral fields and others having very small fields. There are different excitatory-inhibitory sequences. Some cortical neurons give rapid (phasic) responses, others give slow, maintained (tonic) responses. These synaptic actions provide some of the basis for the complex operations the cortex performs in its input-output relations (see below).

RECURRENT EXCITATORY AND INHIBITORY ACTIONS   Synaptic actions in the cortex are also revealed by the antidromic volley in the pyramidal-tract axons that invades collaterals within the cortex. A typical result (Phillips, 1959; Stefanis and Jasper, 1964) is shown in Fig. 16.5 (D). The response consists of the antidromic spike invading the neuron, followed by a long-lasting hyperpolarization. The hyperpolarization can be shown to be due, not to the spike afterpotential, but to an IPSP. The latency of onset is sufficient for at least one synaptic relay, and it has been postulated that there is a circuit from axon collaterals through an inhibitory neuron back onto the pyramidal cells, in analogy with the Renshaw pathway in the spinal cord. This circuit is shown in the diagram of Fig. 16.4.

The inhibitory neurons in this postulated pathway may be basket cells, but the evidence is not conclusive; few cells can be found that discharge a train of impulses as do Renshaw cells in the spinal cord (Brooks, 1967). This might indicate that the inhibition is mediated by graded synaptic action, perhaps through a dendrodendritic pathway from the intrinsic neurons onto pyramidal neurons, in analogy with retinal neurons, olfactory granule cells, and, possibly, the short-axon cells of the thalamus. The finding of dendrodendritic synapses in the neocortex, as described earlier in this chapter, suggests that this possibility deserves serious consideration.

In addition to recurrent inhibition, depolarizing sequences are also evoked through stimulation of the pyramids, as shown in Fig. 16.5 (E). Although spread of excitation to include afferents from the brain stem to the cortex might be a factor in some experiments, these and other results have indicated the likelihood that pyramidal neurons excite other pyramidal neurons through a direct connection by their recurrent collaterals. This is, therefore, evidence for the re-excitation loops previously discussed. It appears that these actions are mainly directed from smaller, superficial neurons to larger, deep ones, providing a possible mechanism for rapid enhancement of phasic drives by the largest output neurons to the motoneurons (Oshima, 1969; Purpura, 1972).

MOTOR CONTROL   In the century following the discovery of the electrical excitability of the motor cortex, ever more refined methods of stimulation were used, until it was possible to activate single muscle groups and identify the threshold intracellular activity of single pyramidal cells (Phillips, 1956). After the columns were described in sensory cortex (Mountcastle, 1957; Hubel and Wiesel, 1962), Phillips and his colleagues tested for their presence in motor cortex. They determined the extent of cortical surface over which corticospinal pyramidal cells could be stimulated by a single shock to produce minimal monosynaptic EPSPs in a spinal motoneuron (Landgren, Phillips, and Porter, 1962). These and subsequent experiments (Jankowska, Padel, and Tanaka, 1975) have shown that the areas for a given motoneuron vary in size from 1 to 13 μm^2; the areas for both synergistic and antagonistic muscles overlap; and there may be multiple areas projecting to a single motoneuron. The results suggest that the corticospinal fibers originate in clusters, or colonies, of pyramidal cells that vary in extent from narrow cylinders (e.g., columns) of cells to more widely distributed populations.

The synaptic organization of pyramidal cells has been further studied by intracortical microstimulation, introduced by Asanuma and Sakata in 1967. They found that the low-threshold points for facilitation of a given monosynaptic reflex were confined within a vertically oriented segment of cortex that ranged in diameter down to 0.5 mm i.e., similar to the narrowest columns of Phillips and his co-workers. Subsequent studies have demonstated the intracortical mono- and polysynaptic connections onto pyramidal cells within these segments (Asanuma and Rosén, 1973) and the types of afferent inputs to the segments serving particular muscles (Asanuma and Rosén, 1972). An example from the latter study is shown in Fig. 16.6. The cortical cells in a given segment receive afferent inputs from proprioceptors in the corresponding joints and muscles, and also from tactile receptors in the overlying skin.

At present, the precise nature of the columnar organization of motor cortex remains uncertain (see reviews by Asanuma, 1975, and Phillips and Porter, 1977). However, there is agreement on the principles involved. Anatomically, the organization of neurons and circuits is primarily radial (Lorente de Nó, 1938); the input-output arrangements are in terms of modules of neuronal elements (Scheibel and Scheibel, 1970); and there is a mosaic of overlapping modules, columns, or other neuronal or cytoarchitectonic entities (Colonnier and Rossiginol, 1969). Physiologically, several types of functional units can be identified (Fig. 16.7). The minimal input-output module is the single pyramidal cell with its several sources of afferent inputs, associated intrinsic circuits, and particular output targets (cf. Brooks and Stoney, 1971). The next level of organization is a colony or column of pyramidal cells; this can be specified with regard to the sharing of a type of input, or a common output target. It is this level which is equivalent to the column of sensory cortex, and is the hardest to define in motor cortex. Perhaps this should be expected, in view of the differing character of sensory inputs and motor outflow. The modules which project to a particular motoneuron pool are collected into larger aggregates termed "projection areas" (see Phillips and Porter, 1977).

In the analysis of cortical organization relative to motor control, an important development has been the ability to record the activity of pyramidal tract neurons in an awake animal as it performs specific tasks. This approach, in the awake monkey, has been pioneered by Evarts (1969). These studies have begun to provide information about the timing of impulse output in relation to movement. In the experiment illus-

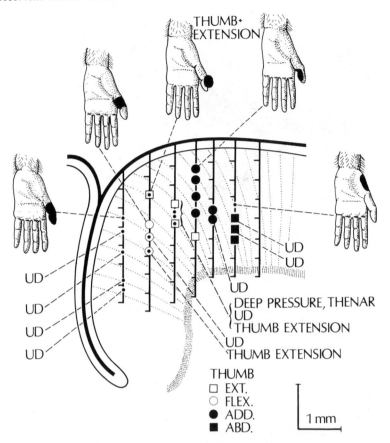

FIG. 16.6. Input-output relations in thumb area of monkey motor cortex. Electrode penetrations, indicated by vertical numbered lines, passed through several efferent zones projecting to different thumb muscles. Weak intracortical shocks (5 μA) evoked motor effects shown by large symbols. The shocks did not evoke effects at sites shown by short horizontal bars. Dots show sites of recorded cells, connected to descriptions of receptive fields and adequate stimuli. (Redrawn from Asanuma and Rosén, 1972.)

trated in Fig. 16.8, the monkey has been trained to depress a telegraph key and then release it promptly when a light appears. As can be seen, the motor cortex begins to fire impulses in advance (some 60 msec) of the onset of muscle contraction. We have previously seen that cell activity in both cerebellum and basal ganglia also precedes muscle movement. From these studies it appears that, in contrast to the traditional view of motor

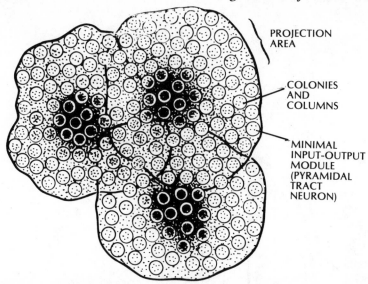

PROJECTION
AREA

COLONIES
AND
COLUMNS

MINIMAL
INPUT-OUTPUT
MODULE
(PYRAMIDAL
TRACT
NEURON)

FIG. 16.7. Postulated levels of organization in motor cortex. Each dot indicates a minimal input-output module centered on a single pyramidal tract neuron which forms its core and discharges its integrated output. Modules are grouped into colonies and columns (medium-size circles), perhaps with different thalamocortical inputs. The three largest circles indicate overlapping projection areas. (From Phillips and Porter, 1977.)

cortex being placed at the highest level of motor integration and subcortical regions at lower levels, all three regions participate in the early stages of motor programming (see Evarts, 1975).

One of the most relevant studies for the synaptic organization of the cortex has been addressed to the problem of whether the impulse output of a cortical neuron is correlated with the distance over which a particular movement is carried out, or the force necessary to move over that distance. The results have shown (Evarts, 1969) that there is a high correlation between impulse frequency and the force exerted to move a limb. These experiments indicate that there is not a simple mapping from impulse frequency to linear displacement.

These results carry the implication that feedback from the muscle spindles is a necessary input to the cortex in order to keep it informed of the progress of a movement under different conditions of loading. From this it has been inferred that there must be some type of servo-loop through the cortex, superimposed on the reflex arc or loop at the seg-

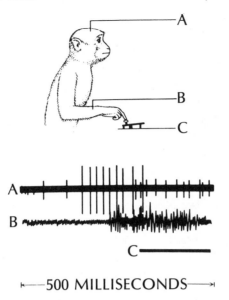

⊢―500 MILLISECONDS―→

FIG. 16.8. Relation of unit activity in motor cortex to movement. (A) Single unit activity in arm area of cortex. Trace starts when a light comes on; monkey trained to release key within 350 msec. (B) Electromyograph, showing onset of contraction of arm muscles. (C) Telegraph key open. Note that cortical unit activity leads muscle activity. Compare with unit recordings in similar experiments on cerebellum (Fig. 10.7) and basal ganglia (Fig. 12.7). (From Evarts, 1975.)

mental level in the spinal cord. The relation between the two loops can be seen in the diagram of Fig. 1.1. Phillips (1969) has shown that there is, in fact, a correlation in the synaptic organization at the two levels, in that the spinal motoneurons that innervate the hand are those that not only receive the most monosynaptic (Ia) input from the muscle spindles, but also the most monosynaptic input through the corticospinal fibers from the motor cortex. In his words:

> It is almost as if these particular spinal motoneurons had been transplanted into the cerebral cortex: as if the dendrites of the corticospinal pyramids were acting vicariously for the dendrites of the alpha motoneurons as antennae sensitive to intracortical synaptic activities.

RHYTHMIC POTENTIALS   The synaptic actions that have been described thus far have been produced by single electrical shocks or by discrete natural stimuli; the responses have taken the form of relatively simple synaptic potentials and impulse discharges that have their counterparts in the spinal cord and in other brain regions. But all cortical responses are not of this stereotyped nature. For example, stimulation of a nonspecific thalamic nucleus produces the responses shown in Fig. 16.5 (F). The response consists of an EPSP that has a long latency, a long duration, and a low amplitude; in the first response of Fig. 16.5 (F), the depolarization is below threshold for impulse initiation. This has been characterized as a *conditional* type of response, in contrast to the powerful *unconditional* response to specific thalamic nuclei (Purpura, Schofer, and Musgrave, 1964). We have noted in Chapter 14 that the responses of hippocampal pyramidal cells can also be characterized by their conditional and unconditional nature.

During *repetitive stimulation* the response in Fig. 16.5 (F) changes, building up from a subthreshold depolarization to one that triggers three impulses; the EPSPs are superimposed on a gradually increasing hyperpolarization. The buildup in the responses bears some resemblance to that elicited by repetitive stimulation of the hippocampus and dentate fascia, although it is less dramatic. As in the latter cases, some of the buildup may be due to an increased potency of the synapses. In the cortex, however, much of this effect is believed to be due to spread of activity within the circuits of the thalamus itself (see Purpura, 1972). This reflects the fact that the cortex and the thalamus are closely related, and it is a reminder that cortical function must be viewed within the context of corticothalamic organization.

As is well known, the *resting activity* of the cortex, recorded by electrodes on the scalp, takes the form of potential waves occurring at 8–12/sec, the so-called *alpha rhythm*. The rhythm is somewhat faster than that of the theta waves of the hippocampus. We have discussed in Chapter 11 the postulated mechanism whereby the cortex is driven by input from the thalamus; the activity of the thalamus is rhythmically generated by a combination of membrane excitability changes and an inhibitory phasing of impulse discharge through recurrent feedback circuits. Similar mechanisms within the cortex itself may also contribute to the rhythmicity of the cortex. The potentials recorded from the scalp are due to summed currents generated by the entire ensemble of active neurons. To discuss this complex subject would take us far afield. For an extensive discussion of the mechanisms of the alpha rhythm, the reader is referred to Andersen and Andersson (1968).

We have noted the tendency of the hippocampus to develop *seizure activity*, and the neocortex shares in this property. One form of activity consists of large depolarizing waves that generate a burst of impulses, the *paroxysmal depolarizing shift*. As in the case of the hippocampus, the factors that contribute to the development of such activity include altered excitability of the neuronal membrane and abnormal balance of activity in synaptic circuits. The re-excitatory axon collaterals in cortical regions would appear to be a potent source of excessive excitatory drive that is absent in most of the other regions we have considered. Another factor is the accumulation of ions in the intercellular spaces; we have mentioned some of the effects this may have on neuronal excitability in Chapter 4, and there is current interest in the possible role of extracellular K in producing long-lasting depolarizations of both neurons and glial cells in the cortex. These and other aspects of synaptic organization as they relate to the mechanisms of epileptic seizures are discussed by Ayala et al. (1973) and Jasper, Ward, and Pope (1969).

DENDRITIC PROPERTIES

In our studies of other regions of the brain, we have seen that an understanding of synaptic organization requires knowledge of dendritic properties. This is particularly true for the neocortex, in which the apical dendrites of the pyramidal neurons constitute the main vertical elements of the cortical framework and the major substrate for synaptic connections. Cortical dendrites may have presynaptic as well as postsynaptic positions, as noted previously; the evidence for the former is still tentative, however, and attention may be confined for present interests to the postsynaptic functions. We first consider the electrical parameters, then the transfer through the apical dendritic trunk; local dendritic properties, with special reference to dendritic spines, have been discussed in the previous chapter.

ELECTRICAL PARAMETERS   The whole neuron resistance (R_N) of a pyramidal neuron to the flow of current injected through an intracellular electrode in the cell body has been found to lie in the range of 4–15 MΩ, with an average of about 8 MΩ (Takahashi, 1965; Lux and Pollen, 1966). The charging time constant (τ_N) has been found to be approximately 8 msec. Both these values are similar to those for hippocampal neurons and several times greater than those for spinal motoneurons.

To obtain values for the specific membrane resistance (R_m) an estimate of dendritic dominance (ρ) is needed (cf. Chapter 5). Under assumptions of a range for this factor of from 3 to 10, a range of 1500–4000 Ω cm^2 was obtained (Lux and Pollen, 1966). This is somewhat higher than the estimates for the spinal motoneuron. The higher resistance and the longer time constant enhance the spread of synaptic current through the dendritic tree of the pyramidal neuron. Similar observations have been made with regard to the hippocampal pyramidal neurons.

In using these figures to estimate electrotonic lengths of apical dendrites, we must take into account the fact that the dendrites vary in both diameter and length, and therein emerges an interesting fact. We have discussed in Chapter 5 the point that the characteristic length (λ) varies with the square root of the diameter (d), with the consequence that electrotonic spread is relatively effective even in thin dendrites. Thus, even though the larger dendrite provides for more effective current flow over a given distance, the longer length produces more severe attenuation over the whole extent. If we compare the diameter and length of the apical dendrites of small pyramidal cells in the superficial layers of the center and large cells in the deep layers, it appears that not only does the scaling principle (introduced in Chapter 7) apply but that it may favor the smaller ones.

SYNAPTIC TRANSFER AND LAMINATION We are now in a position to discuss the sites of different synaptic inputs to the pyramidal dendritic tree. The locus of generation of a synaptic potential has been assessed, using the same criteria as used for neurons of other regions: the relative amplitude of the synaptic potential, its shape index (see Chapter 5), its sensitivity to currents and to ions injected into the cell body. Many of these studies have been discussed by Purpura (1972), and Fig. 16.9 provides a schematic summary, similar to that presented for the spinal motoneuron (Fig. 4.10).

The essential results are, first, that monosynaptic and disynaptic inputs from the specific thalamic relay nuclei (see typical responses in Fig. 16.5) are sited proximally on the dendritic tree and cell body. The excitatory inputs are, thus, in a position to trigger impulses in the axon hillock, the inhibitory inputs are in an optimal position to oppose impulse generation; and the overlap in the distribution of the two types of input provides for maximum dynamic interaction between them. Pre-

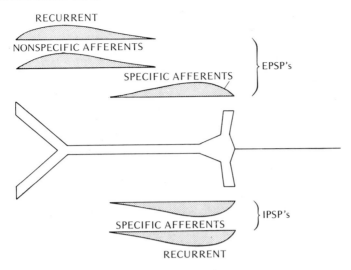

FIG. 16.9. Distribution of some synaptic inputs to the pyramidal cell of the neocortex.

sumably, there is a complex summing of many individual inputs that leads up to the initiation and control of impulse generation. In these aspects, synaptic integration in the cortical pyramidal cell is similar to the spinal motoneuron.

The cortical pyramidal cell also has inputs preferentially sited on the distal branches of the apical dendrite; among the inputs that have thus far been identified are excitatory synaptic actions by the nonspecific thalamic nuclei and the re-excitatory collaterals of the pyramidal cell axons (see Fig. 16.9). The question then arises: How can these distal inputs have any effect on the integrative activity of the pyramidal cell?

In order to answer this question, calculations of the electrotonic properties of the apical dendrites have been made by Jacobson and Pollen (1968) using the methods of Rall. Starting with the values of whole neuron resistance previously obtained (see above), a study was made of Golgi-stained neurons in the cat neocortex in order to determine first the contribution of the apical as distinct from the basal part of the dendritic tree. The first major branch point in the apical shaft was found to be about 250 μm from the cell body. It was calculated that a steady synaptic potential at that point would decrement to 25–40% in spreading to the cell body. A depolarization of 20 mV throughout the dendritic tree distal to that point would therefore produce 5–8 mV of depolarization at the cell body; such depolarizations are, in fact, produced by strong stimulation of the nonspecific afferents from the thalamus, which are believed to have the majority of their terminals on the superficial dendrites (see Fig. 16.9).

What then of inputs to the most distal branches? It was calculated that synaptic potentials in apical dendrites 750 μm from the cell body would decrement to only 2–3%; thus, a 20-mV depolarization at that distance would produce less than 1 mV of change in the cell body. Although this is only a fraction of the total depolarization needed to raise the membrane potential to the threshold for impulse discharge (5–10 mV), studies have shown that such small depolarizations can have marked effects on impulse frequency when the neuron is near the threshold level (Nacimiento, Lux, and Creutzfeldt, 1964). Thus, a modulating role of distal dendrites could consist of a refinement in the firing rates of neurons already brought close to firing level by the afferent systems that terminate closer to the cell body (Jacobson and Pollen, 1968).

We may also note that, with respect to transfer through the dendritic tree, the apical dendrite can be viewed as a series of loci for local integration, each locus having its maximum effect on its immediate neighbors. By this means, a given locus can bias or modulate the effect of an input to neighboring loci, an effect that takes on added significance if it is of a long-lasting or plastic nature such as might underlie learning or memory. A dendritic site can also have a local output function through a dendro-dendritic synapse; it remains to be determined how important such functions are in the cerebral cortex, in comparison with the olfactory bulb, retina, and thalamus.

In the course of this book we have seen that there are various mechanisms by which the transfer of signals through a dendritic tree can be enhanced. One is a *higher membrane resistance*, which provides for increased passive spread of electrical current; we have already noted the evidence for this in apical dendrites of both hippocampal cells and neocortical cells. A second mechanism is the presence of *active spots* or patches, which serve as booster zones. We have noted that these appear to be present in chromatolytic motoneurons, Purkinje cells, and hippocampal pyramidal cells. Fast prepotentials and dendritic spikes generated by such zones have not been reported in cortical neurons of adult animals; they have been observed, however, in recording from immature cortex of very young animals (see Purpura, 1972). A third mechanism is the *potentiation* of synaptic potentials to give larger amplitude responses upon repetitive stimulation; as we have seen, this is a characteristic that synapses in the neocortex share with synapses in the hippocampus; it is also found, to a certain extent, in the synapses that neocortical cells make onto spinal motoneurons. Potentiation, in effect, brings a given synapse nearer, functionally, to the axon hillock, and is therefore an important means by which an input could dominate a pyramidal neuron impulse output. Whether such a mechanism is operative during normal functioning awaits further investigation.

REFERENCES

Adam, G. and M. Delbruck. 1964. Reduction of dimensionality in biological diffusion processes.

Adrian, E.D. 1950. The electrical activity of the mammalian olfactory bulb. Electroencephalog. Clin. Neurophysiol. 2: 377–388.

Adrian, E.D. 1953. Sensory messages and sensation: The response of the olfactory organ to different smells. Acta physiol. scand. 29: 5–14.

Agduhr, E. 1934. Vergleich der Neuritenanzahl in dem Wurzeln der Spinalnerven bei Kröte, Maus, Hund und Mensch. Z. Anat. 102: 194–210.

Aghajanian, G.K. and B.S. Bunney. 1976. Dopamine "autoreceptors": pharmacological characterization by microiontophoretic single cell recording studies. Naunyn-Schmiedeberg's Arch. Pharmacol. 297: 1–7.

Aitken, J. and J. Bridger. 1961. Neuron size and neuron population density in the lumbosacral region of cat spinal cord. J. Anat. (London) 95: 38–53.

Aitken, L.M. and C.W. Dunlop. 1969. Inhibition in the medial geniculate body of the cat. Exp. Brain Res. 7: 68–83.

Akert, K., K. Pfenninger, C. Sandri, and H. Moore. 1972. Freeze etching and cytochemistry of vesicles and membrane complexes in synapses of the central nervous system. In Structure and Function of Synapses (G.D. Pappas and D.P. Purpura, eds.). New York: Raven, pp. 67–86.

Albers, R.W. and R.O. Brady. 1959. The distribution of glutamate decarboxylase in the nervous system of the rhesus monkey. J. Biol. Chem. 234: 926–928.

Allen, R.A. 1969. The retinal bipolar cells and their synapses in the inner plexiform layer. In The Retina: Morphology, Function and Clinical Characteristics (B.R. Straatsma, M.O. Hall, R.A. Allen and F. Crescitelli, eds.). UCLA Forum in Medical Sciences No. 8. pp. 101–143.

Allison, A.C. 1953. The morphology of the olfactory system in the vertebrates. Biol. Rev. 28: 195–244.

Allison, A.C. and R.T.T. Warwick. 1949. Quantitative observations on the olfactory system of the rabbit. Brain 72: 186–197.

Amassian, V.E. and H. Weiner. 1966. Monosynaptic and polysynaptic activation of pyramidal tract neurons by thalamic stimulation. In The Thalamus

(D.P. Purpura and M.D. Yahr, eds.). New York: Columbia University Press. pp. 255–282.

Anden, N.E., K. Fuxe, B. Hamberger, and T. Hökfelt. 1966. A quantitative study on nigro-neostriatal dopamine neuron system in the rat. Acta Physiol. Scand. 67: 306–312.

Andersen, P. and S.A. Andersson. 1968. Physiological Basis of the Alpha Rhythm. New York: Appleton-Century-Crofts.

Andersen, P., T.W. Blackstad, and T. Lømo. 1966. Location and identification of excitatory synapses on hippocampal pyramidal cells. Exp. Brain Res. 1: 236–248.

Andersen, P., B.H. Bland, and J.D. Dudar. 1973. Organization of the hippocampal output. Exp. Brain Res. 17: 152–168.

Andersen, P., T.V.P. Bliss, and K.K. Skrede. 1971. Lamellar organization of hippocampal excitatory pathways. Exp. Brain Res. 13: 222–238.

Andersen, P. and J.C. Eccles. 1962. Inhibitory phasing of neuronal discharge. Nature 196: 645–647.

Andersen, P., J.C. Eccles, and Y. Løyning. 1964. Location of postsynaptic synapses on hippocampal pyramids. J. Neurophysiol. 27: 592–607.

Andersen, P., J.C. Eccles, and T.A. Sears. 1964. The ventro-basal complex of the thalamus: types of cells, their responses and their functional organization. J. Physiol. 174: 370–399.

Andersen, P., B. Holmquist, and P.E. Voorhoeve. 1966. Excitatory synapses on hippocampal apical dendrites activated by entorhinal stimulation. Acta physiol. scand. 66: 461–472.

Andersen, P., S.H. Sundberg, O. Sveen, and H. Wigström. 1977. Specific long-lasting potentiation of synaptic transmission in hippocampal slices. Nature 266: 736–737.

Andres, K.H. 1965. Der Feinbau des Bulbus Olfactorius der Ratte unter besonderer Berücksichtigung der synaptischen Verbindungen. Z. Zellforsch. 65: 530–561.

Andres, K.H. 1970. Anatomy and ultrastructure of the olfactory bulb in fish, amphibia, reptiles, birds and mammals. *In* CIBA Foundation Symposium on Taste and Smell in Vertebrates (G.E.W. Wolstenholme and Julie Knight, eds.). pp 177–194.

Angaut, P. and C. Sotelo. 1973. The fine structure of the cerebellar central nuclei in the cat. II. Synaptic organization. Exp. Brain Res. 16: 431–454.

Armstrong, C.M., F. Bezanilla, and E. Rojas. 1974. Charge movement associated with the opening and closing of the activation gates of Na channels. J. Gen. Physiol. 63: 533–552.

Asanuma, H. 1975. Recent developments in the study of the columnar arrangement of neurons within the motor cortex. Physiol. Rev. 55: 143–156.

Asanuma, H., J. Fernandez, M.E. Schiebel, and A.B. Schiebel. 1974. Characteristics of projections from the nucleus ventralis lateralis to the motor cortex in cats: an anatomical and physiological study. Exp. Brain Res. 20: 315–330.

Asanuma, H. and I. Rosén. 1972. Topographical organization of cortical efferent zones projecting to distal forelimb muscles in the monkey. Exp. Brain Res. 14: 243–256.

Asanuma, H. and I. Rosén. 1973. Spread of mono- and polysynaptic connections within cat's motor cortex. Exp. Brain Res. 16: 507–520.

Asanuma, H. and H. Sakata. 1967. Functional organization of a cortical efferent system examined with focal depth stimulation. J. Neurophysiol. 30: 35–54.

Ayala, G.F., M. Dichter, R.J. Gummit, H. Matsumoto, and W.A. Spencer. 1973. Genesis of epileptic interictal spikes. New knowledge of cortical feedback systems suggests a neurophysiological explanation of brief paroxysms. Brain Res. 52: 1–17.

Baker, P.F., A.L. Hodgkin, and E.B. Ridgeway. 1971. Depolarization and calcium entry in squid giant axons. J. Physiol. 218: 709–755.

Baker, R. and R. Llinás. 1971. Electrotonic coupling between neurones in the rat mesencephalic nucleus. J. Physiol. 212: 45–63.

Barber, R. and K. Saito. 1976. Light microscopic visualization of GAD and GABA-T in immunocytochemical preparations of rodent CNS. *In* GABA in Nervous System Function. (E. Roberts, T.W. Chase, and D.B. Tower, eds.). New York: Raven. pp. 113–132.

Barber, R., J.E. Vaughn, K. Saito, B.J. McLaughlin, and E. Roberts. 1978. GABAergic terminals are presynaptic to primary afferent terminals in the substantia gelatinosa of the rat spinal cord: morphological substrates for presynaptic modification of cutaneous afferent activity. Brain Res. 141: 35–50.

Barlow, H.B. 1953. Summation and inhibition in the frog's retina. J. Physiol. 119: 69–88.

Barrett, E.F. and J.N. Barrett. 1976. Separation of two voltage-sensitive potassium currents, and demonstration of a tetrodotoxin-resistant calcium current in frog motoneurones. J. Physiol. 255: 737–774.

Barrett, J.N. and W.E. Crill. 1974. Specific membrane properties of cat motoneurones. J. Physiol. 239: 301–324.

Baylor, D.A., M.G.F. Fuortes, and P.M. O'Bryan. 1971. Receptive fields of cones in the retina of the turtle. J. Physiol. 214: 265–294.

Baylor, D.A. and J.G. Nicholls. 1969. After-effects of nerve impulses on signalling in the central nervous system of the leech. J. Physiol. 203: 571–589.

Belcher, G. and R.W. Ryall. 1977. Substance P and Renshaw cells: a new concept of inhibitory synaptic interactions. J. Physiol. 272: 105–119.

Bennett, M.V.L. 1973. Function of electrotonic junctions in embryonic and adult tissues. Fed. Proc. 32: 65–75.

Bennett, M.V.L. 1978. Electrical transmission: a functional analysis and comparison to chemical transmission. *In* Handbook of Physiology, Sect. 1: The Nervous System, vol. 1: Cellular Biology of Neurons (E.R. Kandel, ed.). Bethesda: Am. Physiol. Soc. pp. 367–416.

Biedenbach, M.A. and C.F. Stevens. 1969. Synaptic organization of cat olfactory cortex as revealed by intracellular recording. J. Neurophysiol. 32: 204–214.

Bird, S.J. and G.K. Aghajanian. 1975. Denervation supersensitivity in the cholinergic septo-hippocampal pathway: a microiontophoretic study. Brain Res. 100: 355–370.

Biscoe, T.J., A. Lall, and S.R. Sampson. 1970. Electron microscopic and electrophysiological studies on the carotid body following intracranial section of the glossopharyngeal nerve. J. Physiol. 208: 133–152.

Bishop, G.H. 1956. Natural history of the nerve impulse. Physiol. Rev. 36: 376–399.

Bjorklund, A. and O. Lindvall. 1975. Dopamine in dendrites of substantia nigra neurons: suggestions for a role in dendritic terminals. Brain Res. 83: 531–537.

Blackman, J.G., B.L. Ginsborg, and C. Ray. 1963. Synaptic transmission in the sympathetic ganglion of the frog. J. Physiol. 167: 355–373.

Blackstad, T.W. 1967. Cortical grey matter. A correlation of light and electron microscopic data. *In* The Neuron (H. Hydén, ed.). Amsterdam: Elsevier, pp. 49–118.

Blackstad, T.W. 1975. Electron microscopy of experimental axonal degeneration in photochemically modified Golgi preparations: a procedure for precise mapping of nervous connections. Brain Res. 95: 191–210.

Blackstad, T.W. and A. Kjaerheim. 1961. Special axo-dendritic synapses in the hippocampal cortex: Electron and light microscopic studies on the layer of mossy fibers. J. Comp. Neur. 117: 133–159.

Blakemore, C. and G.F. Cooper. 1970. Development of the brain depends on the visual environment. Nature 228: 477–478.

Bland, B.H., G.K. Kostopoulos, and J.W. Phillis. 1974. Acetylcholine sensitivity of hippocampal formation neurons. Can. J. Physiol. Pharm. 52: 966–971.

Bliss, T.V.P. and A.R. Gardner-Medwin. 1973. Long-lasting potentiation of synaptic transmission in the dentate area of the unanesthetized rabbit following stimulation of the perforant pathway. J. Physiol. 232: 357–374.

Bliss, T.V.P. and T. Lømo. 1973. Long-lasting potentiation of synaptic transmission in the dentate area of the anaesthetized rabbit following stimulation of the perforant path. J. Physiol. 232: 331–356.

Bloom, F.E. 1971. Norepinephrine as a CNS transmitter. *In* Brain Monoamines and Endocrine Function (R.J. Wurtman, ed.), NRP Bull. 9: 212–213.

Bloom, F.E. 1975. Central adrenergic synaptic mechanisms. *In* The Nervous System (D.B. Tower, ed.), vol. I: The Basic Neurosciences. New York: Raven. pp. 373–380.

Bloom, F.E., E. Costa, and G.C. Salmoiraghi. 1965. Anesthesia and the responsiveness of individual neurons of the caudate nucleus of the cat to acetylcholine, norepinephrine and dopamine administered by microelectrophoresis. J. Pharmacol. Exp. Therap. 150: 244–252.

Bloom, F.E., B.J. Hoffer, and G.R. Siggins. 1971. Studies on norepinephrine-containing afferents to Purkinje cells of rat cerebellum. I. Localization of the fibers and their synapses. Brain Res. 25: 501–521.

Bodian, D. 1966. Synaptic types on spinal motoneurons: An electron microscopic study. Bull. Johns Hopkins Hosp. 119: 16–45.

Bodian, D. 1972. Synaptic diversity and characterization by electron microscopy. In Structure and Function of Synapses (G.D. Pappas and D.P. Purpura, eds.). New York: Raven. pp. 45–66.

Boycott, B.B. and J.E. Dowling. 1969. Organization of the primate retina: Light microscopy. Phil. Trans. Roy. Soc. Lond. B. 255: 109–184.

Boycott, B.B. and H. Kolb. 1973. The horizontal cells of the rhesus monkey retina. J. Comp. Neur. 148: 115–140.

Boycott, B.B. and H. Wässle. 1974. The morphological types of ganglion cells of the domestic cat's retina. J. Physiol. 240: 397–419.

Brand, S., A.-L. Dahl, and E. Mugnaini. 1976. The length of parallel fibers in the cat cerebellar cortex. An experimental light and electron microscopic study. Exp. Brain Res. 26: 39–58.

Braitenberg, V. and R.P. Atwood. 1958. Morphological observations on the cerebellar cortex. J. Comp. Neur. 109: 1–27.

Brightman, M.W. and T.S. Reese. 1969. Junctions between intimately apposed cell membranes in the vertebrate brain. J. Cell Biol. 40: 648–677.

Broadwell, R.D. 1978. Neurotransmitter pathways in the olfactory system. In Society for Neuroscience Symposia III (J.A. Ferrendelli, ed.). Bethesda: Soc. for Neurosci. pp. 131–166.

Brodal, A. 1947. The hippocampus and the sense of smell. A review. Brain 70: 179–222.

Brodal, A. 1969. Neurological Anatomy. New York: Oxford University Press.

Brooks, V.B. and S.D. Stoney Jr. 1971. Motor mechanisms: the role of the pyramidal system in motor control. Ann. Rev. Physiol. 33: 337–392.

Brown, A.G. and R.E.W. Fyffe. 1978. The morphology of group Ia afferent fibre collaterals in the spinal cord of the cat. J. Physiol. 274: 111–127.

Brownstein, J.H.J., M Saavedia, J. Axelrod, G.H. Zeman, and D.O. Carpenter. 1974. Coexistence of several putative neurotransmitters in single identified neurons of Aplysia. Proc. Nat. Acad. Sci. 71: 4662–4665.

Bruesch, S.R. and L.B. Arey. 1942. The number of myelinated and unmyelinated fibers in the optic nerve of vertebrates. J. Comp. Neur. 77: 631–665.

Buchwald, N.A., D.D. Price, L. Vernon, and C.D. Hull. 1973. Caudate intracellular response to thalamic and cortical inputs. Exp. Neurol. 38: 311–323.

Bullock, T.H. 1976. Introduction to Nervous Systems. San Francisco: Freeman.

Bunney, B.S. and G.K. Aghajanian. 1976a. Dopaminergic influence in the basal ganglia: evidence for striatonigral feedback regulation. In The Basal Ganglia (M.D. Yahr, ed.). New York: Raven. pp. 249–266.

Bunney, B.S. and G.K. Aghajanian. 1976b. The precise localization of nigral afferents in the rat as determined by a retrograde tracing technique. Brain Res. 117: 423–435.

Burke, R.E. 1971. Control systems operating on spinal reflex mechanisms. In

Central Control of Movement (E.V. Evarts, ed.). Neurosci. Res. Prog. Bull. 9 (No. 1). pp. 60–85.

Burke, R.E. and G. ten Bruggencate. 1971. Electrotonic characteristics of alpha motoneurones of varying size. J. Physiol. 212: 1–20.

Burke, W. and A.J. Sefton. 1966. Discharge patterns of principal cells in lateral geniculate nucleus of rat. J. Physiol. 187: 201–212.

Burt, D.R., I. Creese and S.H. Snyder. 1976. Properties of [³H] Haloperidol and [³H] Dopamine binding associated with dopamine receptors in calf brain membranes. Molec. Pharmacol. 12: 800–812.

Busis, N.A., F.F. Weight, and P.A. Smith. 1978. Synaptic potentials in sympathetic ganglia: are they mediated by cyclic nucleotides? Science 200: 1079–1081.

Cajal, S. Ramón y. 1891. Sur la structure de l'écorce cerebrale de quelques mammifères. La Cellule 7: 124–176.

Cajal, S. Ramón y. 1911. Histologie du Système Nerveux de l'Homme et des Vertébrés. Paris: Maloine.

Cajal, S. Ramón y. 1955. Studies on the Cerebral Cortex. London: Lloyd-Luke.

Calleja, C. 1896. La region olfactoria del cerebro. Madrid: N. Moya

Calvin, W.H. and C. Graubard. 1979. Styles of neuronal computation. *In* The Neurosciences: Fourth Study Program (F.O. Schmitt and F.G. Worden, eds.) Cambridge: M.I.T. pp. 513–524.

Carlsson, A. W. Kehr, M. Lindquist, T. Magnusson, and C. Atack. 1972. Regulation of monoamine metabolism in the central nervous system. Pharmacol. Rev. 24: 371–384.

Carlsson, A. and M. Lindquist. 1963. Effect of chlorpromazine or haloperidol on formation of 3-methoxy tyramine and nor-metanephrine in mouse brain. Acta Pharmacol. 20: 140–144.

de Castro, F. 1932. Sympathetic ganglia, normal and pathological. *In* Cytology and Cellular Pathology of the Nervous System, vol. I (W. Penfield, ed.). New York: Hoeber. pp. 317–379.

Chan-Palay, V. 1971. The recurrent collaterals of Purkinje cell axons: a correlated study of the rat's cerebellar cortex with electron microscopy and the Golgi method. Z. Anat. Entwickl.-Gesch. 134: 200–234.

Chan-Palay, V. 1973. Neuronal circuitry in the nucleus lateralis of the cerebellum. Zeit. Anat. Entwickl.-Gesch. 142: 259–265.

Chan-Palay, V. and S.L. Palay, 1971a. Tendril and glomerular collaterals of climbing fibers in the granular layer of the rat's cerebellar cortex. Z. Anat. Entwickl.-Gesch. 133: 247–273.

Chan-Palay, V. and S.L. Palay. 1971b. The synapse *en marron* between Golgi II neurons and mossy fibers in the rat's cerebellar cortex. Z. Anat. Entwickl.-Gesch. 133: 274–287.

Charlton, B.T. and E.G. Gray. 1966. Comparative electron microscopy of synapses in the vertebrate spinal cord. J. Cell Sci. 1: 67–80.

Chiu, S.Y., J.M. Ritchie, R.B. Rogart, and D. Stagg. 1979. A quantitative description of membrane currents in mammalian myelinated nerve. J. Physiol. (in press).

Christensen, B.N. and F.F. Ebner. 1978. The synaptic architecture of neurons in opossum somatic sensory-motor cortex: a combined anatomical and physiological study. J. Neurocytol. 7: 39–60.

Chujo, T., Y. Yamada, and C. Yamamoto. 1975. Sensitivity of Purkinje cell dendrites to glutamic acid. Exp. Brain Res. 23: 293–300.

Clark, W.E. le Gros. 1951. The projection of the olfactory epithelium on the olfactory bulb in the rabbit. J. Neurol. Neurosurg. Psychiat. 14: 1–10.

Clark, W.E. le Gros. 1957. Inquiries into the anatomical basis of olfactory discrimination. Proc. Roy. Soc. B 146: 299–319.

Cleland, B.G. and W.R. Levick. 1974. Brisk and sluggish concentrically organized ganglion cells in the cat's retina. J. Physiol. 240: 421–456.

Cohen, A.I. 1972. Rods and cones. *In* Physiology of Photoreceptor Organs (M.G.F. Fuortes, ed.). Handbook of Sensory Physiology (Vol. VII/1B). Berlin: Springer. pp. 63–110.

Coggeshall, R.E., J.D. Coulter, and W.D. Willis. 1974. Unmyelinated axons in the ventral roots of the cat lumbosacral enlargement. J. Comp. Neurol. 153: 39–58.

Colonnier, M. 1968. Synaptic patterns on different cell types in the different laminae of the cat visual cortex. An electron microscopic study. Brain Res. 9: 268–287.

Colonnier, M. and S. Rossignol. 1969. Heterogeneity of the cerebral cortex. *In* Basic Mechanisms of the Epilepsies (H.H. Jasper, A.A. Ward, and A. Pope, eds.). Boston: Little Brown. pp. 29–40.

Colquhoun, D., R. Henderson, and J.M. Ritchie. 1972. The binding of labelled tetrodotoxin to non-myelinated nerve fibers. J. Physiol. 227: 95–126.

Connor, J.A. and C.F. Stevens. 1971. Prediction of repetitive firing behaviour from voltage clamp data on an isolated neurone soma. J. Physiol. 213: 31–53.

Conradi, S. 1909. On motoneuron synaptology in adult cats. Acta physiol. scand. Suppl. 332.1–115.

Cooper, J.R., F.E. Bloom, and R.H. Roth. 1978. The Biochemical Basis of Neuropharmacology. New York: Oxford University Press.

Coulter, J.D., L. Ewing, and C. Carter. 1976. Origin of primary sensorimotor cortical projections to lumbar spinal cord of cat and monkey. Brain Res. 103: 366–372.

Cowan, W.M. 1970. Centrifugal fibres to the avian retina. Brit. Med. Bull. 26: 112–118.

Creutzfeldt, O. and M. Ito. 1968. Functional synaptic organization of primary visual cortex neurones in the cat. Exp. Brain 6: 324–352.

Crill, W.E. 1970. Unitary multi-spiked responses in cat inferior olive nucleus. J. Neurophysiol. 33: 199–209.

Csillik, B., C. Toth, and S. Karesh. 1973. Acetylcholinesterase activity of dendritic elements and Renshaw bulbs. A light- and electron-microscopical histochemical study. J. Neurocytol. 2: 441–455.

Curtis, D.R. and D. Felix. 1971. The effect of bicuculline upon synaptic inhibition in the cerebral and cerebellar cortices of the cat. Brain Res. 34: 301–321.

Curtis, D.R., D. Felix, and H. McLennan. 1970. GABA and hippocampal inhibition. Br. J. Pharmacol. 40: 881–883.

Curtis, D.R., C.J.A. Game, D. Lodge, and R.M. McCulloch. 1976. A pharmacological study of Renshaw cell inhibition. J. Physiol. 258: 227–242.

Curtis, D.R. and R.W. Ryall. 1964. Nicotinic and muscarinic receptors of Renshaw cells. Nature 203: 652.

Daitz, H.M. and T.P.S. Powell. 1954. Studies of the connexions of the fornix system. J. Neurol. Neurosurg. Psychiat. 17: 75–82.

Dale, H.H. 1935. Pharmacology and nerve endings. Proc. Roy. Soc. Med. 28: 319–332.

Deiters. O. 1865. Untersuchungen uber Gehirn und Ruckenmark. Braunschweig: Vieweg.

DeLong, M.R. and P.L. Strick. 1974. Relation of basal ganglia, cerebellum, and motor cortex units to ramp and ballistic limb movements. Brain Res. 71: 327–335.

Descarries, L., K.C. Watkins, and Y. Lapierre. 1977. Noradrenergic axon terminals in the cerebral cortex of the rat. III. Topometric ultrastructural analysis. Brain Res. 133: 197–222.

Diamond, J., E.G. Gray, and G.M. Yasargil. 1970. The function of the dendritic spine: An hypothesis. *In* Excitatory Synaptic Mechanisms (P. Andersen and J.K.S. Jansen, eds.). Oslo: Universitets-forlag. pp. 213–222.

Dodge, F.A. Jr. and J.W. Cooley. 1973. Action potential of the motoneuron. IBM J. Res. Div. 17: 219–229.

Douglas, W.W. 1977. Calcium and exocytosis in endocrine, exocrine, neurosecretory, and mast cells. *In* Depolarization-Release Coupling Systems in Neurons (R.R. Llinás and J.E. Heuser, eds.). NRP Bulletin 15. Cambridge: M.I.T. pp. 591–602.

Dowling. J.E. 1968. Synaptic organization of the frog retina. An electron microscopic analysis comparing the retinas of frogs and primates. Proc. Roy. Soc. B. 170: 205–228.

Dowling, J.E. 1970. Organization of vertebrate retinas. Invest. Ophth. 9: 655–680.

Dowling, J.E. and B.B. Boycott. 1966. Organization of the primate retina: Electron microscopy. Proc. Roy. Soc. B. 166: 80–111.

Dowling, J.E., B. Ehinger, and W.L. Hedden. 1976. The interplexiform cell: a new type of retinal neuron. Invest. Opthal. 15: 916–926.

Dowling, J.E. and H. Ripps. 1973. Effect of magnesium on horizontal cell activity in the Skate retina. Nature 242: 101–103.

Dreifuss, J.J., J.S. Kelly, and K. Krnjevic. 1969. Cortical inhibition and γ-aminobutyric acid. Exp. Brain Res. 9: 137–154.

Droz, B. 1975. Synthetic machinery and axoplasmic transport: maintenance of neuronal connectivity. *In* The Nervous System, vol. I: Basic Neurosciences (D.B. Tower, ed.). New York: Raven. pp. 111–127.

Dun, N. and S. Nishi. 1974. Effects of dopamine on the superior cervical ganglion of the rabbit. J. Physiol. 239: 155–164.

Eccles, J.C. 1953. The Neurophysiological Basis of Mind. Oxford: Clarendon Press.

Eccles, J.C. 1957. The Physiology of Nerve Cells. Baltimore: Johns Hopkins University Press.

Eccles, J.C. 1964. The Physiology of Synapses. Berlin: Springer.

Eccles, J.C. 1969. The Inhibitory Pathways of the Central Nervous System. Springfield: Thomas.

Eccles, J.C. 1973. The cerebellum as a computer: Patterns in space and time. J. Physiol. 229: 1–32.

Eccles, J.C., P. Fatt, and K. Koketsu. 1954. Cholinergic and inhibitory synapses in a pathway from motor-axon collaterals to motoneurones. J. Physiol. 216: 524–562.

Eccles, J.C., M. Ito, and J. Szentágothai. 1967. The Cerebellum as a Neuronal Machine. Berlin: Springer.

Eccles, J.C., B. Libet, and R.R. Young. 1958. The behavior of chromatolyzed motoneurons studied by intracellular recording. J. Physiol. 143: 11–40.

Eccles, R.M. 1955. Intracellular potentials recorded from mammalian sympathetic ganglion. J. Physiol. 130: 572–584.

Edwards, C. and D. Ottoson. 1958. The site of impulse initiation in a nerve cell of a crustacean stretch receptor. J. Physiol. 143: 138–148.

Ehinger, B., B. Falck, and A.M. Laties. 1969. Adrenergic neurons in teleost retina. Z. Zellforsch. Mikro. Anat. 97: 285–297.

Elfvin, L.-G. 1963. The ultrastructure of the superior cervical sympathetic ganglion of the cat. II. The structure of the preganglionic end fibers and the synapses as studied by serial sections. J. Ultrastr. Res. 8: 441–476.

Elfvin, L.-G. 1971. Ultrastructural studies on the synaptology of the inferior mesenteric ganglion of the cat. III. The structure and distribution of the axodendritic and dendrodendritic contacts. J. Ultrastr. Res. 37: 432–448.

Emson, P.C. and O. Lindvall. 1979. Distribution of putative neurotransmitters in the neocortex. Neurosci. 4: 1–30.

Engberg, I. and K.C. Marshall. 1971. Mechanism of noradrenalin hyperpolarization in spinal cord motoneurones of the cat. Acta Physiol. Scand. 83: 142–144.

Enroth-Cugell, C. and J.C. Robson. 1966. The contrast sensitivity of retinal ganglion cells of the cat. J. Physiol. 187: 517–522.

Eränkö, O. 1955. Distribution of adrenaline and noradrenaline in the adrenal medulla. Nature 175: 88.

Eränkö, O. and M. Härkönen. 1965. Monoamine-containing small cells in the superior cervical ganglion of the rat and an organ composed of them. Acta Physiol. Scand. 63: 511–512.

Erulkar, S.D., C.W. Nichols, M.B. Popp, and G.B. Koelle. 1968. Renshaw elements: Localization and acetylcholinesterase content. J. Histochem. Cytochem. 16: 128–135.

Erulkar, S.D. and R. Rahamimoff. 1978. The role of calcium ions in tetanic and post-tetanic increase of miniature end-plate potential frequency. J. Physiol. 278: 501–511.

Erulkar, S.D., and F.F. Weight. 1977. Extracellular potassium and transmitter release at the giant synapse of squid. J. Physiol. 266: 209–218.

Erulkar, S.D. and J.K. Woodward. 1968. Intracellular recording from mammalian superior cervical ganglion *in situ*. J. Physiol. 199: 189–203.

Evarts, E.V. 1968. Relation of pyramidal tract activity to force exerted during voluntary movement. J. Neurophysiol. 31: 14–27.

Evarts, E.V. 1971. Feedback and corollary discharge. A merging of the concepts. *In* Central Control of Movement (E.V. Evarts, ed.). Neurosci. Res. Prog. Bull. 9 (No. 1). pp. 86–112.

Evarts, E.V. 1975. Activity of cerebral neurons in relation to movement. *In* The Nervous System (D.B. Tower, ed.). vol 1: The Basic Neurosciences. New York: Raven. pp. 221–233.

Evarts, E.V. and W.T. Thach. 1969. Motor mechanisms of the CNS: cerebro-cerebellar interrelations. Ann. Rev. Physiol. 31: 451–498.

Fadiga, E. and J.M. Brookhart. 1960. Monosynaptic activation of different portions of the motor neuron membrane. Am. J. Physiol. 198: 693–703.

Fairén, A., A. Peters, and J. Saldanha. 1977. A new procedure for examining Golgi impregnated neurons by light and electron microscopy. J. Neurocytol. 6: 311–337.

Falck, B., N.-A. Hillarp, G. Thieme, and A. Torp. 1962. Fluorescence of catecholamines and related compounds condensed with formaldehyde. J. Histochem. Cytochem. 10: 348–354.

Famiglietti, E.V., Jr. 1970. Dendro-dendritic synapses in the lateral geniculate nucleus of the cat. Brain Res. 20: 181–191.

Famiglietti, E.V., Jr., and A. Peters. 1972. The synaptic glomerulus and the intrinsic neuron in the dorsal lateral geniculate nucleus of the cat. J. Comp. Neur. 144: 285–334.

Feltz, P. and M. Rasminsky. 1974. A model for the mode of action of GABA on primary afferent terminals: depolarizing effects of GABA applied iontophoretically to neurons of mammalian dorsal root ganglia. Neuropharmacol. 13: 553–563.

Fifkova, E. and A. van Harreveld. 1977. Long-lasting morphological changes in dendritic spines of dentate granular cells following stimulation of the entorhinal area. J. Neurocytol. 6: 211–230.

Fonnum, F., I. Grofova, E. Rinvik, J. Storm-Mathisen, and F. Walberg. 1974. Origin and distribution of glutamate decarboxylase in substantia nigra of the cat. Brain Res. 71: 77–92.

Forbes, A. 1922. The interpretation of spinal reflexes in terms of present knowledge of nerve conduction. Physiol. Rev. 2: 361–414.

Fox, C.A., A.N. Andrade, D.E. Hillman, and R.C. Schwyn. 1971. The spiny neurons in the primate striatum: a Golgi and electron microscopic study. J. Hirnforsch. 13: 181–201.

Fox, C.A. and J.W. Barnard. 1957. A quantitative study of the Purkinje cell dendritic branchlets and their relationship to afferent fibers. J. Anat. 91: 299–313.

Fox, C.A. and J.A. Rafols. 1976. The striatal efferents in the globus pallilus and in the substantia nigra. *In* The Basal Ganglia (M.D. Yahr, ed.). New York: Raven. pp. 37–55.

Frank, K. and M.G.F. Fuortes. 1956. Stimulation of spinal motoneurones with intracellular electrodes. J. Physiol. 134: 451–470.

Frank, K. and M.G.F. Fuortes. 1957. Presynaptic and postsynaptic inhibition of monosynaptic reflex. Fed. Proc. 16: 39–40.

Freeman, W.J. 1964. A linear distributed feedback model for prepyriform cortex. Exp. Neurol. 10: 525–547.

Freeman, W.J. 1968. Patterns of variation in waveform of averaged evoked potentials from prepyriform cortex of cats. J. Neurophysiol. 31: 1–13.

Fujita, Y. 1968. Activity of dendrites of single Purkinje cells and its relationship to so-called inactivation response to rabbit cerebellum. J. Neurophysiol. 31: 131–141.

Fulton, J.F. 1938. Physiology of the Nervous System. London: Oxford.

Furshpan, E.J. and D.D. Potter. 1959. Transmission at the giant motor synapses of the crayfish. J. Physiol. 145: 289–325.

Furukawa, T. and E.J. Furshpan. 1963. Two inhibitory mechanisms in the Mauthner neurons of goldfish. J. Neurophysiol. 26: 140–176.

Fuxe, K. 1965. Evidence for the existence of monoamine neurons in the central nervous system. III. The monoamine nerve terminal. Zeit. Zellforsch. 65: 573–596.

Gallagher, J.P., H. Higashi, and S. Nishi. 1978. Characterization and ionic basis of GABA-induced depolarizations recorded *in vitro* from cat primary afferent neurones. J. Physiol. 275: 263–282.

Garey, L.J. 1971. A light and electron microscopic study of the visual cortex of the cat and monkey. Proc. Roy. Soc. B. 179: 21–40.

Garey, L.J. and T.P.S. Powell. 1971. An experimental study of the lateral geniculo-cortical pathway in the cat and monkey. Proc. Roy. Soc. B. 179: 41–63.

Gelfan, S. 1963. Neurone and synapse populations in spinal cord: indication of role in total integration. Nature 198: 162–163.

Gerschenfeld, H.M. and M. Piccolino. 1977. Muscarinic antagonists block cone to horizontal cell transmission in turtle retina. Nature 268: 257–259.

Getchell, T.V. and G.M. Shepherd. 1975a. Synaptic actions on mitral and tufted cells elicited by olfactory nerve volleys in the rabbit. J. Physiol. 251: 497–522.

Getchell, T.V. and G.M. Shepherd. 1975b. Short-axon cells in the olfactory bulb: dendrodendritic synaptic interactions. J. Physiol. 251: 523–548.

Gilbert, C.D. 1977. Laminar differences in receptive field properties of cells in cat primary visual cortex. J. Physiol. 268: 391–421.

Gilbert, C.D. and J.P. Kelly. 1975. The projections of cells in different layers of the cat's visual cortex. J. Comp. Neurol. 163: 81–106.

Globus, A. and A.B. Scheibel. 1967. The effect of visual deprivation on cortical neurons: A Golgi study. Exp. Neurol. 19: 331–345.

Gogan, P., J.P. Gueritand, G. Horcholle-Bossavit, and S. Tyc-Dumont. 1977. Direct excitatory interactions between spinal motorneurones of the cat. J. Physiol. 272: 755–767.

Goldman, P.S. and W.J.H. Nauta. 1977. An intricately patterned prefronto-caudate projection in the rhesus monkey. J. Comp. Neur. 171: 369–385.

Gottlieb, D.I. and W.M. Cowan. 1972. On the distribution of axonal terminals containing spheroidal and flattened synaptic vesicles in the hippocampus and dentate gyrus of the rat and cat. Z. Zeilforsch. 129: 413–429.

Graham, L.T. Jr. and M.H. Aprison. 1975. Putative transmitters in denervated olfactory cortex. J. Neurochem. 24: 445–449.

Granit, R. 1955. Receptors and Sensory Perception. New Haven: Yale University Press.

Granit. R. and C.G. Phillips. 1956. Excitatory and inhibitory processes acting upon individual Purkinje cells of the cerebellum in cats. J. Physiol. 133: 520–547.

Gray, E.G. 1959. Axo-somatic and axo-dendritic synapses of the cerebral cortex: An electron-microscope study. J. Anat. 93: 420–433.

Gray, E.G. 1962. A morphological basis for presynaptic inhibition? Nature 193: 82–83.

Graybiel, A.M. and C.W. Ragsdale. 1978. Histochemically distinct compartments in the striatum of human being, monkey, and cat demonstrated by acetylcholinesterase staining method. Proc. Nat. Acad. Sci. 75, 11: 5723–5726.

Green, J.D. 1964. The hippocampus. Physiol. Rev. 44: 561–608.

Greengard, P. 1976. Possible role for cyclic nucleotides and phosphorylated membrane proteins in postsynaptic actions of neurotransmitters. Nature 260: 101–108.

Greengard, P. 1978. Cyclic Nucleotides, Phosphorylated Proteins and Neuronal Function. New York: Raven.

Greengard, P. and Ritchie, J.M. 1971. Electrogenic ion pumping in nervous tissue. *In* Current Topics in Bioenergetics (vol. 4) pp. 327–356.

Grillner, S. 1975. Locomotion in vertebrates—central mechanisms and reflex interaction. Physiol. Rev. 55: 247–304.

Grillo, M.A., L. Jacobs, and J.H. Comroe, Jr. 1974. A combined fluorescence, histochemical and electron microscopic method for studying special mono-amino-containing cells (SIF cells). J. Comp. Neurol. 153: 1–14.

Grofova, I. 1975. The identification of striatal and pallidal neurons projecting to substantia nigra. An experimental study by means of retrograde axonal transport of horseradish peroxidase. Brain Res. 91: 286–291.

Grossman, A., A.R. Lieberman, and K.E. Webster. 1973. A Golgi study of the rat dorsal lateral geniculate nucleus. J. Comp. Neur. 150: 441–466.

Groves, P.M., C.J. Wilson, S.J. Young, and G.V. Rebec. 1975. Self-inhibition by dopaminergic neurons. Science 190: 522–529.

Guillery, R.W. 1971. Patterns of synaptic interconnections in the dorsal lateral geniculate nucleus of cat and monkey: A brief review. Vision Res. Suppl. no. 3: 211–227.

Haberly, L.B. 1969. Single unit responses to odor in the prepyriform cortex of the rat. Brain Res. 12: 481–484.

Haberly, L.B. 1973a. Unitary analysis of opossum prepyriform cortex. J. Neurophysiol. 36: 762–787.

Haberly, L.B. 1973b. Summed potentials evoked in opossum prepyriform cortex. J. Neurophysiol. 36: 775–788.

Haberly, L.B. and J.L. Price. 1978. Association and commissural fiber systems of the olfactory cortex of the rat. I. Systems originating in the piriform cortex and adjacent, caudal areas. J. Comp. Neurol. 178: 711–740.

Haberly, L.B. and G.M. Shepherd. 1973. Current density analysis of summed evoked potentials in opossum prepyriform cortex. J. Neurophysiol. 36: 789–802.

Halasz, N., Å. Llungdahl, and T. Hökfelt. 1978a. Transmitter histochemistry of the rat olfactory bulb. II. Fluorescence histochemical, autoradiographic and electron microscopic localization of monoamines. Brain Res. 154: 253–271.

Halasz, N., A. Llungdahl, and T. Hökfelt. 1978b. Transmitter histochemistry of the rat olfactory bulb. III. Autoradiographic localization of ^{3}H-GABA, glycine and leucine. Brain Res. (in press).

Halasz, N., A. Llungdahl, T. Hökfelt, O. Johansson, M. Goldstein, D. Park, and P. Biberfeld. 1977. Transmitter histochemistry of the rat olfactory bulb. I. Immunohistochemical localization of monoamine synthesizing enzymes. Support for intrabulbar, periglomerular dopamine neurons. Brain Res. 126: 455–474.

Hamlyn, L.H. 1963. An electron microscope study of pyramidal neurons in the Ammon's horn of the rabbit. J. Anat. 97: 189–201.

Hamori, J. and E. Mezey. 1977. Serial and triadic synapses in the cerebellar nuclei of the cat. Exp. Brain Res. 30: 259–273.

Harding, B.N. 1971. Dendro-dendritic synapses, including reciprocal synapses, in the ventrolateral nucleus of the monkey thalamus. Brain Res. 34: 181–185.

Hattori, T., H.C. Fibiger, P.L. McGeer, and L. Maler. 1973. Analysis of the fine structure of the dopaminergic nigrostriatal projection by electron microscopic autoradiography. Exp. Neurol. 41: 599–611.

Hattori, T., P.L. McGeer, H.C. Fibirger, and E.G. McGeer. 1973. On the source of GABA-containing terminals in the substantia nigra. Electron microscopic, autoradiographic, and biochemical studies. Brain Res. 54: 103–114.

Hebb. D.O. 1961. The Organization of Behavior. New York: Wiley.

Heimer, L. 1968. Synaptic distribution of centripetal and centrifugal nerve fibres in the olfactory system of the rat. An experimental anatomical study. J. Anat. 103: 413–432.

Henneman, E. 1968. Organization of the spinal cord. *In* Medical Physiology (V.B. Mountcastle, ed.) vol. II. St. Louis: Saunders. pp. 1717–1732.

Herrick, C.J. 1948. The Brain of the Tiger Salamander. Chicago: Chicago University Press.

Heuser, J.E. and T.S. Reese. 1973. Evidence for recycling of synaptic vesicle membrane during transmitter release at the frog neuromuscular junction. J. Cell Biol. 57: 315–344.

Heuser, J.E. and T.S. Reese. 1977. Vesicle membrane retrieval and recycling after exocytosis. *In* Depolarization-Release Coupling Systems in Neurons (R.R. Llinas and J.E. Heuser, eds.). NRP Bulletin 15. Cambridge: M.I.T. pp. 656–659.

Hild, W. and I. Tasaki. 1962. Morphological and physiological properties of neurons and glial cells in tissue culture. J. Neurophysiol. 25: 277–304.

Hirata, Y. 1964. Some observations on the fine structure of the synapses in the olfactory bulb of the mouse, with particular reference to the ayptical synaptic configuration. Arch. Histol. Japan. 24: 293–302.

Hjorth-Simonsen, A. 1973. Some intrinsic connections of the hippocampus in the rat: an experimental analysis. J. Comp. Neur. 147: 145–162.

Hjorth-Simonsen, A. and B. Jeune. 1972. Origin and termination of the hippocampal perforant path in the rat studied by silver impregnation. J. Comp. Neur. 144: 215–232.

Hodgkin, A.L. 1964. The Conduction of the Nervous Impulse. Springfield, Ill. Thomas.

Hodgkin, A.L. 1972. Recent work on visual mechanisms. Proc. Roy. Soc. B. 180: X–XX.

Hodgkin, A.L. and A.F. Huxley. 1952. A quantitative description of membrane current and its application to conduction and excitation in nerve. J. Physiol. 117: 500–544.

Hoffman, K.-P. 1973. Conduction velocity in pathways from retina to superior colliculus in the cat: a correlation with receptive-field properties. J. Neurophysiol. 36: 409–424.

Hoffman, K.-P. and J. Stone. 1971. Conduction velocity of afferents to cat visual cortex: a correlation with cortical receptive field properties. Brain Res. 32: 460–466.

Hore, J., J. Meyer-Lohmann, and V.B. Brooks. 1977. Basal ganglia cooling disables learned arm movements of monkeys in the absence of visual guidance. Science 195: 584–586.

Hökfelt, T., J.O. Kellerth, G. Nilsson, and B. Pernow. 1975. Experimental immunohistochemical studies on the localization and distribution of substance P in cat primary sensory neurons. Brain Res. 100: 235–252.

Hökfelt, T. and A. Llungdahl. 1972. Autoradiographic identification of cerebellar and cerebral cortical neurons accumulating labelled gamma-aminobutyric acid [^{3}H]-GABA. Exp. Brain Res. 14: 354–362.

Hubel, D.H. and T.N. Wiesel. 1962. Receptive fields, binocular interaction and functional architecture in the cat's visual cortex. J. Physiol. 160: 106–154.

Hubel, D.H. and T.N. Wiesel. 1968. Receptive fields and functional architecture of monkey striate cortex. J. Ph, c'ol. 195: 215–243.

Hubel, D.H. and T.N. Wiesel. 1974. Sequence regularity and geometry of orientation columns in the monkey striate cortex. J. Comp. Neurol. 158: 267–294.

Hubel, D.H., T.N. Wiesel, and M.P. Stryker. 1978. Anatomical demonstration of orientation columns in macaque monkey. J. Comp. Neurol. 177: 361–380.

Hultborn, H., E. Jankowska, and S. Lindström. 1971. Recurrent inhibition of interneurones monosynaptically activated from group la afferents. J. Physiol. 215: 613–636.

Hunt, S. and J. Schmidt. 1978. Are mitral cells cholinergic? *In* Society for Neuroscience Symposia III (J.A. Ferrendelli, ed.). Bethesda: Soc. for Neurosci. pp. 204–218.

Iansek, R. and S.J. Redman. 1973. The amplitude, time course and charge of unitary excitatory post-synaptic potentials evoked in spinal motoneurone dendrites. J. Physiol. 234: 665–688.

Ibata, Y. and N. Otsuka. 1969. Electron microscopic demonstration of zinc in the hippocampal formation using Timm's sulphide-silver technique. J. Histochem. Cytochem. 17: 171–175.

Iles, J.F. 1976. Central terminations of muscle afferents on motoneurones in the cat spinal cord. J. Physiol. 262: 91–117.

Isaacson, R.L. and K.H. Pribram (eds.). 1975. The Hippocampus. New York: Plenum.

Iverson, L.L. 1970. Neurotransmitters, neurohormones and other small molecules in neurons. *In* The Neurosciences: Second Study Program (F.O. Schmitt, ed.-in-chief) New York: Rockefeller. pp. 768–781.

Iversen, L.L. and F.E. Bloom. 1972. Studies on the uptake of [^{3}H] GABA and [^{3}H] glycine in slices and homogenates of rat brain and spinal cord by electron microscopic autoradiography. Brain Res. 41: 131–143.

Jack, J.J.B. 1979. Introduction to linear cable theory. *In* The Neurosciences: Fourth Study Program (F.O. Schmitt and F.G. Worden, eds.). Cambridge: M.I.T. pp. 423–437.

Jack, J.J.B., S. Miller, R. Porter, and S. J. Redman. 1971. The time course of minimal excitatory post-synaptic potentials evoked in spinal motoneurones by group Ia afferent fibers. J. Physiol. 215: 353–380.

Jack, J.J.B. and S.J. Redman. 1971. An electrical description of the motoneurone, and its application to the analysis of synaptic potentials. J. Physiol. 215: 321–352.

Jackowski, A., J.G. Parnevalas, and A.R. Lieberman. 1978. The reciprocal synapse in the external plexiform layer of the mammalian olfactory bulb. Brain Res. 159: 17–28.

Jacobson, S. and D.A. Pollen. 1968. Electrotonic spread of dendritic potentials in feline pyramidal cells. Science 164: 1351–1353.

Jankowska, E. and S. Lundström. 1971. Morphological identification of Renshaw cells. Acta Physiol. Scand. 81: 428–430.

Jankowska, E. and S. Lindström. 1972. Morphology of interneurones mediating Ia reciprocal inhibition of motoneurones in the spinal cord of the cat. J. Physiol. 226: 805–823.

Jankowska, E., Y. Padel, and R. Tanaka. 1975. Projections of pyramidal tract cells to α motoneurones innervating hind-limb muscles in the monkey. J. Physiol. 249: 637–667.

Jansen, J.K.S. and J.G. Nicholls. 1973. Conductance changes, an electrogenic pump and the hyperpolarization of leech neurones following impulses. J. Physiol. 229: 635–655.

Jansen, J.K.S. and L. Walløe. 1970. Signal transmission between successive neurons in the dorsal spinocerebellar pathway. *In* The Neurosciences: Second Study Program (F.O. Schmitt, ed.-in-chief). New York: Rockefeller. pp. 617–629.

Jasper, H.H., A.A. Ward, and A. Pope. 1969. Basic Mechanisms of the Epilepsies. Boston: Little, Brown.

Jones, E.G. 1975. Lamination and differential distribution of thalamic afferents within the sensory-motor cortex of the squirrel monkey. J. Comp. Neurol. 160: 167–204.

Jones, E.G., J.D. Coulter, H. Burton, and R. Porter. 1977. Cells of origin and terminal distribution of corticostriatal fibers arising in the sensory-motor cortex of monkeys. J. Comp. Neurol. 173: 53–80.

Jones, E.G. and T.P.S. Powell. 1969. Electron microscopy of synaptic glomeruli in the thalamic relay nuclei of the cat. Proc. Roy. Soc. B 172: 153–171.

Jones, E.G. and T.P.S. Powell. 1970a. Electron microscopy of the somatic sensory cortex of the cat. I. Cell types and synaptic organization. Phil. Trans. Roy. Soc. B 257: 1–11.

Jones, E.G. and T.P.S. Powell. 1970b. An electron microscopic study of the laminar pattern and mode of termination of afferent fibre pathways in the somatic sensory cortex of the cat. Phil. Trans. Roy. Soc. B 257: 45–62.

Jones, E.G. and S.P. Wise. 1977. Size, laminar and columnar distribution of efferent cells in the sensory-motor cortex of monkeys. J. Comp. Neurol. 175: 391–438.

Kalil, R.E. and R. Chase. 1970. Corticofugal influence on activity of lateral geniculate neurons in the cat. J. Neurophysiol. 33: 459–474.

Kandel, E.R. 1976. Cellular Basis of Behavior. San Francisco: Freeman.

Kandel, E.R. and W.A. Spencer. 1961. Electrophysiology of hippocampal neurons. II. After-potentials and repetitive firing. J. Neurophysiol. 24: 243–259.

Kandel, E.R., W.A. Spencer, and F.J. Brinley Jr. 1961. Electrophysiology of hippocampal neurons. I. Sequential invasion and synaptic organization. J. Neurophysiol. 24: 225–242.

Kandel, E.R. and W.A. Spencer. 1968. Cellular neurophysiological approaches in the study of learning. Physiol. Rev. 48: 65–134.

Kane, E.C. 1973. Octopus cells in the cochlear nucleus of the cat: heterotypic synapses upon homeotypic neurons. Intern. J. Neuroscience 5: 251–279.

Kaneko, A. 1970. Physiological and morphological identification of horizontal, bipolar and amacrine cells in goldfish retina. J. Physiol. 207: 623–633.

Katz, B. 1962. The transmission of impulses from nerve to muscle, and the subcellular unit of synaptic action. Proc. Roy. Soc. B 155: 455–477.

Katz, B. 1966. Nerve, Muscle and Synapse. New York: McGraw-Hill.

Katz, B. 1969. The Release of Neural Transmitter Substances. Liverpool: Liverpool University.

Katz, B. and R. Miledi. 1967. A study of synaptic transmission in the absence of nerve impulses. J. Physiol. 192: 407–436.

Katz, B. and R. Miledi. 1972. The statistical nature of the acetylcholine potential and its molecular components. J. Physiol. 224: 665–669.

Kauer, J.S. 1974. Response patterns of amphibian olfactory bulb neurones to odour stimulation. J. Physiol. 243: 675–715.

Kauer, J.S. and D.G. Moulton. 1974. Responses of olfactory bulb neurones to odour stimulation of small nasal areas in the salamander. J. Physiol. 243: 717–737.

Kauer, J.S. and G.M. Shepherd. 1977. Analysis of the onset phase of olfactory bulb unit responses to odour pulses in the salamander. J. Physiol. 272: 495–516.

Kebabian, J.W. and P. Greengard. 1971. Dopamine-sensitive adenyl cyclase: possible role in synaptic transmission. Science 174: 1346–1349.

Kebabian, J.W., G.L. Petzold, and P. Greengard. 1971. Dopamine-sensitive adenylate cyclase in caudate nucleus of rat brain and its similarity to the "dopamine receptor". Proc. Nat. Acad. Sci. 69: 2145–2149.

Kelly, J.P. and D.C. van Essen. 1974. Cell structure and function in the visual cortex of the cat. J. Physiol. 238: 515–547.

Kelly, J.S. and K. Krnjevic. 1969. The action of glycine on cortical neurones. Exp. Brain Res. 9: 155–163.

Kemp, J.M. and T.P.S. Powell. 1971a. The structure of the caudate nucleus of the cat: light and electron microscopy. Proc. Roy. Soc. B 262: 383–402.

Kemp, J.M. and T.P.S. Powell. 1971b. The synaptic organization of the caudate nucleus. Proc. Roy. Soc. B 262: 403–412.

Kemp, J.M. and T.P.S. Powell. 1971c. The site of termination of afferent fibres in the caudate nucleus. Proc. Roy. Soc. B 262: 413–427.

Kemp. J.M. and T.P.S. Powell. 1971d. The termination of fibres from the cerebral cortex and thalamus upon dendritic spines in the caudate nucleus: a study with the Golgi method. Proc. Roy. Soc. B 262: 429–439.

Kemp, J.M. and T.P.S. Powell. 1971e. The connexions of the striatum and globus pallidus: synthesis and speculation. Proc. Roy. Soc. B 262: 441–457.

Kennedy, C., M.H. Des Rosiers, J.W. Jehle, M. Reivich, F.R. Sharp, and L. Sokoloff. 1975. Mapping of functional neural pathways by autoradiographic survey of local metabolic rate with [14C] deoxyglucose. Science 187: 850–853.

Kennedy, C., M.H. Des Rosiers, O. Sakurada, M. Shinoham, M. Reivich, J.W. Jehle, and L. Sokoloff. 1976. Metabolic mapping of the primary visual system of the monkey by means of the autoradiographic [14C] deoxyglucose technique. Proc. Nat. Acad. Sci. 73: 4230–4234.

Keynes, R.D. 1975. Organization of the ionic channels in nerve membranes. *In* The Nervous System, vol. 1: Basic Neurosciences (D.B. Tower, ed.). New York: Raven. pp. 165–175.

Kidd, M. 1962. Electron microscopy of the inner plexiform layer of the retina in the cat and pigeon. J. Anat. 96: 179–187.

Kirby, A.W. and C. Enroth-Cugell. 1976. The involvement of gamma-aminobutyric acid in the organization of cat retinal ganglion cell receptive fields. J. Gen. Physiol. 68: 465–484.

Kitai, S.T., M. Sugimori, and J.D. Kocsis. 1976. Excitatory nature of dopamine in the nigro-caudate pathway. Exp. Brain Res. 24: 351–363.

Kocsis, J.D. and S.T. Kitai. 1977. Dual excitatory inputs to caudate spiny neurons from substantia nigra stimulation. Brain Res. 138: 271–283.

Kocsis, J.D., M. Sugimori, and S.T. Kitai. 1977. Convergence of excitatory synaptic inputs to caudate spiny neurons. Brain Res. 124: 403–413.

Kolb, H. 1970. Organization of the outer plexiform layer of the primate retina: electron microscopy of Golgi-impregnated cells. Proc. Roy. Soc. B 258: 261–283.

Kolb, H. 1977. The organization of the outer plexiform layer in the retina of the cat: electron microscopic observations. J. Neurocytol. 6: 131–153.

Kolb, H. and R.W. West. 1977. Synaptic connections of the interplexiform cell in the retina of the cat. J. Neurocytol. 6: 155–170.

Korn, H. and D.S. Faber. 1979. Electrical interactions between vertebrate neurons: field effects and electrotonic coupling. *In* The Neurosciences: Fourth Study Program (F.O. Schmitt and F.G. Worden, eds.). Cambridge: M.I.T. pp. 333–358.

Korn, H., C. Sotelo, and F. Crepel. 1973. Electrotonic coupling between neurons in rat lateral vestibular nucleus. Exp. Brain. Res. 16: 255–275.

Kornhuber, H.H. 1974. Cerebral cortex, cerebellum and basal ganglia: an introduction to their motor functions. *In* the Neurosciences: Third Study Program (F.O. Schmitt and F.G. Worden, eds.). Cambridge: M.I.T. pp. 267–280.

Krieger, N.R. and J.S. Heller. 1978. Glutamic acid decarboxylase within laminae of the olfactory tubercle. Neurosci. Abstr. 1414.

Krieger, N.R., J.S. Kauer, G.M. Shepherd, and P. Greengard. 1977. Dopamine-sensative adenylate cyclase within laminae of the olfactory tubercle. Brain Res. 131: 303–312.

Kreutzberg, G.W., P. Schubert, and H.D. Lux. 1975. Neuroplasmic transport in axons and dendrites. *In* Golgi Centennial Symposium (M. Santini, ed.). New York: Raven. pp. 161–166.

Kristensson, K., Y. Olsson, and J. Sjöstrand. 1971. Axon uptake and retrograde transport of exogenous proteins in the hypoglossal nerve. Brain Res. 32: 399–406.

Krnjevic, K. 1970. Central excitatory transmitters in vertebrates. *In* Excitatory Synaptic Mechanisms (P. Andersen and J.K.S. Jansen, eds.). Oslo, Universitetsforlag. pp. 95–104.

Krnjevic, K. 1974. Chemical nature of synaptic transmission in vertebrates. Physiol. Rev. 54: 418–540.

Kuffler, S.W. 1953. Discharge patterns and functional organization of mammalian retina. J. Neurophysiol. 16: 37–68.

Kuffler, S.W. and J.G. Nicholls. 1976. From Neuron to Brain. Sunderlund, Massachusetts: Sinauer.

Kuno, M. 1971. Quantum aspects of central and ganglionic synaptic transmission in vertebrates. Physiol. Rev. 51: 647–678.

Kuno, M. and R. Llinás. 1970. Alterations of synaptic action in chromatolysed motoneurones of the cat. J. Physiol. 210: 823–838.

Laatsch, R.H. and W.M. Cowan. 1966. Electron microscopic studies of the dentate gyrus of the rat. I. Normal structure with special reference to synaptic organization. J. Comp. Neur. 128: 359–396.

Ladman, A.J. 1958. The fine structure of the rod-bipolar cell synapse in the retina of the albino rat. J. Biophys. Biochem. Cytol. 4: 459–466.

Lake, M. and L.M. Jordan. 1974. Failure to confirm cyclic AMP as second messenger for norepinephrine in rat cerebellum. Science 183: 663–664.

Lam, D.M.K. 1972. Biosynthesis of acetylcholine in turtle photoreceptors. Proc. Nat. Acad. Sci. 69: 1987–1991.

Land, L.J. and G.M. Shepherd. 1974. Autoradiographic analysis of olfactory receptor projections in the rabbit. Brain Res. 70: 506–510.

Landgren, S., C.G. Phillips, and R. Porter. 1962. Cortical fields of origin of the monosynaptic pyramidal pathways to some alpha motoneurones of the baboon's hand and forearm. J. Physiol. 161: 112–125.

Landis, D.M.D. and T.S. Reese. 1974. Differences in membrane structure between excitatory and inhibitory synapses in the cerebellar cortex. J. Comp. Neur. 155: 93–126.

Laporte, Y. and R. Lorente de Nó. 1950. Properties of sympathetic B ganglion cells. J. Cell Comp. Physiol. 35 Suppl. 2: 41–60.

Larramendi, L.M.H. and T. Victor. 1967. Synapses on the Purkinje cell spines in the mouse. An electron microscopic study. Brain Res. 5: 15–30.

LeVay, S. 1971. On the neurons and synapses of the lateral geniculate nucleus of the monkey, and the effects of eye enucleation. Z. Zellforsch. 113: 396–419.

LeVay, S. 1973. Synaptic patterns in the visual cortex of the cat and monkey. Electron microscopy of Golgi preparations. J. Comp. Neur. 150: 53–86.

Leventhal, A.G. and H.V.B. Hirsch. 1978. Receptive-field properties of neurons in different laminae of visual cortex of the cat. J. Neurophysiol. 41: 948–962.

Leveteau, J. and P. MacLeod. 1966. Olfactory discrimination in the rabbit olfactory glomerulus. Science 153: 175–176.

Levinson, S.R. and H. Meves. 1975. The binding of labelled tetrodotoxin to nonmyelinated nerve fibres. J. Physiol. 227: 95–126.

Levitt, P. and R.Y. Moore. 1978. Noradrenaline neuron innervation of the neocortex in the rat. Brain Res. 139: 219–231.

Libet, B. 1970. Generation of slow inhibitory and excitatory post-synaptic potentials. Fed. Proc. 29: 1945–1956.

Libet, B. 1976. The SIF cell as a functional dopamine-releasing interneuron in the rabbit superior cervical ganglion. *In* SIF Cells (O. Eranko, ed.). DHEW Publication No. (NIH) 76–942. Washington, D.C.: U.S. Govt. Printing Office. pp. 163–179.

Lieberman, A.R. and K.E. Webster. 1974. Aspects of the synaptic organization of intrinsic neurons in the dorsal lateral geniculate nucleus. J. Neurocytol. 3: 677–710.

Llinás, R. 1975. Electrical synaptic transmission in the mammalian central neurons system. *In* Golgi Centennial Symposium. (M. Santini, ed.). New York: Raven. pp. 379–386.

Llinás, R. 1977. Calcium and transmitter release in squid synapse. *In* Society for Neuroscience Symposia II. (W.M. Cowan and J.A. Ferendelli, eds.). Bethesda: Soc. for Neurosci. pp. 139–160.

Llinás, R., R. Baker, and C. Sotelo. 1974. Electrotonic coupling between neurons in the cat inferior olive. J. Neurophysiol. 37: 560–571.

Llinás, R. and R. Hess. 1976. Tetrodotoxin-resistant dendritic spikes in avian Purkinje cells. Proc. Nat. Acad. Sci. 73: 2520–2523.

Llinás, R. and D.E. Hillman. 1969. Physiological and morphological organization of the cerebellar circuits in various vertebrates. *In* Neurobiology of Cerebellar Evolution and Development (R. Llinás, ed.). Chicago: Am. Med. Assoc. pp. 43–73.

Llinás, R. and C. Nicholson, 1971. Electrophysiological properties of dendrites and somata in alligator Purkinje cells. J. Neurophysiol. 34: 532–551.

Lloyd, D.P.C. 1943. Reflex action in relation to patterns and peripheral source of afferent stimulation. J. Neurophysiol. 6: 111–120.

Lorente de Nó, R. 1922. La corteza cerebral del raton. Trab. Lab. Invest. Biol. (Madrid) 20: 41–78.

Lorente de Nó, R. 1934. Studies on the structure of the cerebral cortex. II. Continuation of the study of the Ammonic system. J. Psychol. Neurol. 46: 113–177.

Lorente de Nó, R. 1938. The cerebral cortex: Architecture, intracortical connections and motor projections. *In* Physiology of the Nervous System (J.F. Fulton). London: Oxford University Press. pp. 291–325.

Lorente de Nó, R. and C.A. Condouris. 1959. Decremental conduction in peripheral nerve. Integration of stimuli in the neuron. Proc. Nat. Acad. Sci. 45: 592–617.

Lund, J.S. 1973. Organization of neurons in the visual cortex, area 17, of the monkey (*Macaca mulatta*) J. Comp. Neur. 147: 455–496.

Lund, J.S., R.D. Lund, A.E. Hendrickson, A.H. Burt, and A.F. Fuchs. 1975. The origin of the efferent pathways from the primary visual cortex, area 17, of the macaque monkey as shown by retrograde transport of horseradish peroxidase. J. Comp. Neurol. 164: 287–304. *

Lund, R.D. 1978. Development and Plasticity of the Brain. New York: Oxford.

Lund, R.D. and L.E. Westrum. 1966. Synaptic vesicle differences after primary formalin fixation. J. Physiol. 185: 7–9P.

Lundberg, A. 1970. The excitatory control of the Ia inhibitory pathway. *In* Excitatory Synaptic Mechanisms (P. Andersen and J.K.S. Jansen, eds.). Oslo: Universitetsforlag. pp. 333–340.

Lundberg, A. 1975. Control of spinal mechanisms from the brain. *In* The Nervous System, vol. I: The Basic Neurosciences (D.B. Tower, ed.). New York: Raven. pp. 253–265.

Lundberg, A., K. Malmgren, and E.D. Schomburg. 1977. Cutaneous facilitation of transmission in reflex pathways from Ib afferents to motoneurons. J. Physiol. 265: 763–780.

Lux, H.D. and D.A. Pollen. 1966. Electrical constants of neurons in the motor cortex of the cat. J. Neurophysiol. 29: 207–220.

Lux, H.D, P. Schubert and G.W. Kreutzberg. 1970. Direct matching of morphological and electrophysiological data in cat spinal motoneurones. *In* Excitatory Synaptic Mechanisms (P. Andersen and J.K.S. Jansen, eds.). Oslo: Universitetsforlag. pp. 189–198.

Lynch, G.S., T. Dunwiddie, and V. Gribkoff. 1977. Heterosynaptic depression: a postsynaptic correlate of long-term potentiation. Nature 266: 737–739.

MacLean, P.D. 1972. Implications of microelectrode findings on exteroceptive inputs to the limbic cortex. *In* Limbic System Mechanisms and Autonomic Function (C.H. Hockman, ed.). Springfield: Ill.: Thomas. pp. 115–136.

Makowski, L., D.L.D. Caspar, W.C. Phillips, and D.A. Goodenough. 1977. Gap junction structure. II. Analysis of the X-ray diffraction data. J. Cell Biol. 74: 629–645.

Margolis, F.L. 1978. Biochemical studies of the primary olfactory pathway. *In* Society for Neuroscience Symposia III (J.A. Ferrendelli, eds.). Bethesda: Soc. for Neurosci. pp. 167–188.

Marin-Padilla, M. 1972. Double origin of the pericellular baskets of the pyramidal cells of the human motor cortex: a Golgi study. Brain Res. 38: 1–12.

Marin-Padilla, M. 1974. Three-dimensional reconstruction of the pericellular nests (baskets) of the motor (area 4) and visual (area 17) areas of the human cerebral cortex. A Golgi study. Z. Anat. Entwickl. 144: 123–135.

Marmarelis, P.Z. and K. Naka. 1972. Spatial distribution of potential in a flat cell. Application to the catfish horizontal cell layers. Biophys. J. 12: 1515–1532.

Marr, D. 1969. A theory of cerebellar cortex. J. Physiol. 202: 437–470.

Marshall, J. and M. Voaden. 1975. Autoradiographic identification of the cells accumulating ^{3}H -aminobutyric acid in mammalian retinae: a species comparison. Vision Res. 15: 459–461.

Marshall, L.M. and F.S. Werblin. 1978. Synaptic transmission to the horizontal cells in the retina of the larval tiger salamander. J. Physiol. 279: 321–346.

Martin, A.R. 1966. Quantal nature of synaptic transmission. Physiol. Rev. 46: 51–66.

Matsumoto, H. and C. Ajmone-Marsan. 1964. Cortical cellular phenomena in experimental epilepsy: interictal manifestations. Exp. Neurol. 9: 286–304.

Matthews, M.A., W.D. Willis, and V.F. Williams. 1971. Dendrite bundles in lamina IX of cat spinal cord: a possible source for electrical interaction between motoneurons? Anat. Rec. 171: 313–328.

Matthews, M.R. and G. Raisman. 1969. The ultrastructure and somatic efferent synapses of small granule-containing cells in the superior cervical ganglion. J. Anat. 105: 255–282.

Matthews, P.B.C. 1972. Mammalian Muscle Receptors and their Central Actions. Baltimore: Williams & Wilkins.

Maturana, H.R., J.Y. Lettvin, W.S. McCulloch, and W.H. Pitts. 1960. Anatomy and physiology of vision of the frog (*Rana pipiens*) J. Gen. Physiol. 43: 129–175.

Maynard, C.W., R.B. Leonard, J.D. Coulter, and R.E. Coggeshall. 1977. Central connections of ventral root efferents as demonstrated by the HRP method. J. Comp. Neurol. 172: 601–608.

McAfee, D.A., M. Schorderet, and P. Greengard. 1971. Adenosine 3′,5′-monophosphate in nervous tissue: increase associated with synaptic transmission. Science 171: 1156–1158.

McDonald, D.M. and R.A. Mitchell. 1975. The innervation of glomus cells, ganglion cells and blood vessels in the rat carotid body: a quantitative ultrastructural analysis. J. Neurocytol. 4: 177–220.

McIlwain, J.T. and O.D. Creutzfeldt. 1967. Microelectrode study of synaptic excitation and inhibition in the lateral geniculate nucleus of the cat. J. Neurophysiol. 30: 1–21.

McLardy, T. 1962. Zinc enzymes and the hippocampal mossy fibre system. Nature 194: 300–302.

McLaughlin, B.J. 1972a. The fine structure of neurons and synapses in the motor nuclei of the cat spinal cord. J. Comp. Neur. 144: 429–460.

McLaughlin B.J. 1972b. Dorsal root projections to the motor nuclei in the cat spinal cord. J. Comp. Neur. 144: 461–474.

McLaughlin, B.J., R. Barber, K. Saito, E. Roberts, and J.Y. Wu. 1975. Immunocytochemical localization of glutamate decarboxylase in rat spinal cord. J. Comp. Neurol. 164: 305–322.

McLaughlin, B.J. J.G. Wood, K. Saito, R. Barber, J.E. Vaughn, E. Roberts, and J.Y. Wu. 1974. The fine structural localization of glutamate decarboxylase in synaptic terminals of rodent cerebellum. Brain Res. 76: 377–391.

McLennan, H. 1971. The pharmacology of inhibition of mitral cells in the olfactory bulb. Brain Res. 29: 177–184.

McMahan, U.J. and D. Purves. 1976. Visual identification of two kinds of nerve cells and their synaptic contacts in a living autonomic ganglion of the mud puppy (*Necturus maculosus*). J. Physiol. 254: 405–426.

Meech, R.W. 1972. Intracellular calcium injection causes increased potassium conductance in *Aplysia* nerve cells. Comp. Biochem. Physiol. 42A: 493–499.

Mendell, L.M. and E. Henneman. 1968. Terminals of single Ia fibers: distribution within a pool of 300 homonymous motor neurons. Science 160: 96–98.

Michael, C.R. 1969. Retinal processing of visual images. Sci. Am. 220: 104–114.

Missotten, L. 1965. The Ultrastructure of the Human Retina. Brussels: Arscia Uitgaven.

Moore, R.Y. and F.E. Bloom. 1978. Central catecholamine neuron systems: anatomy and physiology of the dopamine systems. Ann. Rev. Neurosci. 1: 129–169.

Moore, R.Y. and A.E. Halaris. 1975. Hippocampal innervation by serotonin neurons of the midbrain raphé in the rat. J. Comp. Neurol. 164: 171–184.

Morest, D.K. 1971. Dendrodendritic synapses of cells that have axons: the fine structure of the Golgi type II cell in the medial geniculate body of the cat. Z. Anat. Entwickl.-Gesch. 133: 216–246.

Mori, K. and S.F. Takagi. 1978a. An intracellular study of dendrodendritic inhibitory synapses on mitral cells in the rabbit olfactory bulb. J. Physiol. 279: 569–588.

Mori, K. and S.F. Takagi. 1978b. Activation and inhibition of olfactory bulb neurones by anterior commissure volleys in the rabbit. J. Physiol. 279: 589–604.

Mountcastle, V.B. 1957. Modality and topographic properties of single neurons of cat's somatic sensory cortex. J. Neurophysiol. 20: 408–434.

Mountcastle, V.B. (ed.). 1974. Medical Physiology. St. Louis: Mosby.

Mountcastle, V.B. 1978. An organizing principle for cerebral function: the unit module and the distributed system. *In* The Mindful Brain (G.E. Edelman and V.B. Mountcastle, eds.). Cambridge: M.I.T. pp.7–50.

Mountcastle, V.B. and T.P.S. Powell. 1959. Central neutral mechanisms subserving position sense and kinaesthesia. Bull. Johns Hopkins Hosp. 105: 201–230.

Movshon, J.A. 1975. The velocity tuning of single units in cat striate cortex. J. Physiol. 249: 445–468.

Mugnaini, E. 1970. Neurones as synaptic targets. *In* Excitatory Synaptic Mechanisms (P. Andersen and J.K.S. Jansen, eds.). Oslo Universitetsforlag. pp. 149–169.

Müller-Schwartze, D. and M.M. Mozell (eds.). 1977. Chemical Signals in Vertebrates. New York: Plenum.

Murphy, J.T., W.A. MacKay, and F. Johnson. 1973. Responses of cerebellar cortical neurons to dynamic proprioceptive interactions in the cat. Brain Res. 36: 711–723.

Nacimiento, A.C., H.D. Lux, and O.D. Creutzfeldt. 1964. Postsynaptische Potentiale von Nervenzellen des motorischen Cortex nach elektrische Reizung specifischer und unspecifischer Thalamuskerne. Arch. Ges. Physiol. 281: 152–169.

Nadler, J.V., C.W. Cotman, and G.S. Lynch. 1973. Altered distribution of choline acetyltransferase and acetylcholinesterase activities in the developing rat dentate gyrus following entorhinal lesion. Brain Res. 63: 215–230.

Nafstad, P.H.J. 1967. An electron microscope study on the termination of the perforant path fibers in the hippocampus and the fascia dentata. Z. Zellforsch. 76: 532–542.

Naka, K. and W.H. Rushton. 1966. S-potentials from colour units in the retina of fish (*Cyprinidae*). J. Physiol. 185: 536–555.

Nauta, W.J.H. and H.J. Karten. 1970. A general profile of the vertebrate brain, with sidelights on the ancestry of cerebral cortex. *In* The Neurosciences: Second Study Program (F.O. Schmitt, ed.-in-chief). New York: Rockefeller. pp. 7–25.

Neal, M.J. and L.L. Iversen. 1972. Autoradiographic localization of ^{3}H-GABA in rat retina. Nature New Biol. 235: 217–218.

Negishi, K., S. Kato, T. Teranishi, and M. Laufer. 1978. An electrophysiological study on the cholinergic system in the carp retina. Brain Res. 148: 85–93.

Neher, E. and J.H. Steinbach. 1978. Local anaesthetics transiently block currents through single acetylcholine-receptor channels. J. Physiol. 227: 153–176.

Nelson, P.G. and S.D. Erulkar. 1963. Synaptic mechanisms of excitation and inhibition in the central auditory pathway. J. Neurophysiol. 26: 908–923.

Nelson, R. 1973. A comparison of electrical properties of neurons in *Necturus* retina. J. Neurophysiol. 36: 519–535.

Nelson, R. A.V. Lützow, H. Kolb, and P. Gouras. 1975. Horizontal cells in cat retina with independent dendritic systems. Science 189: 137–139.

Nicoll, R.A. 1969. Inhibitory mechanisms in the rabbit olfactory bulb: Dendrodendritic mechanisms. Brain Res. 14: 157–172.

Nicoll, R.A. 1971. Pharmacological evidence for GABA as a transmitter in granule cell inhibition in the olfactory bulb. Brain Res. 35: 137–149.

Nicholls, C.W. and G.B. Koelle. 1968. Comparison of the localization of acetylcholine-esterase and non-specific cholinesterase activities in mammalian and avian retinas. J. Comp. Neurol. 133: 1435–1442.

Nicholls, J.G. and D. Purves. 1972. A comparison of chemical and electrical synaptic transmission between single sensory cells and a motoneurone in the central nervous system of the leech. J. Physiol. 225: 637–656.

Nieuwenhuys, R. and C. Nicholson. 1969. Aspects of the histology of the cerebellum of mormyrid fishes. In Neurobiology of Cerebellar Evolution and Development (R. Llinás, ed.). Chicago: Am. Med. Assoc. pp. 135–169.

Nishi, S. and K. Koketsu. 1967. Origin of ganglionic inhibitory postsynaptic potential. Life Sci. 6: 2049–2055.

Noble, D., J.J.B. Jack, and R. Tsien. 1974. Electric Current Flow in Excitable Cells. Oxford: Clarendon Press.

Nowycky, M.C. and R.H. Roth. 1978. Dopaminergic neurons: role of presynaptic receptors in the regulation of transmitter biosynthesis. Progr. Neuro-Psychopharm. 2: 139–158.

Nygren, L.-G. and L. Olson. 1977. A new major projection from locus coeruleus: the main source of noradrenergic terminals in the ventral and dorsal columns of the spinal cord. Brain Res. 132: 85–93.

O'Leary, J.L. 1937. Structure of the primary olfactory cortex of the mouse. J. Comp. Neur. 67: 1–31.

Olson, L. and K. Fuxe. 1971. On the projections from the locus coeruleus noradrenaline neurons: the cerebellar innervation. Brain Res. 28: 165–171.

Oscarsson, O., I. Rosén, and I. Sulg. 1966. Organization of neurones in the cat cerebral cortex that are influenced from group I muscle afferents. J. Physiol. 183: 189–210.

Oshima, T. 1969. Studies of pyramidal tract cells. In Basic Mechanisms of the Epilepsies (H.H. Jasper, A.A. Ward, and A. Pope, eds.). Boston: Little, Brown. pp. 253–262.

Ottoson, D. and G.M. Shepherd. 1972. Transducer properties and integrative mechanisms in the frog's muscle spindle. In Principles of Receptor Physiology (W.R. Lowenstein, ed.). Handbook of Sensory Physiology, vol. I. New York: Springer. pp. 442–499.

Palay, S.L. 1967. Principles of cellular organization in the nervous system. In The Neurosciences: A Study Program (G.C. Quarton, T. Melnechuck, and F.O. Schmitt, eds.). New York: Rockefeller. pp. 24–31.

Palay, S.L. and V. Chan-Palay. 1973. Cerebellar Cortex: Cytology and Organization. Berlin: Springer.

Palay, S.L. and G.E. Palade. 1955. The fine structure of neurons. J. Biophys. Biochem. Cytol. 1: 69–88.

Palkovitz, M., P. Magyar, and J. Szentágothai. 1971. Quantitative histological analysis of the cerebellar cortex in the cat. I. Number and arrangement in space of the Purkinje cells. Brain Res. 32: 1–14.

Pasik, P., T. Pasik, and M. Di Figlia. 1976. Quantitative aspects of neuronal organization in the neostriatum of the Macaque monkey. In The Basal Ganglia (M.D. Yahr, ed.). New York: Raven. pp. 57–90.

Pasik, P., T. Pasik, J. Hámori, and J. Szentágothai. 1973. Golgi type II interneurons in the neuronal circuit of the monkey lateral geniculate nucleus. Exp. Brain Res. 17: 18–34.

Pearson, K. 1976. Nerve cells without action potentials. *In* Simpler Networks and Behavior (J.C. Fentress, ed.). Sunderland, Massachusetts: Sinauer. pp. 99–110.

Pellionisz, A. and R. Llinás. 1977. A computer model of cerebellar Purkinje cells. Neurosci. 2: 37–48.

Penn, R.D. and W.A. Hagins. 1972. Kinetics of the photocurrent of retinal rods. Biophys. J. 12: 1073–1094.

Peters, A. and M.L. Feldman. 1977. The projection of the lateral geniculate nucleus to area 17 of the rat cerebral cortex. IV. Terminations upon spiny dendrites. J. Neurocytol. 6: 669–689.

Peters, A. and I.R. Kaiserman-Abramof. 1969. The small pyramidal neuron of rat cerebral cortex. The synapses upon dendritic spines. Z. Zellforsch. 100: 487–506.

Peters, A. and S.L. Palay. 1966. The morphology of laminae A and A₁ of the dorsal nucleus of the lateral geniculate body of the cat. J. Anat. 100: 451–486.

Peters, A., S.L. Palay, and H. de F. Webster. 1976. The Fine Structure of the Nervous System, 2nd ed. New York: Harper & Row.

Peters, A., C.C. Proskauer, and I.R. Kaiserman-Abramof. 1968. The small pyramidal neuron of the rat cerebral cortex. The axon hillock and initial segment. J. Cell Biol. 39: 604–619.

Phillips, C.G. 1956. Intracellular records from Betz cells in the cat. Quart. J. Exp. Physiol. 41: 58–69.

Phillips, C.G. 1959. Actions of antidromic pyramidal volleys on single Betz cells in the cat. Quart. J. Exp. Physiol. 44: 1–25.

Phillips, C.G. 1969. Motor apparatus of the baboon's hand. Proc. Roy. Soc. B. 173: 141–174.

Phillips, C.G. 1971. Evolution of the corticospinal tract in primates with special reference to the hand. Proc. 3rd Int. Congr. Primat. 2: 2–23.

Phillips, C.G. and R. Porter. 1964. The pyramidal projections to motoneurones of some muscle groups of the baboon's forelimb. Prog. Brain. Res. 12: 222–242.

Phillips, C.G. and R. Porter. 1977. Corticospinal Neurones. Their Role in Movement. London: Academic.

Phillips, C.G., T.P.S. Powell, and G.M. Shepherd. 1963. Responses of mitral cells to stimulation of the lateral olfactory tract in the rabbit. J. Physiol. 168: 65–88.

Phillis, J.W. 1970. The Pharmacology of Synapses. New York: Pergamon.

Pickel, V.M., M. Segal, and F.E. Bloom. 1974. An autoradiographic study of the efferent pathways of the nucleus locus coeruleus. J. Comp. Neurol. 155: 15–42.

Pinching, A.J. 1971. Myelinated dendritic segments in the monkey olfactory bulb. Brain Res. 29: 133–138.

Pinching, A.J. and T.P.S. Powell. 1971. The neuropil of the glomeruli of the olfactory bulb. J. Cell Sci. 9: 347–377.

Plum, F., A. Gjedde, and F.E. Sampson. 1976. Neuroanatomical Functional Mapping by the Radioactive 2-deoxy-D-glucose Method. NRP Bull. 14: 457–518.

Polyak, S.L. 1941. The Retina. Chicago: Chicago University Press.

Porter, R. and J. Hore. 1969. Time course of minimal corticomotoneuronal excitatory postsynaptic potentials in lumbar motoneurones of the monkey. J. Neurophysiol. 32: 443–451.

Powell, T.P.S., W.M. Cowan, and G. Raisman. 1965. The central olfactory connexions. J. Anat. 99: 791–813.

Powell, T.P.S., R.W. Guillery, and W.M. Cowan. 1957. A quantitative study of the fornix-mammillo-thalamic system. J. Anat. 91: 419–437.

Pribram, K.H. and L. Kruger. 1954. Functions of the "Olfactory Brain." Ann. N.Y. Acad. Sci. 58: 109–138.

Price, J.L. 1973. An autoradiographic study of complementary laminar patterns of termination of afferent fibers to the olfactory cortex. J. Comp. Neur. 150: 87–108.

Price, J.L. and T.P.S. Powell. 1970a. The synaptology of the granule cells of the olfactory bulb. J. Cell Sci. 7: 125–155.

Price, J.L. and T.P.S. Powell. 1970b. An electron-microscopic study of the termination of the afferent fibres to the olfactory bulb from the cerebral hemispheres. J. Cell Sci. 7: 157–187.

Price, J.L. and T.P.S. Powell. 1971. Certain observations on the olfactory pathway. J. Anat. 110: 105–126.

Price, J.L. and W.W. Sprich. 1975. Observations on the lateral olfactory tract of the rat. J. Comp. Neurol. 162: 321–336.

Purpura, D.P. 1967. Comparative physiology of dendrites. In The Neurosciences: A Study Program (G.C. Quarton, T. Melnechuck, and F.O. Schmitt, eds.). New York: Rockefeller. pp. 372–392.

Purpura, D.P. 1972. Intracellular studies of synaptic organization in the mammalian brain. In Structure and Function of Synapses (G.D. Pappas and D.P. Purpura, eds.). New York: Raven. pp. 257–302.

Purpura, D.P. 1976. Physiological organization of the basal ganglia. In The Basal Ganglia (M.D. Yahr, ed.). New York: Raven. pp. 91–114.

Purpura, D.P. and B. Cohen. 1962. Intracellular recording from thalamic neurons during recruiting responses. J. Neurophysiol. 25: 621–635.

Purpura, D.P. and A. Malliani. 1967. Intracellular studies of the corpus striatum. I. Synaptic potentials and discharge characteristics of caudate neurons activated by thalamic stimulation. Brain Res. 6: 325–340.

Purpura, D.P., R.J. Shofer, and F.S. Musgrave. 1964. Cortical intracellular potentials during augmenting and recruiting responses. II. Patterns of synaptic activities in pyramidal and nonpyramidal tract neurons. J. Neurophysiol. 27: 133–151.

Rafols, J.A. and F. Valverde. 1973. The structure of the dorsal lateral geniculate nucleus in the mouse. A Golgi and electron microscopic study. J. Comp. Neur. 150: 303–332.

Raisman, G. 1969. Neuronal plasticity in the septal nuclei of the adult rat. Brain Res. 14: 25–48.

Raisman, G., W.M. Cowan, and T.P.S. Powell. 1965. The extrinsic afferent, commissural and association fibres of the hippocampus. Brain 88: 963–996.

Rakić, P. (ed.). 1975. Local Circuit Neurons. NRP Bull. 3: 291–446.

Rakić, P. 1979. Genetic and epigenetic determinants of local neuronal circuits in the mammalian nervous system. *In* The Neurosciences: Fourth Study Program (F.O. Schmitt and F.G. Worden, eds.). Cambridge: M.I.T. pp. 109–127.

Rakić, P. and R.L. Sidman. 1973. Organization of cerebellar cortex secondary to deficit of granule cells in Weaver mutant mice. J. Comp. Neur. 139: 473–500.

Rall, W. 1957. Membrane time constant of motoneurons. Science 126: 454–455.

Rall, W. 1959a. Dendritic current distribution and whole neuron properties. Naval Med. Res. Inst., Research Report NM 01-05-00.01.02.

Rall, W. 1959b. Branching dendritic trees and motoneuron membrane resistivity. Exp. Neurol. 1: 491–527.

Rall, W. 1960. Membrane potential transients and membrane time constant of motoneurons. Exp. Neurol. 2: 503–532.

Rall, W. 1962. Theory of physiological properties of dendrites. Ann. N.Y. Acad. Sci. 96: 1071–1092.

Rall, W. 1964. Theoretical significance of dendritic trees for neuronal input-output relations. *In* Neural Theory and Modelling (R.F. Reiss, ed.). Palo Alto: Stanford University Press. pp. 73–97.

Rall, W. 1967. Distinguishing theoretical synaptic potentials computed for different soma-dendritic distributions of synaptic input. J. Neurophysiol. 30: 1138–1168.

Rall, 1969. Time constants and electrotonic lengths of membrane cylinders and neurons. Biophys. J. 9: 1483–1508.

Rall, W. 1970. Cable properties of dendrites and effects of synaptic location. *In* Excitatory Synaptic Mechanisms (P. Andersen and J.K.S. Jansen, eds.). Oslo: Universitetsforlag. pp. 175–187.

Rall, W. 1977. Core conductor theory and cable properties of neurons. *In* Handbook of Physiology, Sect. 1: The Nervous System, vol. 1: Cellular Biology of Neurons (E.R. Kandel, ed.). Bethesda: Am. Physiol. Soc. pp. 39–98.

Rall, W., R.E. Burke, T.G. Smith, P.G. Nelson, and K. Frank. 1967. Dendritic location of synapses and possible mechanisms for the monosynaptic EPSP in motoneurons. J. Neurophysiol. 1967: 1169–1193.

Rall, W. and J. Rinzel. 1971. Dendritic spine function and synaptic attenuation calculations. Soc. Neurosci. Abstracts. 64.

Rall, W. and J. Rinzel. 1973. Branch input resistance and steady attenuation for input to one branch of a dendritic neuron model. Biophys. J. 13: 648–688.

Rall, W. and G.M. Shepherd. 1968. Theoretical reconstruction of field potentials and dendrodendritic synaptic interactions in olfactory bulb. J. Neurophysiol. 31: 884–915.

Rall, W., G.M. Shepherd. T.S. Reese, and M.W. Brightman, 1966. Dendrodendritic synaptic pathway for inhibition in the olfactory bulb. Exp. Neurol. 14: 44–56.

Ralston, H.J. III. 1968. The fine structure of neurons in the dorsal horn of the cat spinal cord. J. Comp. Neur. 132: 275–302.

Ralston, H.J. III. 1971. Evidence for presynaptic dendrites and a proposal for their mechanism of action. Nature 230: 585–587.

Ralston, H.J. III. 1979. Neuronal circuitry of the ventrobasal thalamus: the role of presynaptic dendrites. *In* The Neurosciences: Fourth Study Program (F.O. Schmitt and F.G. Worden, eds.). Cambridge: M.I.T. pp. 373–379.

Ralston, H.J. III, and M.M. Herman. 1969. The fine structure of neurons and synapses in the ventrobasal thalamus of the cat. Brain Res. 14: 77–97

Ramón-Moliner, E. 1962. An attempt at classifying nerve cells on the basis of their dendritic patterns. J. Comp. Neur. 119: 211–227.

Ramón-Moliner, E. 1977. The reciprocal synapses of the olfactory bulb: questioning the evidence. Brain Res. 128: 1–20.

Reese, T.S. and M.W. Brightman. 1970. Olfactory surface and central olfactory connections in some vertebrates. *In* CIBA Foundation Symposium on Taste and Smell in Vertebrates (G.E.W. Wolstenholme and Julie Knight, eds.). London: Churchill. pp. 115–149.

Reese, T.S. and G.M. Shepherd. 1972. Dendro-dendritic synapses in the central nervous system. *In* Structure and Function of Synapses (G.D. Pappas and D.P. Purpura, eds.). New York: Raven. pp. 121–136.

Rexed, B. 1954. A cytoarchitectonic atlas of the spinal cord in the cat. J. Comp. Neur. 100: 297–379.

Ribak, C.E. 1977. Aspinous and sparsely-spinous stellate neurons in the visual cortex of rats contain glutamic acid decarboxylase. J. Neurocytol. 7: 461–478.

Ribak, C.E., J.E. Vaughn, K. Saito, R. Barber, and E. Roberts. 1976. Immunocytochemical localization of glutamate decarboxylase in rat substantia nigra. Brain Res. 116: 287–298.

Ribak, C.E., J.E. Vaughn, K. Saito, R. Barber, and E. Roberts. 1977. Glutamate decarboxylase localization in neurons of the olfactory bulb. Brain Res. 126: 1–18.

Rinvik, E. and I. Grofova. 1970. Observations on the fine structure of the substantia nigra in the cat. Exp. Brain Res. 11: 229–248.

Roberts, E. 1975. GABA in nervous system function—an overview. *In* The Nervous System (D.B. Tower, ed.). vol. I: The Basic Neurosciences. New York: Raven. pp. 541–552.

Roper, S. 1976. An electrophysiological study of chemical and electrical synapses on neurones in the parasympathetic cardiac ganglion of the mudpuppy, *Necturus maculosus:* evidence for intrinsic ganglionic innervation. J. Physiol. 254: 427–454.

Rose, D. 1977. Responses of single units in cat visual cortex to moving bars of light as a function of bar length. J. Physiol. 271: 1–23.

Ross, C.D. and D.B. McDougal Jr. 1976. The distribution of choline acetyl transferase activity in vertebrate retina. J. Neurochem. 26: 521–526.

Ryall, R.W., M.F. Piercey, and C. Polosa. 1971. Intersegmental and intrasegmental distribution of mutual inhibition of Renshaw cells. J. Neurophysiol. 34: 700–707.

Salmoiraghi, G.C. and C.N. Stefanis. 1965. Patterns of central nervous responses to suspected transmitters. Arch. Ital. Biol. 103: 705–724.

Sandoval, M.E. and C.W. Cotman. 1978. Evaluation of glutamate as a neurotransmitter of cerebellar parallel fibers. Neurosci. 31: 199–206.

Schaffer, K. 1892. Beitrag zur Histologie der Ammonshornformation. Arch. Mikr. Anat. 39: 611–632.

Scheibel, M.E., T.L. Davies, and A.B. Scheibel. 1972. An unusual axonless cell in the thalamus of the adult cat. Exp. Neurol. 36: 512–518.

Scheibel, M.E. and A.B. Scheibel. 1966. Spinal motoneurons, interneurons and Renshaw cells. A Golgi study. Arch. Ital. Biol. 104: 328–353.

Scheibel, M.E. and A.B. Scheibel. 1970. Elementary processes in selected thalamic and cortical subsystems—the structural substrates. *In* The Neurosciences: Second Study Program (F.O. Schmitt, ed.-in-chief). New York: Rockefeller. pp. 443–457.

Schmidt, R.F. 1971. Presynaptic inhibition in the vertebrate central nervous system. Ergebn. Physiol. 63: 19–101.

Schmitt, F.O., P. Dev, and B.H. Smith. 1977. Electrotonic processing of information by brain cells. Science 193: 114–120.

Schultz, S.G. and P.F. Curran, 1970. Coupled transport of sodium and organic solutes. Physiol. Rev. 50: 637–718.

Schwartzkroin, P.A. 1977. Further characteristics of hippocampal CA1 cells *in vitro*. Brain Res. 128: 53–68.

Schwartzkroin, P.A. and P. Andersen. 1975. Glutamic acid sensitivity of dendrites in hippocampal slices *in vitro*. *In* Properties of Dendrites, vol. 12: Adv. Neurol. (G. Kreutzberg, ed.). New York: Raven. pp. 45–51.

Schwartzkroin, P.A. and M. Slawsky. 1977. Probable calcium spikes in hippocampal neurons. Brain Res. 135: 157–161.

Sharp, F.R., J.S. Kauer, and G.M. Shepherd. 1975. Local sites of activity-related glucose metabolism in rat olfactory during olfactory stimulation. Brain Res. 98: 596–600.

Sharp, F.R., J.S. Kauer, and G.M. Shepherd. 1977. Laminar analysis of 2-deoxyglucose uptake in olfactory bulb and olfactory cortex of rabbit and rat. J. Neurophysiol. 40: 800–813.

Shepherd, G.M. 1963. Neuronal systems controlling mitral cell excitability. J. Physiol. 168: 101–117.

Shepherd. G.M. 1970. The olfactory bulb as a simple cortical system: Experimental analysis and functional implications. *In* The Neurosciences: Second Study Program (F.O. Schmitt, ed.-in-chief). New York: Rockefeller. pp. 539–552.

Shepherd, G.M. 1971. Physiological evidence for dendrodendritic synaptic interactions in the rabbit's olfactory glomerulus. Brain Res. 32: 212–217.

Shepherd, G.M. 1972a. Synaptic organization of the mammalian olfactory bulb. Physiol. Rev. 52: 864–917.

Shepherd, G.M. 1972b. The neuron doctrine: a revision of functional concepts. Yale J. Biol. Med. 45: 584–599.

Shepherd, G.M. 1976. Olfactory stimulation. *In* Neuroanatomical Functional Mapping by the Radioactive 2-deoxy-D-glucose Method (F. Plum, A. Gjedde, and F.E. Sampson, eds.). NRP Bull. 14: 457–517.

Shepherd, G.M. 1977. The olfactory bulb: a simple system in the mammalian brain. *In* Handbook of Physiology, Sect. 1: The Nervous System, vol. 1: Cellular Biology of Neurons (E.R. Kandel, ed.). Bethesda: Am. Physiol. Soc. pp. 945–968.

Shepherd, G.M. 1978. Functional analysis of local circuits in the olfactory bulb.. *In* The Neurosciences: Fourth Study Program (F.O. Schmitt and F.G. Worden, eds.). Cambridge: M.I.T. pp. 129–143.

Shepherd, G.M. and R.K. Brayton. 1978. Analysis of a dendrodendritic synaptic circuit by computer simulation. IBM Res. Rep. RC 7344, pp. 1–6.

Sherrington, C.S. 1906. The Integrative Action of the Nervous System. New Haven: Yale University Press.

Sholl, D. 1956. The Organization of the Cerebral Cortex. London: Methuen.

Siggins, G.R., B.J. Hoffer, F.E. Bloom, and U. Ungerstedt. 1976. Cytochemical and electrophysiological studies of dopamine in the caudate nucleus. *In* The Basal Ganglia (M.D. Yahr, ed.). New York: Raven. pp. 227–244.

Sillito, A.M. 1977. Inhibitory processes underlying the directional specificity of simple, complex and hypercomplex cells in the cat's visual cortex. J. Physiol. 271: 699–720.

Singer, W., F. Tretter, and M. Cynader. 1975. Organization of cat striate cortex: a correlation of receptive-field properties with afferent and efferent connections. J. Neurophysiol. 38: 1080–1098.

Sjöstrand, F. 1958. Ultrastructure of retinal rod synapses of the guinea pig eye as revealed by three-dimensional reconstructions from serial sections. J. Ultrastruct. Res. 2: 122–170.

Skrede, K.K. and R.H. Westgaard. 1971. The transverse hippocampal slice: a well-defined cortical structure maintained *in vitro*. Brain Res. 35: 589–593.

Sloper, J.J. 1971. Dendrodendritic synapses in the primate motor cortex. Brain Res. 34: 186–192.

Sloper, J.J. 1973. An electron microscope study of the termination of afferent connections to the primate motor cortex. J. Neurocytol. 2: 361–368.

Smith, P.A. and F.F. Weight. 1979. Synaptic activation of the electrogenic sodium pump and slow synaptic inhibition: a re-evaluation. Nature (in the press).

Sokoloff, L. 1977. Relation between physiological function and energy metabolism in the central nervous system. J. Neurochem. 27: 13–26.

Sotelo, C. and J. Taxi. 1970. Ultrastructural aspects of electrotonic junctions in the spinal cord of the frog. Brain Res. 17: 137–141.

Spencer, W.A. and E.R. Kandel. 1961a. Electrophysiology of hippocampal neurons. III. Firing level and time constant. J. Neurophysiol. 24: 260–271.

Spencer, W.A. and E.R. Kandel. 1961b. Electrophysiology of hippocampal neurons. IV. Fast prepotentials. J. Neurophysiol. 24: 272–285.

Spencer, W.A. and E.R. Kandel. 1968. Cellular and integrative properties of the hippocampal pyramidal cell and the comparative electrophysiology of cortical neurons. Int. J. Neurol. 3–4: 267–296.

Sprague, J.M. 1958. The distribution of dorsal root fibres on motor cells in the lumbrosacral spinal cord of the cat, and the site of excitatory and inhibitory terminals in monosynaptic pathways. Proc. Roy. Soc. B 149: 534–556.

Stefanis, C. and H. Jasper. 1964. Intracellular microelectrode studies of antidromic responses in cortical pyramidal tract neurons. J. Neurophysiol. 27: 828–854.

Stell, W.K. 1964. Correlated light and electron microscope observations on Golgi preparations of goldfish retina. J. Cell Biol. 23: 89 A.

Stell, W.K. 1967. The structure and relationships of horizontal cells and photoreceptor-bipolar synaptic complexes in goldfish retina. Am. J. Anat. 121: 401–424.

Stell, W.K. 1972. The morphological organization of the vertebrate retina. *In* Physiology of Photoreceptor Organs (M.G.F. `Fuortes, ed.). Handbook of Sensory Physiology. VII/1B. Berlin: Springer. pp. 111–214.

Stell, W.K. and P. Witkovsky. 1973. Retinal structure in the smooth dogfish, *Mustelus canis:* general description and light microscopy of giant ganglion cells. J. Comp. Neur. 148: 1–32.

Stevens, C.F. 1969. Structure of cat frontal olfactory cortex. J. Neurophysiol. 32: 184–192.

Stevens, C.S. 1976. Molecular basis for postjunctional conductance increases induced by acetylcholine. Cold Spring Harb. Symp. Quant. Biol. 40: 169–174.

Storm-Mathisen, J. 1977. Localization of transmitter candidates in the brain: the hippocampal formation as a model. Progr. Neurobiol. 8: 119–181.

Storm-Mathisen, J. and T.W. Blackstad. 1964. Cholinesterase in the hippocampal region. Distribution and relation to architectonics and afferent systems. Acta Anat. 56: 216–253.

Strick, P.L. and P. Sterling. 1974. Synaptic termination of afferents from the ventrolateral nucleus of the thalamus in the cat motor cortex. A light and electron microscopic study. J. Comp. Neurol. 153: 77–106.

Svaetichin, G. 1953. The cone action potential. Acta Physiol. Scand. 29 (Suppl. 106): 565–600.

Swanson, L.W. and W.M. Cowan. 1977. An autoradiographic study of the organization of the efferent connections of the hippocampal formation in the rat. J. Comp. Neurol. 172: 49–84.

Swett, J.E. and C.M. Bourassa. 1967. Short latency activation of pyramidal tract cells by Group I afferent volleys in the cat. J. Physiol. 189: 101–117.

Szentágothai, J. 1963. The structure of the synapse in the lateral geniculate body. Acta Anat. 55: 166–185.

Szentágothai, J. 1969. Architecture of the cerebral cortex. *In* Basic Mechanisms of the Epilepsies (H.H. Jasper, A.A. Ward, and A. Pope, eds.). Boston: Little, Brown. pp. 13–28.

Szentágothai, J. 1970. Glomerular synapses, complex synaptic arrangements, and their operational significance. *In* The Neurosciences: Second Study Program (F.O. Schmitt, ed.-in-chief). New York: Rockefeller. pp. 427–443.

Szentágothai, J. 1973. Synaptology of the visual cortex. *In* Handbook of Sensory Physiology, vol. VII/3B (R. Jung, ed.). Heidelberg: Springer. pp. 269–324.

Szentágothai, J. 1979. Local neuron circuits of the neocortex. *In* The Neurosciences: Fourth Study Program (F.O. Schmitt and F.G. Worden, eds.). Cambridge: M.I.T. pp. 399–419.

Takahashi, K. 1965. Slow and fast groups of pyramidal tract cells and their respective membrane properties. J. Neurophysiol. 28: 908–924.

Takahashi, T., S. Konishi, D. Powell, S.E. Leeman, and Otsuka, M. 1974. Identification of the motoneuron depolarizing peptide in bovine dorsal root as hypothalamic substance P. Brain Res. 73: 59–69.

Tanabe, T., M. Iino, and S.F. Takagi. 1975. Discrimination of odors in olfactory bulb, pyriform-amygdaloid areas, and orbitofrontal cortex of the monkey. J. Neurophysiol. 38: 1282–1296.

Tauc, L. and H.M. Gerschenfeld. 1961. Cholinergic transmission mechanisms for both excitation and inhibition in molluscan central synapses. Nature 192: 366–367.

Thach, W.T. 1967. Somatosensory receptive fields of single units in cat cerebellar cortex. J. Neurophysiol. 30: 675–696.

Thach, W.T. 1970. Discharge of Purkinje and cerebellar nuclear neurons during rapidly alternating arm movements in the monkey. J. Neurophysiol. 31: 785–797.

Thach, W.T. 1972. Cerebellar output: properties, synthesis and uses. Brain Res. 40: 89–97.

Tömböl, T. 1967. Short neurons and their synaptic relations in the specific thalamic nuclei. Brain Res. 3: 307–326.

Tomita, T. 1965. Electrophysiological study of the mechanisms subserving color coding in the fish retina. Cold Spr. Harb. Symp. Quant. Biol. 30: 559–566.

Tomita, T. 1972. Light-induced potential and resistance changes in vertebrate photoreceptors. *In* Physiology of Photoreceptor Organs (M.G.F. Fuortes, ed.). Handbook of Sensory Physiology. VII/2B. Berlin: Springer. pp. 483–511.

Towe, A.L., H.D. Patton, and T.T. Kennedy. 1964. Response properties of neurons in pericruciate cortex of cat following electrical stimulation of the appendages. Exp. Neurol. 10: 325–344.

Toyoda, J., H. Nosaki, and T. Tomita. 1969. Light-induced resistance changes in single photoreceptors of *Necturus* and *Gekko.* Vision Res. 9: 453–463.

Toyoma, K., K. Matsunami, T. Ohno, and S. Tokashiki. 1974. An intracellular study of neuronal organization in the visual cortex. Exp. Brain Res. 21: 45–66.

Traub, R.D. and R. Llinás. 1979. Hippocampal pyramidal cells: significance of dendritic ionic conductances for neuronal function and epileptogenesis. J. Neurophysiol. 42: 476–498.

Trifonov, Y.A. 1968. Study of synaptic transmission between photoreceptors and horizontal cells by means of electric stimulation of the retina. Biophysics (Moscow) 13: N 5.

Uchizono, K. 1965. Characteristics of excitatory and inhibitory synapses in the central nervous system of the cat. Nature 207: 642–643.

Uchizono, K. 1966. Excitatory and inhibitory synapses in the cat spinal cord. Jap. J. Physiol. 16: 570–575.

Uchizono, K. 1967. Synaptic organization of the Purkinje cells in the cerebellum of the cat. Exp. Brain Res. 4: 97–113.

Ungerstedt, U. 1971. Stereotaxic mapping of monoamine pathways in the rat brain. Acta Physiol. Scand. Suppl. 367: 1–48.

Valdivia, O. 1971. Methods of fixation and the morphology of synaptic vesicles. J. Comp. Neur. 142: 257–273.

Valverde, F. 1965. Studies on the Pyriform Lobe. Cambridge: Harvard University Press.

Valverde, F. 1967. Apical dendritic spines of the visual cortex and light deprivation in the mouse. Exp. Brain Res. 3: 337–352.

Valverde, F. 1971. Short axon neuronal subsystems in the visual cortex of the monkey. Int. J. Neurosci. 1: 181–197.

van der Loos, H. 1960. On dendro-dendritic junctions in the cerebral cortex. *In* Structure and Function of the Cerebral Cortex D.B. Tower and J.P. Schadé, eds.). Amsterdam: Elsevier. pp. 36–42.

van der Loos, H. and E.M. Glaser. 1972. Autapses in necortex cerebri: synapses between a pyramidal cell's axon and its own dendrites. Brain Res. 48: 355–360.

Van Hoesen, G.W., D.N. Pandya, and N. Butters. 1972. Cortical afferents to the entorhinal cortex of rhesus monkey. Science 175: 1471–1473.

Von Euler, C. 1962. On the significance of the high zinc content in the hippocampal formation. *In* Physiologie de l'hippocampe (P. Passouant, ed.). Coll. Intern. du C.N.R.S. no. 107. Paris: Ed. du Centre Nat. Rech. Scie. pp. 135–145.

Waldeyer, W. 1891. Ueber einige neuere Forschungen im Gebiete der Anatomie des Centralnervensystems. Deutsche Med. Woch. 1352–1356.

Walshe, F.M.R. 1948. Critical Studies in Neurology. Edinburgh: Livingstone.

Watanabe, S., M. Konishi, and O. Creutzfeldt. 1966. Post-synaptic potentials in the cat's visual cortex following electrical stimulation of afferent pathways. Exp. Brain Res. 1: 272–283.

Weight, F. 1968. Cholinergic mechanisms in recurrent inhibition of motoneurons. *In* Psychopharmocology: A Review of Progress, 1957–1967. U.S. Govt. Printing Office, Washington, D.C. pp. 69–75.

Weight, F. 1974. Synaptic potentials resulting from conductance decreases. *In* Synaptic Transmission and Neuronal Interaction (M.V.L. Bennett, ed.). New York: Raven. pp. 141–152.

Weight, F. and A. Padjen. 1973. Slow synaptic inhibition: evidence for synaptic inactivation of sodium conductance in sympathetic ganglion cells. Brain Res. 55: 219–224.

Weight, F. and J. Votova. 1970. Slow synaptic excitation in sympathetic ganglion cells: evidence for synaptic inactivation of potassium conductance. Science 170: 755–758.

Werblin, F.S. and J.E. Dowling. 1969. Organization of the retina of the mudpuppy, Necturus maculosus. II. Intracellular recording. J. Neurophysiol. 32: 339–355.

Werman, R.A. 1966. Criteria for identification of a central nervous system transmitter. Comp. Biochem. Physiol. 18: 745–766.

Werman, R., R.A. Davidoff, and M.H. Aprison. 1968. Inhibitory action of glycine on spinal neurons in the cat. J. Neurophysiol. 31: 81–95.

Wernig, A. and H. Sterner. 1977. Quantum amplitude distributions point to functional unity of the synaptic "active zone." Nature 269: 820–822.

West, R.D. and J.E. Dowling. 1973. Synapses onto different morphological types of retinal ganglion cells. Science 178: 510–512.

Westrum, L.E. 1966. Electron microscopy of degeneration in the prepyriform cortex. J. Anat. 100: 683–685.

Westrum, L.E. 1969. Electron microscopy of degeneration in the lateral olfactory tract and plexiform layer of the prepyriform cortex of the rat. Z. Zellforsch. 98: 157–187.

Westrum, L.E. 1970. Observations on initial segments of axons in the prepyriform cortex of the rat. J. Comp. Neur. 139: 337–356.

Westrum, L.E. and T.W. Blackstad. 1962. An electron microscopic study of the stratum radiatum of the rat hippocampus (regio superior, CA 1) with particular emphasis on synaptology. J. Comp. Neur. 113: 1–42.

White, E.L. 1972. Synaptic organization in the olfactory glomerulus of the mouse. Brain Res. 37: 69–80.

White, E.L. 1973. Synaptic organization of the mammalian olfactory glomerulus: new findings including an intraspecific variation. Brain Res. 60: 299–313.

White, E.L. 1978. The identity of neurons in mouse primary somatosensory cortex which are postsynaptic to degenerating thalamocortical axon terminals. J. Comp. Neurol. 181: 627–662.

Whitten, W.K. and H. Bronson. 1970. The role of pheromones in mammalian reproduction. *In* Communication by Chemical Signals (J.W. Johnston, Jr. D.G. Moulton, and A. Turk, eds.). Advances in Chemoreception, vol. 1. New York: Appleton-Century-Crofts, pp. 309–326.

Williams, T.H., Chiba, A.C. Black Jr., R.C. Bhalla, and J. Jew. 1976. Species variation in SIF cells of superior cervical ganglia: are there two functional types? *In* SIF Cells (O. Eränkö, ed.). DHEW Publication No. (NIH) 76-942. Washington, D.C.: U.S. Govt. Printing Office. pp. 143–162.

Williams. T.H. and S.L. Palay. 1969. Ultrastructure of the small neurons in the superior cervical ganglion. Brain Res. 15: 17–34.

Willis, W.D. 1971. The case for the Renshaw cell. Brain Behav. Evol. 4: 5–52.

Wilson, C.J., P.M. Groves, and E. Fifkova. 1978. Monoaminergic synapses, including dendrodendritic synapses in the rat substantia nigra. Exp. Brain Res. 30: 1–14.

Wilson, S.A.K. 1928. Modern Problems in Neurology. London: Arnold.

Wilson, V.J. and P.R. Burgess. 1962. Disinhibition in the cat spinal cord. J. Neurophysiol. 25: 392–404.

Witkovsky, P. 1971. Peripheral mechanisms of vision. Ann Rev. Physiol. 33: 257–280.

Witkovsky, P. and W.K. Stell. 1971. Gross morphology and synaptic relationships of bipolar cells in the retina of the smooth dogfish, *Mustelus canis.* Anat. Rec. 169: 456–457.

Woolsey, T.A., M.L. Dierker, and D.F. Wann. 1975. Mouse SmI cortex: qualitative and quantitative classification of Golgi-impregnated barrel neurons. Proc. Nat. Acad. Sci. 72: 2165–2169.

Woolsey, T.A. and H. van der Loos. 1970. The structural organization of layer IV in the somatosensory region (S 1) of mouse cerebral cortex. The description of a cortical field composed of discrete cytoarchitectonic units. Brain Res. 17: 205–242.

Yahr, M.D. (ed.). 1976. The Basal Ganglia. New York: Raven.

Yamada, E. and T. Ishikawa. 1965. The fine structure of the horizontal cells in some vertebrate retinae. Cold Spr. Harb. Symp. Quant. Biol. 30: 383–392.

Yamamoto, C. 1967. Pharmacological studies on norepinephrine, acetylcholine and related compounds on neurons in Deiter's nucleus and the cerebellum. J. Pharmacol. Exp. Therap. 156: 39–47.

Yamamoto, C. and K. Iwama. 1962. Intracellular potential recording from olfactory bulb neurones of the rabbit. Jap. J. Physiol. 38: 63–67.

Yamamoto, C., T. Yamamoto, and K. Iwama. 1963. The inhibitory system in the olfactory bulb studied by intracellular recording. J. Neurophysiol. 26: 403–415.

Yokota, T., A.G. Reeves, and P.D. MacLean. 1970. Differential effects of septal and olfactory volleys on intracellular responses of hippocampal neurons in awake, sitting monkeys. J. Neurophysiol. 33: 96–107.

Yoshida, M., A. Rabin, and M. Anderson. 1972. Monosynaptic inhibition of

pallidal neurons by axon collaterals of caudato-nigral fibers. Exp. Brain Res.
15: 333–347.

Young, A.B., M.L. Oster-Granite, R.M. Herndon, and S.H. Snyder. 1974.
Glutamic acid: selective depletion by viral induced granule cell loss in
hamster cerebellum. Brain Res. 73: 1–13.

INDEX